Cambridge History of Medicine
EDITORS: CHARLES WEBSTER AND
CHARLES ROSENBERG

Patients and practitioners

OTHER BOOKS IN THE SERIES

Patients and practitioners

Lay perceptions of medicine in pre-industrial society

Edited by Roy Porter

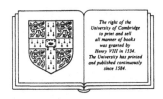

The right of the
University of Cambridge
to print and sell
all manner of books
was granted by
Henry VIII in 1534.
The University has printed
and published continuously
since 1584.

CAMBRIDGE UNIVERSITY PRESS

CAMBRIDGE

LONDON   NEW YORK   NEW ROCHELLE
MELBOURNE   SYDNEY

PUBLISHED BY THE PRESS SYNDICATE OF THE UNIVERSITY OF CAMBRIDGE
The Pitt Building, Trumpington Street, Cambridge, United Kingdom

CAMBRIDGE UNIVERSITY PRESS
The Edinburgh Building, Cambridge CB2 2RU, UK
40 West 20th Street, New York NY 10011–4211, USA
477 Williamstown Road, Port Melbourne, VIC 3207, Australia
Ruiz de Alarcón 13, 28014 Madrid, Spain
Dock House, The Waterfront, Cape Town 8001, South Africa

http://www.cambridge.org

First published 1985
First paperback edition 2002

A catalogue record for this book is available from the British Library

Library of Congress cataloguing in publication data

Main entry under title:
Patients and practitioners.

(Cambridge monographs on the history of medicine)
1. Medicine – Public opinion – History. 2. Health
attitudes – History. 3. Medicine – History. I. Porter,
Roy, 1946–   .II. Series. [DNLM; 1. Attitude to
Health – History. 2. History of Medicine, 17th Cent.
3. History of Medicine, 18th Cent. WZ 56 P298]
R133.P277 1985   362.1′09   85–13257

ISBN 0 521 30915 8 hardback
ISBN 0 521 53061 X paperback

CONTENTS

1

Introduction

ROY PORTER

We have histories of diseases but not of health, biographies of doctors but not of the sick.[1] Admittedly, in recent years in particular, a barrage of attacks has been mounted against the ways scholars have traditionally conceived the history of medicine. The discipline (critics allege) has been too Whiggish, too scientistic, either deliberately fostering or at least unconsciously underwriting myths of the triumphal cavalcade of scientific medicine. And in response strenuous counter-attempts have been made to 'demystify' medical history, and to promote research oriented towards new ways of seeing, in particular examining the socio-cultural construction of medical knowledge and medicine's role within wider networks of ideology and power. As yet, however, these winds of change have rarely led to much attention being paid to the objects of medicine, the recipients of 'the clinical gaze', the sufferers.[2]

[1] For instances of histories of disease see O. Temkin, *The Falling Sickness* (Baltimore, 1945); D. Hopkins, *Princes and Peasants: Smallpox in History* (Chicago, 1983); I. Veith, *Hysteria* (Chicago, 1965); the general point is made in S. Gilman, *Seeing the Insane* (London, 1982). For exceptions see P. L. Entralgo, *Doctor and Patient* (London, 1969) and Charles F. Mullett, 'The lay outlook on medicine in England, *circa* 1800–1850', *Bulletin of the History of Medicine*, xxv (1951), 168–84. Cf. Thomas Szasz's remark that 'A history of psychiatry from the point of view of the "patient" has yet to be written': *The Manufacture of Madness* (St Albans, 1973), p. 155.

[2] For introductions to studies of the social construction of medicine see P. Wright and A. Treacher (eds.), *The Problem of Medical Knowledge* (Edinburgh, 1982); J. Woodward and D. Richards, 'Towards a social history of medicine', in *idem* (eds.), *Health Care and Popular Medicine in Nineteenth Century England* (London, 1977), pp. 15–55; M. Pelling, 'Medicine since 1500', in P. Corsi and P. Weindling (eds.), *Information Sources in the History of Science and Medicine* (London, 1983), pp. 379–410; Charles Webster, 'The historiography of medicine', in *ibid.*, pp. 29–43. For surveys of what has been done see W. F. Bynum, 'Health, disease and medical care', in G. S. Rousseau and Roy Porter (eds.), *The Ferment of Knowledge* (Cambridge, 1980), pp. 211–54; G. S. Rousseau, 'Psychology', in *ibid.*, pp. 143–210.

Indeed, perhaps ironically, these new and critical forays into medical history often end up by silently reinforcing that old stereotype of the sick, i.e. their basic invisibility.[3] Traditional history of medicine simply ignored the patient. After all, it was what the doctor did to, and for, the sick that counted; the patient was just the raw material, the unwitting bearer of a disease or lesion. After all, no one ever suggested that historians of sculpture should concentrate on slabs of marble. Traditional history of medicine thus ignored the patient: he or she was of no interest. Modern critical histories, by contrast, still ignore the patient but often by *design*; for they sometimes argue (as has David Armstrong, following Foucault) that there can be no such material person as the 'patient', directly accessible to the historian. Rather, 'patients' are the constructs of medicine; their self-perceptions are themselves medically contaminated and – the parallel would be with Pygmalion – they can be studied only as they have been rendered visible (which is as much as to say invisible) by the 'medical gaze'. Hence we are now beginning to get sociological projects examining the 'construction' of 'normal patients' or 'defaulting patients', or more broadly dealing with 'the medicalization of life' or 'the expropriation of health'. And it has become a task to show how (as Nicholas Jewson has tellingly put it) the 'sick man' came to disappear from medical cosmology. Indeed this would-be radical current in the history of medicine, which regards patients as being made visible only by medicine's histological staining techniques, runs parallel to much recent medical sociology, with its interest in the role-playing that allegedly governs relations between doctors and patients. Sick people have thus given way to sick roles.[4]

Yet these new directions may actually be historically extremely misleading, the more so, perhaps, the farther back into historical time one searches. Whatever may be true within the 'professional dominance'

[3] See for example M. Foucault, *The Birth of the Clinic* (London, 1972); *idem*, *Discipline and Punish* (London, 1977); D. Armstrong, *The Political Anatomy of the Body* (Cambridge, 1983); T. Szasz, *The Myth of Mental Illness* (New York, 1961).

[4] N. Jewson, 'The disappearance of the sick man from medical cosmology 1770–1870', *Sociology*, x (1976), 225–44; D. Armstrong, 'The invention of the normal child', *The Society for the Social History of Medicine Bulletin*, 27 (1980), 32; J.-P. Goubert (ed.), *La médicalisation de la société française 1770–1830* (Waterloo, Ontario, 1982); I. Illich, *Limits to Medicine* (London, 1976); *idem* (ed.), *Disabling Professions* (London, 1977). For a feminist perspective on the role of medicine see V. Knibiehler and C. Fouquet, *La femme et les médecins* (Paris, 1983).

of today's medical empire,[5] it is not clear that, two or three centuries ago, in that age of weak professionalization before 'the clinic', patients automatically marched to the drum of the medicine man. Indeed, the very word 'patient' may actually be confusing. It is true that in early modern times the term was routinely used – as etymology would suggest – to denote any sick or suffering person, whether or not they had come under medical advice. But nowadays the word 'patient' implies that a person has put himself 'under the doctor', and the term has powerful connotations of passivity. Thus, given today's overtones, it is probably preferable to speak historically of 'sufferers' or 'the sick', some of whom *opted*, in various ways, to put themselves into relations with medical practitioners – relations whose structure and dynamics need exploration.

The aim of this book is to show that the sick in past time constitute important objects of historical study. The contributors have worked on the belief that it is both possible and necessary to study them using techniques that differ from the standard practices current in the history of medicine and of doctors (though it is of course equally crucial that the two approaches should also, where possible, be integrated). Thus the essays in this volume explore different aspects of consciousness of sickness, and of actual experiences of being ill, in pre-industrial society (chiefly, in fact, in seventeenth and eighteenth century England), concentrating on lay beliefs about health and illness, lay self-medication, and lay relations with the various types of medical practice and treatment on offer.

The terrain of the history of the sick is not a total wilderness, but until now it has been cultivated very sparsely.[6] We do possess some valuable

5 For perspectives on the 'professionalization' of modern English medicine drawing on medical sociology, see M. J. Peterson, *The Medical Profession in Mid-Victorian London* (Berkeley, 1978); I. Waddington, 'General practitioners and consultants in early nineteenth century England: the sociology of an intra-professional conflict', in J. Woodward and D. Richards (eds.), *op. cit.* (note 2 above), pp. 164–88; N. Parry and J. Parry, *The Rise of the Medical Profession: A Study of Collective Social Mobility* (London, 1976); and more generally E. Freidson, *Profession of Medicine* (London, 1972); T. J. Johnson, *Professions and Power* (London, 1972); M. S. Larson, *The Rise of Professionalism* (London, 1977); D. Mechanic, *Medical Sociology: A Selective View* (New York, 1968); and the recent reassessment of this literature in R. Dingwall and P. Lewis (eds.), *The Sociology of the Professions* (London, 1983).
6 See D. Guthrie, 'The patient: a neglected factor in the history of medicine', *Proceedings of the Royal Society of Medicine*, xxxvii (1945), 490–4; Mullett, 'The lay outlook on medicine' (note 1 above); and the rather historically sketchy

macro-surveys of the people's health in the past, assessed in biological and material terms, indexed through the use of vital statistics: F. B. Smith's *The People's Health* is a good example.[7] And thanks to the *Annales* school in France, and the popularity of historical demography in Britain, growing numbers of scholars have been exploring morbidity and mortality, incidence of famines and epidemics, nutrition levels and so forth for communities, regions and even nations.[8] The investigations in this collection do not pursue this kind of 'biology of man in history', but to a greater or lesser degree take for granted its background picture of the chances of life in past time.

Studies have also been published of the diseases, disorders, and indeed deaths of particular individuals. These come in several types. On the one hand, medical history buffs have given us plentiful offerings in the 'famous illnesses of famous people' and 'what did Dr Johnson die of?' genres.[9] Paralleling these, we also have studies, inspired by Freud, of the neuroses of writers, artists and celebrities, including the 'was Virginia Woolf really mad?' category, and the ghoulish fascination with the psychopathology of genius.[10] All these approaches can be illuminating, but they rarely explicitly or systematically address the questions foremost in the minds of the contributors to this book. The present studies above all address two broad clusters of issues.

First, they are concerned to uncover what *beliefs* were held (primarily amongst the laity rather than the medical profession) about living and dying, health and sickness and remedies. These essays thus explore such topics as popular conceptions of the workings of the body,

survey by C. Herzlich and J. Pierret, *Malades d'hier, malades d'aujourd'hui* (Paris, 1984).

[7] F. B. Smith, *The People's Health* (London, 1979).

[8] See for instance J.-P. Goubert, *Malades et médecins en Bretagne 1770–1790* (Rennes, 1974); F. Lebrun, *Les hommes et la mort en Anjou aux 17e et 18e siècles* (Paris, 1977). Two volumes of the Johns Hopkins 'Selections from the *Annales*' series present some of this material in translation: *Biology of Man in History* (Baltimore, 1975), and *Medicine and Society in France* (Baltimore, 1980), both ed. by R. Forster and O. Ranum, trans. by E. Forster and P. M. Ranum.

[9] See for example W. B. Ober, *Boswell's Clap and Other Essays* (Carbondale, Ill., 1979); J. Mulhallen and D. J. M. Wright, 'Samuel Johnson: amateur physician', *Journal of the Royal Society of Medicine*, LXXVI (1983), 217–22; or for Pope see M. H. Nicolson and G. S. Rousseau, *This Long Disease My Life* (Princeton, 1968).

[10] See for instance S. Trombley, *'All that Summer She Was Mad': Virginia Woolf and her Doctors* (London, 1981); and G. Pickering, *Creative Malady* (London, 1974). For madness from the sufferers' point of view, see G. Bateson (ed.), *Perceval's Narrative* (New York, 1974); D. Peterson (ed.), *A Mad People's History of Madness* (Pittsburgh, 1982).

of health and disease; they probe the personal and collective meanings of sickness, of suffering and recovery, probing how 'illness experiences' were integrated within the larger meanings of life from the cradle to the grave. And they examine the place of these 'medical' beliefs within and alongside codes of religious faith, socio-political outlooks, philosophies of personal identity and destiny, convictions about man's place within the natural frame of things, and other dimensions of consciousness and culture.

Second they investigate what people did to keep well, and what they then did when they fell sick. In what ways did the healthy seek to fortify themselves and forestall illness by preventive regimes? When sick, did they fatalistically or stoically accept suffering? If not, how did they actively respond? Which sorts of people tried which sorts of self-medication, for which sorts of maladies, under what circumstances? Who sought outside medical aid, and for which conditions? What kinds of practitioners were summoned? How did the sick then manage their doctors, and the practitioners relate to them? By seeking provisional answers to these and other questions we can move towards an understanding of patterns of illness behaviour.

No grand theory animates this book, no grand generalizations emerge. These essays are perhaps best seen as pilot and preliminary studies. And, in any case, it would surely be mistaken to expect to find that attitudes and praxis towards sickness were uniform before the emergence of the 'clinic' (it could be argued that nowadays the dictates of a uniform *medical system* programme some uniformity in patient response). The varieties of sickness experience (these essays show) were mapped upon immensely varying socio-economic circumstances, religious affiliations, levels of education and literacy, class and community perceptions, the availability of skilled professional medical practitioners and a thousand and one other socio-cultural, not to mention individual and personal, circumstances. Thus, at the very time that the Essex clergyman Ralph Josselin was penning his highly 'providentialist' diary of sickness, the metropolitan Samuel Pepys was interpreting his illness experiences in wholly secular terms.

It would be premature to generalize. Michael MacDonald discovered that the early seventeenth century Buckinghamshire physician-parson, Richard Napier, treated few infants. By contrast, Dr George Chalmers, in early eighteenth century Aberdeen, treated lots of them.[11] Does this

---

[11] M. MacDonald, *Mystical Bedlam* (Cambridge, 1981), pp. 40–1; R. Stott, 'The medical practice of George Chalmers, M.D.', *Archivaria*, x (1980), 51–67.

suggest that heightened sense of the value of children's lives which many historians have claimed to recognize in the eighteenth century? Conceivably; but it would be very foolish in our present state of ignorance to venture extrapolations built on such a flimsy basis of evidence.

These essays do not pretend to solve the grand questions about sick people in history, but they do address a common core of questions, and certain themes emerge from the investigations, indicating common patterns of health care and of modulations in them over time. As yet we have only a small and selective mapping, but it is worth drawing attention in this Introduction to some noteworthy contours and landmarks in the terrain that are beginning to appear.

One theme emerging prominently from this collection is the intertwining in past time of sickness experiences and religious experiences; indeed, it forms the central thrust of two papers, Lucinda McCray Beier's 'In sickness and in health: A seventeenth century family's experience', and Andrew Wear's 'Puritan perceptions of illness in seventeenth century England'. There is of course, as Beier and Wear both note, a risk of optical illusion. Back in the seventeenth century it was predominantly the pious who kept diaries and journals. Most of our first-hand records of Sickman's Progress hence derive from them, but we must not assume that they were typical. Yet even so, these two papers, and others, document just how critically important religious beliefs and feelings could be in enabling people to make sense of sickness – their own and other people's – and to face death (and also, as Wear notes, how the ubiquity of illness played a crucial part in bolstering religious convictions themselves). The Reverend Ralph Josselin, the centrepiece of Beier's account, interpreted sickness – his own and his household's, for medicine was very much a family affair – through a rampant providentialism. Yet providentialism certainly did not mean fatalism, for it was one's duty to co-operate with divine providence in the fight against disease – good evidence of how the traditional 'sick role' was that of the 'participant' not the mere passive 'patient', even when God was the physician.

But as Wear stresses, there was more to Christian responses to sickness than a rigid providentialism. For instance, as his analysis of a wide range of autobiographical writings shows particularly well, religion could provide a *language* for expressing and interpreting pain and sickness,[12] while also indicating pious duties, such as visiting the

[12] Cf. K. Keele, *Anatomies of Pain* (Oxford, 1957).

sick, or enacting the proper way to die.[13] Unlike certain later fringe movements such as Christian Science, religious modes of coping with sickness were not at odds with regular medical ones, even if Josselin appears as a man who, though not poor, rarely drew on professional medical advice, and Richard Baxter, though frequently consulting physicians, often swallowed their advice with a generous pinch of salt, and moved eclectically as it suited him between 'medical' and 'religious' modes of explanation for his illnesses.

It might be predicted that predominantly religious ways of making sense of sickness would have lost their grip in the eighteenth century with the popularization of the worldview of the New Science and the advent of Enlightenment naturalism. Indeed, a persuasive and influential current of English historiography does argue that in the post-Restoration period a cultural ambience became dominant which was programmatically secularizing, scientific and rationalizing, and which at best had little sympathy for – and indeed was generally hostile towards – the more traditional cultural amalgam which had encompassed 'magic', popular, oral wisdom and religious healing, all of which came to be dismissed as 'enthusiasm' and vulgar 'superstition'.[14] Such traditional eclectic and pluralistic outlooks, it is alleged, became relegated to the lower orders and to certain Dissenting sects.[15] This is in many ways a fruitful interpretation, not least because it provides a prelude for the emergence in the nineteenth century of 'alternative

[13] For death see J. McManners, *Death and the Enlightenment* (Oxford, 1981); P. Ariès, *The Hour of our Death* (London, 1981); M. Vovelle, *Mourir autrefois: Attitudes collectives devant la mort en XVIIᵉ et XVIIIᵉ siècles* (Paris, 1974); R. Cobb, *Death in Paris 1795–1801* (Oxford, 1978); D. E. Stannard, *The Puritan Way of Death* (New York, 1977); C. Gittings, *Death, Burial and the Individual in Early Modern England* (London, 1984).

[14] See in particular Christopher Hill, *Some Intellectual Consequences of the English Revolution* (London, 1980); and, more globally, M. Berman, *The Re-enchantment of the World* (London, 1981).

[15] M. MacDonald, 'Religion, social change and psychological healing in England 1600–1800', in W. Sheils (ed.), *The Church and Healing* (Oxford, 1982), pp. 101–26. For cultural stratification see U. P. Burke, *Popular Culture in Early Modern Europe* (London, 1978); D. Leith, *A Social History of English* (London, 1983); R. Paulson, *Popular and Polite Art in the Age of Hogarth and Fielding* (London, 1979); R. Darnton, 'In search of the Enlightenment: recent attempts to create a social history of ideas', *Journal of Modern History*, XLIII (1971), 113–32; idem, 'The high Enlightenment and the low life of literature in pre-revolutionary France', *Past and Present*, LI (1971), 81–115; idem, *Mesmerism and the End of the Enlightenment in France* (Cambridge, Mass, 1968); H. C. Payne, 'Elite versus popular mentality in the eighteenth century', *Studies in Eighteenth Century Culture*, VIII (Madison, 1979), 201–37.

medicine', integral to a radical artisan culture coming 'from below', including those traditions of medical botany, holism and plebeian spiritualism illuminated by John Pickstone, Roger Cooter, Logie Barrow and others.[16] But several contributors to this volume also give timely warnings against antedating and overstating the emergence of distinctive and antithetical 'high' and 'low', 'great' and 'small' cultures, and question its usefulness as a device for understanding the configurations of healing traditions before the Industrial Revolution.

For such watertight compartments break down in the teeth of actual examples, as is indicated in Jonathan Barry's 'Piety and the patient: Medicine and religion in eighteenth century Bristol', which draws heavily upon the diaries of an autodidact accountant, William Dyer. As Barry shows, the polarities we might expect to draw as ways of defining distinctive medical traditions – professional versus lay, literate versus oral, secular versus spiritual, commercial versus community, orthodox versus 'quack',[17] and so forth – are simply confounded by Dyer's experience and activities as a layman with deep involvement in interpreting sickness, giving practical medical aid, and practising lively piety. Thus there was nothing incongruous to Dyer about dispensing traditional herbal preparations to his friends, while also deploying proprietary medicines such as Dr James' Fever Powder,[18] and dabbling with fashionable, 'scientific' medical electricity. Similarly

[16] E.g., L. Barrow, 'Democratic epistemology: mid 19th century plebeian medicine', *The Society for the Social History of Medicine Bulletin*, 29 (1981), 25–9; *idem*, 'Anti-establishment healing and spiritualism in England', in W. Shiels (ed.), *The Church and Healing* (Oxford, 1982), pp. 225–48; J. Pickstone, 'Establishment and dissent in nineteenth century medicine: an exploration of some correspondences between religious and medical belief systems in early industrial England', in *ibid.*, pp. 165–90; R. Cooter, 'Deploying "pseudo-science": then and now', in M. P. Hanen, M. J. Osler and R. C. Weyant (eds.), *Science, Pseudo-Science and Society* (Waterloo, Ontario, 1980), pp. 237–72; R. Wallis and P. Morley (eds.), *Marginal Medicine* (London, 1976); J. Whorton, *Crusaders for Fitness* (Princeton, 1982); G. Risse (ed.), *Medicine Without Doctors* (New York, 1977); A. C. and M. Fellman, *Making Sense of Self* (Philadelphia, 1981); R. Cooter, 'Interpreting the fringe', *The Society for the Social History of Medicine Bulletin*, 29 (1981), 33–6; L. M. Beier, 'The creation of the medical fringe', *ibid.*, 29–32.

[17] Obviously the term 'quack' is loaded. For some readings of 'quacks' see G. Williams, *The Age of Agony* (London, 1975), ch. XI; E. Jameson, *The Natural History of Quackery* (London, 1961); A. Corsini, *Medici ciarlatini e ciarlatani medici* (Bologna, 1922); and Grete de Francesco, *Die Macht des Charlatans* (Basle, 1937).

[18] J. Crellin, 'Dr James's Fever Powder', *Transactions of the British Society for the History of Pharmacy*, I (1974), 136–43.

the sicknesses of the body automatically evoked for him sicknesses of the spirit. Attached to Behmen and Wesley as well as to modern science, Dyer integrated the divine and the incarnate, the mystical, spiritual and the medical in a brotherly practice of healing which stood for him as an ecumenical, evangelical expression of practical piety transcending confessional boundaries. Dyer's career, as both a taker and a dispenser of physic, forces us to question ready-made and anachronistic categories and abandon hard-and-fast divides between 'patients' and 'doctors'. At least through to the end of the eighteenth century, medical cultures continued to flourish amongst bourgeois circles which meshed readily with the medicine of the doctors.[19]

Barry's study shows how participation in healing activities could be an expression of practical religious piety. A similar point is central to Johanna Geyer-Kordesch's 'Cultural habits of illness: The Enlightened and the Pious in eighteenth century Germany'. Geyer-Kordesch's study makes a particularly valuable contribution for two reasons. First, it explores patterns of experience outside Britain, and thus translates the question of common contexts and cultural differences onto an international level. Second, it argues that it would be a mistake to study sickness experience and medical activity in isolation from wider belief systems about, and representations of, body, mind and soul, insight, reason and feeling in general.[20] Perhaps for German Pietists in particular, the lived experience of the body became the means of mediating between self and society, thought and action, mortality and transcendence, identity and deity. Encouraged by the 'sentimental movement', and then by Hallerian physiology's preoccupation with the mediating role of the nervous system, Pietists denied clear-cut 'Cartesian' distinctions between mind and body, psyche and soma, health and sickness. Experiencing the body became a dialectical process of psychosomatic exploration and representation, and life became 'psychotherapy', deploying a 'body language' – of anxiety, tribulation and regeneration – which united personal, religious and medical meanings. Quite apart from the role this paradigm of consciousness may have played in the subsequent emergence of psychotherapeutic

[19] For a sympathetic view of the activities of Georgian bourgeois culture see N. McKendrick, J. Brewer and J. H. Plumb, *The Birth of a Consumer Society* (London, 1982).

[20] What counts at a particular time as a '*medical*' experience, or merely as a regular part of the rhythms and expectations of life, is itself, of course, a fascinating issue. See for example P. Crawford, 'Attitudes to menstruation in seventeenth century England', *Past and Present*, XCI (1981), 47–73.

medicine, Geyer-Kordesch's study alerts us to the need for greater sensitivity to *perceptions* of the 'embodied self', in sickness and in health, and thus to the cultural construction of the (sick) 'person'.[21]

A major concern of this book is thus with lay perceptions of the body, of health, and its disturbance. But precisely how sick people then related to professional physicians is also a key theme. Current medical sociology resonates with notions of 'professional dominance'; and recent historical studies have emphasized how the 'birth of the clinic' and the 'therapeutic revolution' in the nineteenth century, and then the forging of a 'political anatomy of the body' during this century, have helped to embed the sufferer into place as 'the patient'. But what was happening before these processes of medical consolidation came to define rational medical action? Our overall grasp of medicine's social relations is patchy. There has been a disproportionate concentration of scholarly endeavour on the inside history of the medical corporations, and particularly upon the elite of physicians in London. Despite recent studies, such as Margaret Pelling's work on Norwich, aiming to grasp the full range of medical services available in traditional communities, we know too little at present about the wider market economics of medical provision. An agenda for research must include investigation of how the supply of medical practitioners adjusted to the demand for them and *vice versa*. We also need to gauge who could afford which

---

[21] For investigations of attitudes towards the body see M. Douglas, *Implicit Meanings* (London, 1975); F. Bottomley, *Attitudes to the Body in Western Christendom* (London, 1979); E. J. Bristow, *Vice and Vigilance: Purity Movements in Britain since 1700* (Dublin, 1977); B. Haley, *The Healthy Body and Victorian Culture* (Cambridge, Mass., 1978); L. Stone, *The Family, Sex and Marriage in England 1500–1800* (London, 1977). For the relations between somatic and psychic illness see G. S. Rousseau, 'Nerves, spirits and fibres: Towards defining the origins of sensibility, with a postscript 1976', in *The Blue Guitar*, vol. 2 (1976), pp. 125–53; *idem*, 'Science and the discovery of the imagination in Enlightenment England', *Eighteenth Century Studies*, III (1969), 108–35; E. Fischer-Homberger, 'Hypochondriasis of the eighteenth century. Neurosis of the present century', *Bulletin of the History of Medicine*, XLVI (1972), 391–401; *idem*, *Hypochondrie, Melancholie bis Neurose: Krankheiten und Zustandsbilder* (Berne, 1970); L. Rather, *Mind and Body in Eighteenth Century Medicine* (Berkeley, 1965); Roy Porter, 'Le prospettive della "folia": Scienza, medicina e letteratura nell'Inghilterra del '700', *Intersezioni*, II (1982), 55–76; M. MacDonald, 'The inner side of wisdom: suicide in early modern England', *Psychological Medicine*, VII (1977), 565–82; L. J. Rather, 'Old and new views of the emotions and bodily changes', *Clio Medica*, I (1965), 1–25; George Vigarello, *Le corps redressé* (Paris, 1978); T. H. Jobe, 'Medical theories of melancholia in the seventeenth and the early eighteenth centuries', *Clio Medica*, XI (1976), 217–31.

kinds of treatment from which kinds of practitioner. Who got medicine free because of gestures of conspicuous philanthropy or Poor Law paternalism? How far were relations between the sick and their physicians governed essentially by a cash nexus, or by norms defined by patronage, professionalism or expertise? How far did patients, as 'consumers', control relations with their practitioners (presumably because they commandeered the power of the purse)? Or did the intrinsic helplessness, even terror, of sickness, together with the practitioner's expertise, create entirely different power relations?[22]

Until now, few scholars have been so bold – one might say foolhardy – as to essay general mappings of the ties between the sick and their doctors. One brave attempt is Jewson's ideal type model for eighteenth century England.[23] Jewson has suggested that in Georgian England patients were able to exercise a control over their physicians analogous to the sway which grandee political patrons held over their clients, i.e. a relationship more or less the reverse of current 'professional dominance'. But could Jewson's schema of 'lay dominance' apply to more than a small elite of wealthy sufferers? (It is worth noting, though, as Barry points out, that these hypothetical relationships are rather similar to those obtaining between William Dyer and his *apothecaries*.) But Jewson's views remain rather embryonic, and scholars have not joined the fray to confirm or confute his interpretation.

One thing seems clear, however. Patient/doctor relations in early

[22] For studies of the medical profession in society see C. Webster (ed.), *Health, Medicine and Mortality in the Sixteenth Century* (Cambridge, 1979); T. Gelfand, *Professionalizing Modern Medicine* (Westpoint, Conn., 1980); G. Holmes, *Augustan England: Professions, State, and Society 1680–1730* (London, 1982); J. F. Kett, 'Provincial medical practice in England, 1730–1815', *Journal of the History of Medicine*, XIX (1964), 17–29; R. S. Roberts, 'The personnel and practice of medicine in Tudor and Stuart England', *Medical History*, VI (1962), 363–82; M. Pelling, 'Barbers and barber-surgeons: an occupational group in an English provincial town, 1550–1640', *The Society for the Social History of Medicine Bulletin*, 28 (1981), 14–16; idem, 'Medical practice in the early modern period: trade or profession?', *The Society for the Social History of Medicine Bulletin*, 32 (1983), 27–30; I. Waddington, 'Medicine, the market and professional autonomy', *The Society for the Social History of Medicine Bulletin*, 33 (1983), 70; J. Burnby, *A Study of the English Apothecary from 1660 to 1760* (*Medical History* Supplement 3, London, 1983); Joan Lane, 'The medical practitioners of provincial England in 1783', *Medical History*, XXVIII (1984), 353–71.
[23] N. Jewson, 'The disappearance of the sick man from medical cosmology 1770–1870', *Sociology*, X (1976), 225–44; idem, 'Medical knowledge and the patronage system in eighteenth century England', *Sociology*, VIII (1974), 369–85.

modern England probably more more resemblance to those characteristic of classical antiquity – ones surviving thereafter, in transmuted
forms, through the Middle Ages and the Renaissance – than to current
norms and structures; which is partly due to the fact that physicians
(and, just possibly, patients as well) in later centuries actually *modelled*
their medical behaviour on the example of antiquity. Vivian Nutton's
'Murders and miracles: Lay attitudes towards medicine in classical
antiquity' demonstrates that the medical world of the Greeks and
Romans was essentially an open one. Physicians had no effective
professional organization *de facto* or *de jure*, nor any state monopoly
or protection. With no B.M.A. or G.M.C., and without even a College
of Physicians, a doctor was whoever could individually pass himself
off successfully as one. Medicine was fundamentally a market-place
trade, and the success and rank of individual practitioners and of
medicine as an occupation depended immediately as well as ultimately
on public esteem. This is not to deny that certain doctors were better
(more skilled, more ethical) than others, or that debates raged over
alleged quacks and conmen (influential Romans such as Cato viewed
all medical practitioners as frauds). But it is to stress that antiquity left
as its legacy a body of medical knowledge – including humoralism,
the system of regimen and the non-naturals, etc. – which was perforce
accessible to educated laymen, and aspirations, ethics and etiquette for
the physician through which he strove to elevate himself *up* to the level
of his classier paymasters. Though individual physicians both in
antiquity and in early modern times might be successful, rich and
famous, it would be anachronistic to view them as prototypical of
modern professional dominance and collective upward mobility.

Perhaps surprisingly, similar conclusions are suggested by Ghada
Karmi's paper, 'The colonisation of traditional Arabic medicine'.
Karmi investigates Arabic folk medicine, as it has operated for centuries
and continues to be practised amongst the village communities of the
Near East. She demonstrates (in ways highly illuminating for
understanding vernacular practice in early modern Europe) that
common interests and shared patterns of expectation had existed, time
out of mind, between the sick person, the community and the healer.
Healers (of peasant stock themselves, and often inheriting their
occupation as a family trade) hold their respected position not because
they have undergone formal, academic-scientific training, or possess
personal charisma, esoteric wisdom or dazzling curative powers, but
because they and their clients agree implicitly upon a range of

diagnoses, therapies and services. There is a give and take, a rough parity between sufferers and healers, which allows the sick person some dignity and participation in the healing process. This balance is being totally upset by the injection into peasant communities during the last generation of Western medicine, which has created uniquely high expectations of medicine's Promethean power, patient dependency upon medical authority and, by consequence, high levels of consumer resentment. The traditional bonding and reciprocity between sufferers and healers is thus destroyed – perhaps in a high-speed replay of a process which was occurring in Western Europe over a span of several centuries.

A further interpretative problem raised by Karmi's paper lies in the content of traditional Arabic medical lore. Although passed down within the peasant communities entirely orally, it essentially reproduces centuries-old learned, elite Islamic medicine, which itself mediates the classic Greek philosophical medicine of antiquity. What were the pathways through which this transmission took place? Such problems of grasping how 'great' and 'little' traditions intertwine, how doctors' medicine becomes absorbed into lay minds, must be central to all studies of lay medical belief systems.

Karmi's paper suggests how our historical understanding of Western medicine can be illuminated by current empirical medical anthropology. Adrian Wilson's 'Participant or patient: Seventeenth century childbirth from the mother's point of view' also draws on anthropology, in this case anthropological theory. Applying Van Gennep's[24] interpretation of rites of passage to traditional English childbirth procedures, Wilson offers two important suggestions about patient/healer relations.

The first is that we all too readily assume from the modern clinical order that 'medical encounters' are essentially individual and private.[25] Exploration of traditional childbirth, however, shows something different. Childbirth did not just have a public dimension (it was a community event) but it was positively convivial, ritualistic, almost sacramental. The other concerns medical power. From our present concerns we tend to ask, 'Who has the power, the doctor or the patient?' By contrast, Wilson's paper indicates that we might profitably

[24] A. Van Gennep, *Les rites de passage* (Paris, 1909).
[25] For background explorations which help to explain the valorization of privacy and 'English individualism' see A. Macfarlane, *The Origins of English Individualism* (Oxford, 1978); C. B. MacPherson, *The Political Theory of Possessive Individualism* (Oxford, 1962); H. Perkin, *The Origins of Modern English Society* (London, 1969).

think of *authority*, not power, and see medical rituals as conferring their own authority. Both 'patient' (the mother) and 'practitioner' (in this case the midwife, who indeed exercises most of the moment-to-moment power) operate under the authority of a time-honoured ritual (as also do the 'chorus', the 'gossips'); all are 'under' it, yet are participants in it, even if the ritual also confers power upon the midwife and largely reduces the mother to passivity. It would be interesting to speculate whether childbirth (perhaps like the death-bed) was significantly more 'rule-governed', because a public rite of passage, than routine sickness encounters. And how far, one wants to ask, were the ritualistic aspects of childbirth destroyed by the rise of the man-midwife, or merely replaced by new ones? An interesting parallel would be with the impact upon rituals of death made by the rise of the undertaker.[26]

Implicit in these examples – from antiquity, from modern peasant medicine and from traditional community practice – is the assumption that the rough-and-ready mutuality which obtained between sufferers and healers took place beneath the umbrella of shared knowledge; both parties operated within at least greatly overlapping, if not identical, cognitive worlds. The doctor did not have unique access to esoteric knowledge, either in books or through personal examination – though claims to 'secrets' certainly constituted the lure of the mountebank. Two contributions to this volume specifically address this issue, exploring how the relations between laypeople and doctors are weighted by access to medical knowledge (open or closed?) and its dissemination.[27] In 'Laymen, doctors and medical knowledge in the

[26] For the interpretations of obstetrics, see B. B. Schnorrenberg, 'Is childbirth any place for a woman? The decline of midwifery in eighteenth century England', *Studies in Eighteenth Century Culture*, x (1981), 393–407; J. Donnison, *Midwives and Medical Men: A History of Inter-Professional Rivalries and Women's Rights* (London, 1977); E. Shorter, *A History of Women's Bodies* (Harmondsworth, 1983); B. This, *La Requête des Enfants à Naître* (Paris, 1982); Ann Oakley, 'Wisewomen and medical men: changes in the management of childbirth', in J. Mitchell and A. Oakley (eds.), *The Rights and Wrongs of Women* (London, 1976); R. W. Wertz and D. C. Wertz, *Lying-in: A History of Childbirth in America* (New York, 1977); A. Wilson, 'Childbirth in seventeenth and eighteenth century England' (D.Phil. thesis, University of Sussex, 1983). For undertakers see C. Gittings, *Death, Burial and the Individual in Early Modern England* (London, 1984).

[27] For evaluations of the presentation of popularized medical knowledge by medical men to the public see C. Lawrence, 'William Buchan: medicine laid open', *Medical History*, xix (1975), 20–35; C. Rosenberg, 'Medical text and medical context: explaining William Buchan's *Domestic Medicine*', *Bulletin of the History of Medicine*, lvii (1983), 22–42; L. J. Jordanova, 'Policing public health in France 1780–1815', in T. Ogawa (ed.), *Public Health* (Tokyo, 1981),

eighteenth century: The evidence of the *Gentleman's Magazine'*, Roy Porter explores Jewson's hypothesis of the epistemological parity of patients and doctors in the Enlightenment by conducting a case study of medical communications in one of the leading information channels amongst the educated classes, the *Gentleman's Magazine*.[28] He shows that quite technical and up-to-the-minute elite medical knowledge was being given a wide public airing through this journal. Indeed, many practitioners were themselves keen to participate in medical discussions conducted in the *Magazine*, as a way of bringing their names before, and currying favour with, the educated public. This example suggests that doctors still saw it as good policy to share medical learning with the paymasters rather than guard their own exclusive rights to it. One would like to know whether mutual lay–faculty involvement in diffusing medical knowledge in an organ such as the *Gentleman's Magazine* still remained possible during the nineteenth century.

A parallel study investigating the diffusion of medical knowledge and its implications (did it dominate? did it integrate?) is offered in Ginnie Smith's 'Prescribing the rules of health: Self-help and advice in the late eighteenth century'. In this survey of guides to health, Smith demonstrates how interpreting the flow and functions of popularized medical knowledge poses complex problems, not least because there are fundamental difficulties in knowing who read what, and with what effect. Publication of popular health guides was increasing throughout this period and their scope was probably broadening as well, matters such as diet, cleanliness, and bathing being prominent as well as

pp. 12–30; W. Coleman, 'Health and hygiene: a medical doctrine for the bourgeoisie', *Journal of the History of Medicine*, xxiv (1974), 399–421; P. Slack, 'Mirrors of health and treasuries of poor men: uses of the vernacular medical literature of Tudor England', in Webster (ed.), *Health, Medicine and Mortality* (note 20 above), pp. 237–74. For the important case of the popularization of sexual knowledge, see D'Arcy Power, '*Aristotle's Masterpiece*', in *The Foundations of Medical History* (Baltimore, 1931), lecture VI; J. Blackman, 'Popular theories of generation; the evolution of *Aristotle's Works*. The study of an anachronism', in J. Woodward and D. Richards (eds.), *Health Care and Popular Medicine in Nineteenth Century England* (London, 1977), pp. 56–86; O. T. Beall, Jr, '*Aristotle's Masterpiece* in America: a landmark in the folklore of medicine', *William and Mary Quarterly* (3rd series), xx (1963), 207–22; A. McLaren, 'The pleasures of procreation', in W. F. Bynum and Roy Porter (eds.), *William Hunter and the Eighteenth Century Medical World* (Cambridge, 1985), pp. 323–42. For medical advice to women see B. Ehrenreich and D. English, *For Her Own Good* (London, 1979).

[28] For a parallel, see Fielding H. Garrison, 'Medicine in *The Tatler, Spectator* and *Guardian*', *Bulletin of the History of Medicine*, ii (1934), 477–503.

sickness.[29] A greater proportion of these manuals was being written by doctors. But does all this represent a 'democratization' of knowledge? Or, instead, further steps towards 'medical hegemony' and the 'medicalization' of lifestyles? It is noteworthy that much of the advice dispensed, not least by doctors, centred on self-help, encouraging the layman to be his own physician. But how the spread of do-it-yourself medicine would ultimately affect the dynamics of lay–professional relations is no easy matter to gauge. It may be highly suggestive, however, that the therapeutic advice typically disseminated was congruent with orthodox medical theory (e.g. advice about regimen and the non-naturals).[30] It is not until the next century that 'popular medicine' by contrast increasingly meant 'alternative medicine', because of the emergence of an orthodoxy to be alternative to.

Smith's paper also raises another important issue. Medical historians study disease; hence the temptation, when looking at the patient's experience, might be to concentrate on 'sickness' and 'complaints'. But this would be a mistake. For being and staying 'well' has been at least as important amongst the laity and writers for the laity. We need, thus, to explore the positive pursuit of health in its many modes – hygiene, regimen, temperance, etc. – and this, as Smith shows, necessarily leads us beyond medicine, to purity and morality, to virtue and vice, from healing to wholeness and holiness.

The history of being sick remains largely *terra incognita*. Some of the gaps will be more easily filled than others. As certain of the above-mentioned contributions suggest, personal diaries will often tell us about the medical 'cosmologies' of sufferers, even, as in Beier's study of Josselin, over the period of an entire adult lifespan. And the great deluge of medical advice literature will give clues about what medical knowledge laymen possessed and how they acquired it. Much less readily accessible, however, are the socio-dynamics of interchanges between sufferers and doctors, the fine-textured micropolitics of

---

[29] For some stimulating accounts of attitudes towards dirt and society, see N. Elias, *The Civilizing Process* (Oxford, 1983); S. Schama, 'The unruly realm: appetite and restraint in seventeenth century Holland', *Daedalus*, CVIII (1979), 103–23.

[30] L. J. Rather, 'The six things non-natural: a note on the origins and fate of a doctrine and a phrase', *Clio Medica*, III (1968), 337–47. P. Niebyl, 'The non-naturals', *Bulletin of the History of Medicine*, XLIII (1971), 486–92; C. Rosenberg, 'The therapeutic revolution', in M. Vogel and C. Rosenberg (eds.), *The Therapeutic Revolution* (Philadelphia, 1979), pp. 3–25.

consultations, the 'moral economy' of relations that embraced business, friendship and skill against a backdrop of mortality.[31] Joan Lane's paper, '"The doctor scolds me": The diaries and correspondence of patients in eighteenth century England', helps to lay foundations for such a structure and builds up several courses of the empirical brickwork. Lane's study of published and unpublished archival material shows us where to look for this kind of information, and makes the valuable point that, whereas it would be oversanguine to expect to find in the archives a treasure trove of unknown medical diaries, many other kinds of records, for example the accounts of Overseers of the Poor, properly interrogated, will in fact yield abundant information about the health of the people. Through an evaluation of source materials, she also warns us of some of the pitfalls of the incautious use of evidence, and offers preliminary answers to many of the key questions which examination of journals and diaries raise. Who *called* the doctor? Who by contrast *went to him*? Did doctors always come out if called? Were their instructions obeyed? Were patients loyal to particular physicians, or did they grow dissatisfied and shop around? Could many Georgian physicians pass for gentlemen, or were they automatically dismissed as trumped-up tradesmen? Some of the pieces of the wider social jigsaw begin to interlock in Lane's paper, and her sifting of the evidence of hundreds of diaries points the way towards certain generalizations. For instance she makes it clear that it was still thought perfectly normal for the Quality to summon physicians for second and third opinions without feeling that it was a slur on the profession, and she shows how prescribing by post was still a widespread practice. She also demonstrates the immense power of *repute*. Medicine's great names – Sloane, Hunter, Heberden – were indeed on everyone's lips; their staggering fortunes should come as no surprise.

These papers range widely. But with such a vast uncharted ocean before us, ten articles can no more than put down a few buckets and sample the waters. Many key topics receive no extensive treatment. The book, alas, contains no sustained analysis of medical *language*, of a kind which might reveal how far vocabularies of disease and pain were shared amongst, or differentiated between, laymen and practitioners (though Wear suggests that diaries indicate a growing sophistication of

---

[31] See E. P. Thompson, 'The moral economy of the English crowd in the eighteenth century', *Past and Present*, L (1971), 76–136.

languages of pain).[32] The question of the perdurance, decline or suppression of orally disseminated medical 'folklore' and 'magic' is hardly touched upon.[33] Too little is said about what common people actually took for their complaints, about preparations and popular pharmacy, and how nostrums were recommended and passed down. Many recipe collections survive, but they await study. And the sheer range of lay medical activities needs further exploration. In this volume the focus is essentially on the healthy and the sick as *private individuals*. But collective lay strategies require investigation as well: civic initiatives and 'public health', parish action within the Poor Law, endowed philanthropy, the parts played by legislation and magistrates, and not least the role of Parliament in the literal politics of health.[34]

[32] For suggestive analyses of the interpretation of technical and literary vocabularies, see D. Davie, *The Language of Science and the Language of Literature 1700–1740* (London, 1963); J. Arthos, *The Language of Natural Description in Eighteenth Century Poetry* (New York, 1949); W. K. Wimsatt, *Philosophical Words* (New Haven, 1948); S. Tucker, *Protean Shape* (London, 1967); Roy Porter, 'The doctor and the word', *Medical Sociology News*, IX (1983), 21–8.

[33] See K. V. Thomas, *Religion and the Decline of Magic* (London, 1971); A. Macfarlane, *Witchcraft in Tudor and Stuart England* (London, 1970); E. J. Trimmer, 'Medical folklore and quackery', *Folklore*, LXXVI (1965), 161–75; Neil C. Hultin, 'Medicine and magic in the eighteenth century: the diaries of James Woodforde', *Journal of the History of Medicine*, XXX (1975), 349–66; G. S. Rousseau, 'John Wesley's *Primitive Physick* (1747)', *Harvard Library Bulletin*, XVI (1968), 242–56; J. Gélis, M. Laget and M.-F. Morel, *Entrer dans la vie* (Paris, 1978), and F. Loux, *Le jeune enfant et son corps dans la médecine traditionelle* (Paris, 1978) (both these latter draw upon medical proverbs).

[34] See for some examples R. Palmer, 'The church, leprosy and plague in medieval and early modern Europe', in Sheils (ed.), *Church and Healing* (note 15 above), pp. 79–100; A. W. Russell (ed.), *The Town and State Physician in Europe from the Middle Ages to the Enlightenment* (Wolfenbüttel, 1981); E. Posner, 'Eighteenth-century health and social service in the pottery industry of North Staffordshire', *Medical History*, XVIII (1974), 138–45; M. Bloch, *The Royal Touch* (London, 1973); G. Rosen, *From Medical Police to Social Medicine* (New York, 1974); J. Lane, 'The provincial practitioner and his services to the poor 1750–1800', *The Society for the Social History of Medicine Bulletin*, 28 (1981), 10–14; *idem*, *The Administration of an Eighteenth Century Warwickshire Parish: Butlers Marston* (Dugdale Soc. Occasional Papers XXI, Oxford, 1983); M. C. Buer, *Health, Wealth, and Population in the Early Days of the Industrial Revolution* (London, 1926); Peter Mathias, 'Swords and ploughshares: the armed forces, medicine and public health in the late eighteenth century', in his *The Transformation of England: Essays in the Economic and Social History of England in the Eighteenth Century* (London, 1979). Another gap in this book, as Dr Irvine Loudon has pointed out, is that there is no investigation of patients' experiences of sickness and medicine as recorded by doctors, or indeed of the doctors' own responses. Of course, one should not accept at face value what doctors thought patients experienced: that would be to smuggle back the agenda of traditional medical history. But

All these matters, and many others, are left to entice future researchers. It is at least hoped, however, that the preliminary mappings suggested in this volume will not prove misdirections. We have tried to avoid some of the worst traps. We believe we have resisted the temptation of conjuring up a nostalgic, Rousseauvian myth of a medical world we have lost – olden days, golden days, in which there was less sickness, people coped with it better, or suffered more nobly, and the medical profession hadn't medicalized life or planted anxiety and iatrogenic disorders. Joan Lane's diarists amply prove – we should hardly need telling – that before scientific medicine sickbeds were no beds of roses.[35]

We believe that we have also avoided the trap of viewing lay attitudes towards sickness and medicine as though they formed a hermetically sealed subculture, somehow independent of, and even prior to, the medicine of the faculty. Our investigations suggest it would be quite false to draw sharp boundaries between lay and professional outlooks, oral and literate cures, folk and learned therapeutics. Perhaps such categorical divides have no historical truth whatever (being essentially ideological weapons of war in the contemporary politics of health); perhaps they possess some validity only since some time in the nineteenth century, as medicine has become specialized and esoteric. Drawing such distinctions seems, however, to be a hindrance to understanding the interplay of medical beliefs and social relations before that time.

Until now we have had remarkably few studies of the history of the sick: as F. B. Smith informs us, 'patients loom small in medical history'.[36] And, medical history aside, scholars in other fields have not contributed much. Social historians have given the sick a wide berth, perhaps surprisingly in view of their deep involvement with family and household history, their current interests in childhood and sex, and their associations with the 'morbidity and mortality' interests of historical demographers. Yet the recent reorientation of much social history ought to offer valuable parallels and stimulus. Time was when

to understand the true play of sufferer/doctor relations we must obviously look through both sets of eyes. Michael MacDonald's *Mystical Bedlam* (Cambridge, 1981) offers an important view of seventeenth century patients seen through the eyes of a physician, and a modern account of the doctor himself *as patient* is O. Sacks, *A Leg to Stand On* (London, 1984).

[35] For a critique of these dangers see E. Shorter, *A History of Women's Bodies* (New York, 1982).

[36] Smith, *The People's Health* (note 7 above), p. 5.

'social history' was still mainly 'history from above', viewed as part
of the triumph of 'reform'. But times are changing, and the people
are becoming the subjects, not just the objects, of social history. Thus
old-style 'history of education', traditionally concentrating on schools,
legislation and inspectors, is increasingly giving way to investigations
of how ordinary people acquired knowledge, skills and ideas, leading
to a boom in studies of popular literacy, popular education and cultural
diffusion, and socialization within the family. Similarly the history of
'crime' used to be written in terms of Parliament, police, penology
and prisons; but now 'crime' is increasingly viewed as a function of
the shifting social relations of property, deprivation and repression. The
gaze has been lowered onto the internal dynamics of the community.
The historian studying sickness could learn much from these attempts
to create a people's history 'from below'.[37]

And, it goes without saying, scholarship in other disciplines needs
to be drawn upon. Contemporary medical sociology,[38] particularly the
sociology of doctor/patient relations and communications,[39] will be
valuable, so long as the dangers of anachronistic back-projection are
avoided. The same applies to oral history projects.[40] And the work
of medical anthropologists can help to sensitize us to the symbolic and

[37] For suggestive examples of social history see R. Samuel (ed.), *People's History
and Socialist Theory* (London, 1981); E. Le Roy Ladurie, *Montaillou* (London,
1979); C. Ginzburg, *The Cheese and the Worms* (London, 1980);
E. P. Thompson, 'Eighteenth century English society: class struggle without
class?', *Social History*, III (1978), 133–65; idem, *Whigs and Hunters* (Harmondsworth, 1975); idem, *The Making of the English Working Class* (Harmondsworth, 1968); John Rule, *The Experience of Labour in Eighteenth Century
Industry* (London, 1981).

[38] E. Freidson, *Profession of Medicine* (New York, 1972); D. Mechanic, 'The
concept of illness behaviour', *Journal of Chronic Disease*, xv (1962), 189–94.
And for illuminating surveys, L. J. Jordanova, 'The social sciences and history
of science and medicine', in Corsi and Weindling (eds.), *Information Sources*
(note 2 above), pp. 81–98, and P. W. G. Wright, 'The radical sociology of
medicine', *Social Studies of Science*, x (1980), 103–20.

[39] Valuable are M. Balint, *The Doctor, the Patient and his Illness* (London, 1957);
D. Locker, *Symptoms and Illness: The Cognitive Organization of Disorder*
(London, 1981); Ann Cartwright, *Patients and their Doctors* (London, 1967);
Sir H. Brackenbury, *Patient and Doctor* (London, 1935); G. Gordon, *Role
Theory and Illness* (New Haven, Conn., 1966); G. Stimson and B. Webb,
Going to See the Doctor (London, 1975); M. S. Staum and D. E. Larsen (eds.),
Doctors, Patients and Society (Waterloo, Ontario, 1982). Recent feminist studies
are useful here. See, for example, M. Barrett and Helen Roberts, 'Doctors
and their patients: the social control of women in general practice', in C. and
B. Smart, *Women, Sexuality and Social Control* (London, 1978).

[40] P. Thompson, *The Voice of the Past* (Oxford, 1978).

integrative functions of medical belief systems, as well as revealing the 'magic' and rituals habitually hidden behind the rational-technical mask of *modern* Western therapeutics.[41] There are, moreover, vast collections of medical folklore which remain surprisingly neglected by historians.[42] A great deal may also be learned from religious studies.[43] For, as several of the essays in this volume indicate, religion traditionally provided both rationalizations of the prison-house of the flesh, of 'this long disease, my life', and languages for expressing and coping with the processes of suffering, healing and dying. And the historian of sickness should also listen to literary scholars. For a key feature of imaginative writing has always been relating inner experience to outward symbolic manifestations, feelings to behaviour, soul and body (Tristram Shandy's jerkin and its lining), in ways that provide exemplars for interpreting the subjective and objective realities of sickness experience.[44] Furthermore the skills of literary critics in

[41] See for example C. G. Helman, '"Feed a cold, starve a fever": folk models of infection in an English suburban community, and their relation to medical treatment', *Culture, Medicine and Psychiatry*, II (1978), 107–37; *idem, Culture, Health and Illness* (Bristol, 1984); M. Douglas, *Purity and Danger* (London, 1966); *idem, Cultural Bias* (London, 1978); J. B. Loudon (ed.), *Social Anthropology and Medicine* (London, 1976); A. Kleinman, *Patients and Healers in the Context of Culture* (Berkeley, 1980); J. Comaroff, 'Medicine: symbol and ideology', in P. Wright and A. Treacher (eds.), *The Problem of Medical Knowledge* (Edinburgh, 1982), pp. 49–68. For a medical anthropological approach to modern medicine see T. Posner, 'Magical elements in orthodox medicine', in R. Dingwall *et al.* (eds.), *Health Care and Health Knowledge* (London, 1977), pp. 142–58; and, for a valuable survey, M. MacDonald, 'Anthropological perspectives on the history of science and medicine', in Corsi and Weindling (eds.), *Information Sources* (note 2 above), pp. 81–98.

[42] See for example M. Chamberlain, *Old Wives' Tales* (London, 1981); E. P. Thompson, 'Folklore, anthropology, and social history', *Indian Historical Review*, III (1978), 247–66; G. Lloyd, *Science, Folklore and Ideology* (Cambridge, 1983).

[43] For valuable studies incorporating both religious and anthropological dimensions see T. Ranger, 'Medical science and Pentecost: the dilemma of Anglicanism in Africa', in Sheils, *Church and History* (note 15 above), pp. 333–66; J.-C. Schmitt, *The Holy Greyhound* (Cambridge, 1983); R. Finucane, *Miracles and Pilgrims* (London, 1977). See also R. Heller, '"Priest doctors" as a rural health service in the age of Enlightenment', *Medical History*, xx (1976), 361–83.

[44] For some general reflection see S. Sontag, *Illness as Metaphor* (New York, 1978); and for a survey N. Cousins, *The Physician in Literature* (New York, 1982). For particular investigations of writers' use of illness, see R. Stephanson, 'Defoe's "malade imaginaire": the historical foundations of mental illness in *Roxana*', *Huntingdon Library Quarterly*, xlv (1982), 100–18; R. Erickson, '"Moll's Fate", —Mother Midnight" and *Moll Flanders*', *Studies in Philology*, lxxvi (1979), 75–100; G. S. Rousseau, *Tobias Smollett: Essays of Two Decades*

hermeneutics, in close reading (including reading between lines), and in tracing grids of metaphor, are ones from which historians of the sick could greatly profit.[45]

Particularly if rich and varied resources such as these are drawn upon, the temptation to launch the history of sickness as yet another self-cocooning, and hence sterile, historical subspeciality will be avoided. The stories of the sick deserve to be heard. But they will make best sense – for both medical historians and historians at large – within the collective voicings of the past. A sense of the ambiguities of the flesh, of the tyranny of disease, of the frailty of this mortal coil, dominated the minds of our ancestors to a degree which requires both imagination and patient unravelling to recreate. Health care and medical interventions proved major foci of social interaction, communal ritual, rites of passage, objects of consumption, calls on services, junction-points between private and public worlds. In making and breaking individual lives and social ties, in shaping a sense of the self, sickness was one of life's dominating threats and key experiences. It is the hope of the volume to open eyes more fully to its historical importance.

(Edinburgh, 1982); J. Benthall, *The Body Electric* (London, 1976). For studies of the embodiment of the personality see P. M. Spacks, *Imagining a Self* (Cambridge, Mass., 1976), esp. ch. 5; J. M. Morris, *Versions of the Self* (New York, 1966); and for the Lockean philosophical background to this see H. E. Allison, 'Locke's theory of personal identity: a re-examination', in I. C. Tifton (ed.), *Locke on Human Understanding: Selected Essays* (Oxford, 1977), pp. 105–22. See also S. D. Cox, *The Stranger Within Thee* (Pittsburgh, 1980); P. Delaney, *British Autobiography in the Seventeenth Century* (London, 1969); Joan Webber, *The Eloquent 'I': Style and Self in Seventeenth Century Prose* (Madison, 1968); J. O. Lyons, *The Invention of the Self* (Carbondale, 1978).

[45] For an excellent instance see J. Starobinski, 'The body's moment', in *Montaigne: Essays in Reading* (Yale French Studies no. 64, 1983), pp. 273–305. And for surveys of the field see G. S. Rousseau, 'Science and literature, the state of the art', *Isis*, LXIX (1978), 583–91; *idem*, 'Literature and medicine: the state of the field', *Isis*, LXXII (1981), 406–24.

2

Murders and miracles: Lay attitudes towards
medicine in classical antiquity

VIVIAN NUTTON

The publication in 1724 of Richard Mead's Harveian oration of the
previous year provoked a vigorous and instructive controversy.[1]
Relying largely upon the evidence of a series of coins struck at Smyrna
in Asia Minor, Mead argued that doctors in ancient Rome and its
empire were men of education and high social standing, worthy
precursors of the London College of Physicians. Ancient allegations
of incompetence and corruption he referred to the servile practitioners
of surgery, not to the physicians. Retribution was not long in coming.
Conyers Middleton,[2] theologian, librarian and unstinting contro-
versialist, retorted that, whatever the situation in Greek Smyrna, the
doctor in Rome and Italy was often a slave or an ex-slave, who fully
deserved all the criticism heaped upon him and his fellows. In the
pamphlet war that followed, Middleton more than held his ground,
and there have been few since to question his basic division between
the Greeks and the Romans over their attitudes towards medicine and
physicians, or his assertion of the generally low social status of all

---

[1] Richard Mead, *Oratio anniversaria Harveiana habita 1723; adiecta est dissertatio
de nummis quibusdam in Smyrnaeis in medicorum honorem percussis* (London,
1724). A reprint was issued at Leiden in 1725.

[2] C. Middleton, *De Medicorum apud veteres Romanos degentium conditione quae
contra J. Sponium et R. Meadium servilem atque ignobilem fuisse ostenditur*
(Cambridge, 1726); W. P., *Notae breves in dissertationem de medicorum apud
veteres Romanos degentium conditione* (London, 1726); J. Letherland, *In dissertationem...de medicorum...conditione animadversio brevis* (London, 1727);
J. Ward, *Ad...de medicorum...conditione dissertationem responsio* (London,
1727); C. Middleton, *Dissertationis de medicorum...conditione...defensio, pars
prima* (Cambridge, 1727); J. Ward, *Dissertationis C. Middletoni...defensio
examinata* (London, 1728); J. Lamotte, *An Essay upon the State and Condition
of Physicians* (London, 1728); C. Middleton, *Dissertationis...appendix, seu
defensionis pars secunda, cui accedit ad dominum Lamotte epistula apologetica*
(London, 1761).

medical men in Rome. In the subsequent two and a half centuries scholars have added little to his conclusions and few have commanded his wide range of learning. In their attempts to answer the seductive question of what the Romans thought of their physicians, prejudice has often been canonised as fact, and a traditional commonplace dignified with the title of insight.[3]

Yet past historians of medicine should not be condemned too harshly for their failure in an unavoidable task. The general bias of the surviving medical texts towards theory rather than the realities of day-to-day practice and the fact that they cluster uncomfortably around the years 450–350 B.C., when most of the Hippocratic Corpus was written, and A.D. 100–200, the age of Rufus, Soranus, Aretaeus and Galen, have necessitated a considerable reliance on non-medical sources in the creation of a history of medicine in classical antiquity that is anything more than schematic. Medical history solely from the doctor's point of view is here impossible, yet the alternative is daunting and difficult. The extent and variety of possible sources is vast. They range from imaginary law-court speeches to comic drama, from the tombstones of physicians to the lives of saints, from the dark sayings of pre-Socratic philosophers to the humble fragments of Egyptian papyri recording payments for medical services, from wordy decrees in honour of a departing civic physician to the equally revealing and far more poignant lament of a Hungarian husband for Aurelia Decia 'rarest and most chaste of wives, whose death occurred in my absence, through the fault of those who tried to cure her, and with whom I had lived for twenty-eight years, ten months and twenty-four days'.[4] Each type of evidence presents its own problems of interpretation. It is hard today to understand fully Aristophanes' jokes about the incompetent healer Pittacus, or to decide whether the satirical epigrams of Martial and Lucillius against doctors are an attack on contemporary

---

[3] H. H. Huxley, 'Greek doctor and Roman patient', *Greece and Rome*, XXVI (1957), 132–8; A. Gervais, 'Que pensait-on des médecins dans l'ancienne Rome?', *Bulletin de l'Association Guillaume Budé*, series 4, I (1964), 197–231; J. Scarborough, *Roman Medicine* (London, 1969); G. Baader, 'Der ärztliche Stand in der Antike', *Jahrbuch der Universität Düsseldorf* (1977/8), 301–15; D. W. Amundsen, 'Images of physicians in classical times', *Journal of Popular Culture*, XI (1977), 643–55; K. D. Fischer, 'Zur Entwicklung des ärztlichen Standes im römischen Kaiserreich', *Medizin-historisches Journal*, XIV (1979), 165–75; F. Kudlien, *Der griechische Arzt im Zeitalter des Hellenismus* (Mainz, 1979), who attempts a very detailed investigation of the different groups of healers.   [4] *Corp. Inscr. Lat.* III.3355.

practitioners or merely variations on an age-old theme.[5] The evidence of archaeology, whether it is for Roman military hospitals or the so-called Gallo-Roman oculists, is no less difficult to interpret.[6] It is no wonder, then, that historians have preferred to use only a few of the available texts and to hope that their choice has been a significant one, rather than carry out a detailed comparison and examination of all the evidence, even for a particular topic.

To fulfil such a task adequately would require a lengthy monograph, and even so it is doubtful whether the assemblage of information from diverse authors, regions and centuries could compensate for the absence of any long series of revelations about the health of a single individual. Neither Cicero nor Libanius, the most voluminous correspondents to survive from antiquity, says much about health and illness, and the *Confessions* of St Augustine are not the diary of Ralph Josselin. In their place historians have set the musings of the hypochondriac philosopher Seneca and, in particular, the *Sacred Tales* of Aelius Aristeides. But Seneca's elegant rhetoric often disguises rather than reveals the truth, and Aristeides' orations, which are prime documents for the interaction of religious belief and medicine in the second century A.D., remain enigmatic, even after they have been confronted with the evidence of cure inscriptions from other healing shrines and with the testimony of a medical contemporary, Galen.[7] To base the patient's view of medicine largely on such evidence is to build a house on sand.

Instead, I shall exploit the plurality of the non-medical evidence to investigate two questions where the convergence of data drawn from inscriptions, art, philosophy, theology and other literature offers the possibility of a sound and reliable generalisation. I shall first examine

[5] L. Gil and I. R. Alfageme, 'La figura de médico en la comedia Atica', *Cuadernos de filología clásica*, III (1972), 35–91; J. D. Rolleston, 'Medical aspects of the Greek anthology', *Proceedings of the Royal Society of Medicine*, VII (1914), 2–13, 30–56.

[6] R. Watermann, *Medizinisches und hygienisches aus Germania Inferior* (Neuss, 1974), pp. 111–27; V. Nutton, 'Roman oculists', *Epigraphica*, XXXIV (1972), 16–29, cf. H. Lieb, 'Nachträge zu den römischen Augenärzten und den Collyria', *Zeitschrift für Papyrologie und Epigraphik*, XLIII (1981), 207–15; G. C. Boon, 'Potters, oculists and eye troubles', *Britannia*, XIV (1983), 1–12.

[7] K. F. H. Marx, 'Uebersichtliche Anordnung der die Medizin betreffenden Aussprüche des Philosophen Lucius Annäus Seneca', *Abhandlungen der königlichen Gesellschaft der Wissenschaften zu Göttingen*, XXII (1877); C. A. Behr, *Aelius Aristeides and the Sacred Tales* (Amsterdam, 1968); Galen, *In Platonis Timaeum comment.*, Corp. Med. Graec., Suppl. I (Leipzig, Berlin, 1934), pp. 33, 83–4.

who in classical antiquity were called 'doctors', the standard translation of the Greek '*iatroi*' and the Latin '*medici*', and, secondly, I shall review some of the objections raised by laymen against medicine and medical men. The results of these investigations have a more than antiquarian interest, for the dicta of the classical authors helped to mould the responses of later educated laymen, particularly in the sixteenth, seventeenth and eighteenth centuries, to the medicine of their own day. The words of classical poets, orators, historians and philosophers then took on a universal meaning and were used to illustrate contemporary medical problems and debates. The future Bishop Atterbury's *Reflections on Antonius Musa's character represented by Virgil in the person of Iapis* can thus be read on more than one level: as a display of erudition and as a tract for the times.[8] The identification was made all the more easy because of the continued survival of the therapeutics, and of much of the theory, of the Greeks and Romans well into the nineteenth century. If the medical ideas and practices of antiquity were thus allowed some validity, then it could be argued that the reactions of the ancient consumers, of the Greek or Roman patient, also had something important to offer as a model for later conduct. Above all this could be set the Scriptures, whose eternal significance masked the fact that they were in part written within a Hellenistic framework of ideas about illness and medicine. The resurgence of interest in the fathers of the early Church, which began in the Renaissance, also helped to foster the belief in a unity of Christian and classical culture that had been somehow broken in the Middle Ages, and which had now been restored.[9] Richard Mead and William Heberden in the eighteenth century saw themselves as the heirs of Galen and Hippocrates, and their patients agreed.

Yet this, often subconscious, identification of ancient and modern obscured one crucial difference. In antiquity, the decision as to who was or was not to be called a doctor was, with very few exceptions, made either by the layman or by the individual doctor himself. It is true that there existed societies, colleges and clubs (*scholae*) of physicians, but not until A.D. 368, with the foundation by the emperor Valentinian of the Rome college of physicians, can doctors be shown

---

[8] London, 1740, and several times reprinted along with his translation of Virgil. It was perhaps composed in the 1690s.

[9] C. L. Stinger, *Humanism and the Church Fathers: Ambrogio Traversari (1386–1439) and Christian Antiquity in the Italian Renaissance* (Albany, 1977); J. C. Olin, *Six Essays on Erasmus* (New York, 1979), pp. 33–47.

beyond doubt to have played any role in the selection and approbation of physicians for public practice.[10] But the Roman college was no General Medical Council. It was not concerned with the setting of any initial qualification for practice; it had no general oversight over medical men in the capital; and its numbers, a mere fourteen of the physicians active in the city, would not have helped greatly the emperor's wish that it should aim to provide medical assistance freely to all those who needed it most. His injunction that the members of the college should prefer a humble service to the poor over craven attendance on the rich was little more than a pious hope, and, as the subsequent history of the college shows, it remained an elite body, concerned with the status, privileges and, occasionally, obligations of a select few. It is, of course, possible, given the fragmentary nature of the surviving evidence, that doctors regularly passed judgement on the competence of their fellows in other ways. Galen had a man who claimed to have learned a dubious technique from him hauled off to punishment by a magistrate, and he informed on a medical man whose knowledge of local plants had led him to dabble in murder.[11] At Ephesus and Smyrna in the second century A.D. the corporate activities of doctors also involved contests of medical skill whose results were inscribed in stone as a public record, but it would be unwise to posit an otherwise unrecorded proliferation of medical Olympics elsewhere.[12] As far as our evidence goes, it is safe to conclude that, with these few late exceptions, doctors in classical antiquity played little or no part in deciding who was to be called a physician. In this the verdict of the layman was decisive.

His canons of judgement were straightforward. A doctor was a person, male or female, who carried out medical treatment for a fee, or who, like Galen, devoted much of his time to healing, even if he

---

[10] *Cod. Theodos.* 13.3.8–9 and 13. See also V. Nutton, 'Archiatri and the medical profession in Antiquity', *Papers of the British School at Rome*, XLV (1977), 207–10, 217f; *idem*, 'Continuity or rediscovery? The city physician in classical Antiquity and mediaeval Italy', in A. W. Russell (ed.), *The Town and State Physician from the Middle Ages to the Enlightenment* (Wolfenbüttel, 1981), pp. 17–21.

[11] M. Meyerhof, 'Autobiographische Bruchstücke Galens aus arabischen Quellen', *Sudhoffs Archiv*, XXII (1929), 83; Galen, XI.336–9 K.

[12] *Die Inschriften von Ephesos*, 1160–1170, 4101; D. Knibbe, 'Neue Inschriften aus Ephesos', *Jahresheft der österreichischen archäologischen Instituts*, LIII (1981–2), p. 136, no. 46; P. Lebas and W. H. Waddington, *Voyage archéologique* (Paris, 1870), vol. III, 1523, an inscription associating a doctor with a president of the games.

never actually made any monetary charge but merely received presents.[13] It is this association of medicine with gain (*questus*) that unites the doctor with the humble Egyptian peasant-physician, farming his land and supplementing his income by his services as a healer. He was a craftsman, just like the village carpenter or the potter. If he resided in one place, he needed to have extra income from land, for the local community was rarely so large or so rich as to support him entirely on his medical activities. On the other hand he might, like the author of the Hippocratic *Epidemics*, be forced to travel in search of patients. Whatever course he chose, his social status was not of the highest, except in the rarest of circumstances. Medicine, like architecture, might be termed by theoreticians a liberal art, and on a higher plane than cobbling, but even so it was suitable, in Cicero's damning phrase, only for those of an appropriate rank in society. The practice of medicine for gain was for tradesmen, not for gentlemen.[14]

The ubiquity of this view can be seen also from the life and writings of Galen (129–*c*. 210), the leading physician of his age. His naive delight in being addressed as a gentleman by the emperor Marcus Aurelius, and his insistence on his own financial independence of his substantial medical practice, a claim accepted and turned against him by jealous opponents, bespeak a reluctance to be classed alongside the average doctor with a living to make.[15] Galen's own justification of medicine is a desperate attempt to raise it to the level and status of philosophy, an art fully worthy of the truly free man. His convoluted argument links a doctor's detailed knowledge of the internal organs of the body with the possession of all the moral virtues, and turns the doctor into a super-saint. This is obvious special pleading, and it becomes still more so when placed alongside Vitruvius' similar claims for architecture or the satirist Lucian's defence of solo dancing. These writers are all using the same language and arguments in an attempt

---

[13] Meyerhof, 'Autobiographische Bruchstücke', p. 84, cf. Galen, XIV.647 K. The importance of '*questus*' as a motive is underlined by Celsus, *De medicina*, III.4.10.

[14] Cicero, *De officiis*, I.72; this sort of argument goes back a long way, cf. Aristotle, *Nic. Eth.*, I.13.7. One should not interpret this disdain as reducing every physician to the same humble level. Doctors, when viewed by writers at the summit of the social scale (and these, in general, are our main source), might well appear less than acceptable; when seen from the bottom of society, the scribblers of Egyptian papyri, their social status often appears considerably elevated.

[15] Galen, XIV.660 K.; X.561 K., a feeble denial by Galen of the obvious truth of his wealthy background.

to suggest that their own individual speciality is somehow on a higher social and intellectual plane. They endeavour to replace mundane reality by a high ideal. Money enters into medicine, Galen cannot deny, but its sordidity is masked by the claim that its getting merely involves the true doctor in the practice of temperance; his charges are never excessive.[16]

Yet, paradoxically, it was precisely this monetary aspect of medical practice that involved non-medical authors in defining clearly and precisely who was a doctor. From perhaps 42 B.C. onwards in the Roman Empire, and possibly even earlier in the cities of the Greek East, doctors were eligible for certain tax concessions and exemptions from such obligations as military call-up and billetting.[17] These immunities were confirmed by a series of emperors until at least the sixth century, and the legal discussions on the appropriate qualification for them called forth a substantial body of case law which, at least in theory, might seem to have defined the ancient doctor. The great lawyer, Ulpian, writing in the early years of the third century, declared that one might perhaps accept as a doctor one who promised to cure only one part of the body or only one ailment – for example an ear doctor, a dentist or a specialist in fistulae. But he drew the line at a man who used incantations, imprecations and exorcisms, for they were not 'types of medicine, even though there would be some to swear that they had derived benefit therefrom'.[18] In other words, any person carrying out medical treatment for money could claim to be a doctor for tax purposes, unless he relied entirely on exorcism and the like.

This legal approach to the definition of a doctor, however, has its own limitations. It was designed to settle a problem about status and taxation, not specifically about the efficacy of medicine. The decision

---

[16] Galen, I.53–63 K. See further, E. Wenkebach, 'Der hippokratische Arzt als das Ideal Galens', *Quellen und Studien zur Geschichte der Naturwissenschaft und der Medizin*, III.4 (1935), 155–75; P. Bachmann, 'Galens Abhandlung darüber, dass der vorzügliche Arzt Philosoph sein muss', *Nachrichten von der Akademie der Wissenschaften in Göttingen, philologisch-historische Klasse* (1965), 1–67; P. Brain, 'Galen on the ideal of the physician', *South African Medical Journal*, LII (1977), 936–8. Cf. also Vitruvius, *De archit.*, I.1ff; Lucian, *De Salt.* 35.81; and Onasander's praise of the moral and philosophical qualities of the general, *Strat.* 1–2.

[17] D. Knibbe, 'Neue Inschriften', pp. 136–40 (= *Zeitschrift für Papyrologie und Epigraphik*, XLIV (1981), 1–10); this corrects and extends V. Nutton, 'Two notes on immunities: *Digest* 27, 1, 6, 10 and 11', *Journal of Roman Studies*, LXI (1971), 52–63.

[18] *Digest*, 50.13.3. Cf. *ibid.* 2, for Ulpian's acceptance of obstetrices with a knowledge of medicine.

was made by a layman, a magistrate, but from the viewpoint of the Roman or local administration, not from that of the consumer. Ulpian's definition is admirably clear and precise, but even he recognises the difficulties it involves in leaving out several reportedly effective healers. Furthermore, if the only surviving detailed decision from an individual case can be taken as typical, fitness to practice played only a minor part in the operation of this legal ruling. In October A.D. 142 a local doctor, Psasnis, appeared at Alexandria before the governor of Egypt, Valerius Eudaemon. He had appealed against the actions of his fellow villagers, who had compelled him against his will to undertake duties from which as a doctor he was legally exempt. Eudaemon's response was cutting. He suggested that perhaps they had found that Psasnis' therapies were no good. Nevertheless, he ruled that Psasnis must return to his region, and declare personally before the local magistrate that he was a proper doctor, and his immunity would then be confirmed.[19] There is here no examination, no qualifying-test or oral, only the doctor's own attestation before a magistrate that he is a doctor. This self-proclamation is acceptable, even though patients might complain of the doctor's incompetence, and even though it was in the town and state's interest to have as many tax-payers as possible, and to reduce the number of those in possession of tax immunities.

It is thus clear that the change, beloved of epigrammatists, from cobbler, carpenter, weaver and even undertaker to doctor could be managed without difficulty.[20] All that was required was the individual's own affirmation that he was now a doctor. The transition would further have been eased by the fact that medical ideas and therapies were by no means confined to a limited group of medical men. In Greece in the sixth and fifth centuries B.C. the pre-Socratic philosophers wrote and argued on medical themes, and the debates reflected in the Hippocratic Corpus were conducted by doctors and laymen alike.[21] The Hippocratic Oath, with its attempt to restrict the knowledge of medicine to a small group, was a dead letter even as it was being

[19] P. Oxyrrhynchus 40, with the re-edition of H. C. Youtie, 'A reconsideration of P. Ox. I, 40', *Festschrift F. Oertel* (Bonn, 1964), pp. 20–9.

[20] Cf. Amundsen, 'Images', pp. 646–8. It should also be noted that the distinction between quacks, charlatans and physicians is impossible to determine, except on the basis of results, and, even here, mistakes might be made, cf. Galen, *In Epid. II comm. VI: Corp. Med. Graec.* V.10.1; pp. 401–2. It is hard to see on what charge the quack revealed by Galen was punished (Meyerhof, 'Autobiographische Bruchstücke', p. 83).

[21] G. E. R. Lloyd, *Magic, Reason and Experience* (Cambridge, 1979), esp. pp. 38–47.

written. If medicine and medical discourse were part of the public domain in Greece, the situation was even more favourable to lay medicine in Rome. The historian Cassius Hemina (fl. 200 B.C.) claimed, according to Pliny, that the first doctor reached Rome only in 219 B.C. – undoubtedly an exaggeration, but one that was reflected in the belief of the elder Cato that Rome had survived for centuries on a system of patriarchal self-help.[22] But the introduction of Greek medical ideas did not end lay involvement in medical debates and practice. The two encyclopaedists, Celsus and Pliny, both laymen with an interest in medicine and therapeutics, made available in Latin a vast range of Greek medical learning, and there is no doubt that Celsus himself put some of it into practice on his landed estates.[23] The theory of humours and its later rival, that of atoms and pores, could be easily understood by anyone with a modicum of interest, intelligence and a smattering of philosophy. Indeed, it was precisely the claims of the Methodists that their atomist medicine could be taught within a mere six months that aroused Galen's greatest wrath: not surprisingly, for his ten-year study of medicine with teachers at Pergamum, Smyrna and Alexandria represents the other extreme of medical education.

An easy interchange between doctors and laymen was further facilitated by the absence of a specifically medical terminology for most aspects of medicine. A Hippocratic writer and the historian Thucydides could use the same words to describe symptoms of plague, fever and hoarseness; Seneca (d. A.D. 65), a life-long sufferer from asthma and other complaints, wrote so vividly about his illness that he convinced a nineteenth century savant that here was a medical man;[24] and the great Alexandrian anatomist Herophilus (fl. 280 B.C.) drew his coinages for his new discoveries from everyday life. 'The wine-press', 'the pen-like process', 'the little pine-cone' – denoting, respectively, the torcular Herophili, the styloid process and the pineal gland – are three examples of Herophilus' graphic style of nomenclature, and they would

---

[22] Pliny, *Hist. Nat.*, XXIX.6.12–13.

[23] See the passages assembled by W. G. Spencer in the *Introduction* to his Loeb translation of Celsus (London, 1935), pp. xi–xii.

[24] Adam Parry, 'The language of Thucydides' description of the plague', *Bulletin of the Institute of Classical Studies*, XVI (1969), 106–18; Marx, 'Seneca', p. 16 ('Die Bemerkungen scheinen nicht von einem Nichtarzte oder Dilettanten, sondern von einem erfahrenen gediegenen Praktiker herzurühren'). Marx's comment reflects the opinion of a very competent medical man, whose sole error lay in underestimating the extent of medical knowledge it was possible for a 'layman' to gain in antiquity.

have been comprehensible to the layman who had looked at a body.[25] Attempts by later authors to forge a more exact and a more specifically medical terminology for sores and ulcers were derided by fellow doctors like Galen, who sought precision in the use of the old words, not a confusion of neologisms.[26]

The accessibility of medical ideas and the relative absence of any strictly medical language enabled medicine to take a prominent place in general literary culture. Medical jokes were made by satirists and comic poets, while the genesis of new diseases formed an apt topic of conversation at a Greek dinner table. Polite society might even regard an acquaintance with medicine as a shibboleth to distinguish the man of culture from the boor. About A.D. 100 Plutarch pleaded passionately for the close interrelation of medicine and philosophy, and fifty years later Aulus Gellius considered it the grossest of solecisms for a man of learning to be so ignorant of medical terms as to confuse his veins with his arteries.[27] At almost the same date, in Roman Africa, the orator Apuleius produced a string of medical arguments as part of his defence against a charge of sorcery. The purpose of his citation of the opinions of Plato, Aristotle and Theophrastus on the true causes of epilepsy was not in any way scientific. It was to suggest to his judge, the proconsul Claudius Maximus, that the ignorance of his accusers in such matters proved them to be country-bumpkins or worse, and that their testimony was thus unreliable and inferior to that of a man of true learning, like the proconsul himself.[28] In Rome Galen was a lion of society; senators, intellectuals and imperial officials accompanied him on his visits, watched his anatomical demonstrations, and argued with him on medical minutiae.[29] Medicine was a part of upper-class culture.

---

[25] P. Potter, 'Herophilus of Chalcedon: an assessment of his place in the history of anatomy', *Bulletin of the History of Medicine*, I (1976), 46–8. No ancient source gives the naming of the pineal gland to him (or to anyone else), but as the analogy is so like what we know of his style, and since he was among the first to investigate the brain, I see no reason to deny him this honour.

[26] Galen, X.423–6. On the relationship between technical and ordinary language in Greek (as opposed to Latin or more modern) medical texts, see the eminently sane discussion of G. F. Moore, in H. J. Cadbury, *The Style and Literary Method of Luke* (Cambridge, Mass., 1919), pp. 53–4, relying in part on U. v. Wilamowitz-Moellendorff, *Die Kultur der Gegenwart*, 2nd edn. (Berlin, 1907), p. 59.

[27] Plutarch, *De sanitate tuenda*; note also the important medical discussion at *Symp.* VIII.5. Gellius, *Noct. Att.*, XVIII.10.1.

[28] Apuleius, *Apolog.*, 48–52.

[29] G. W. Bowersock, *Greek Sophists in the Roman Empire* (Oxford, 1969), pp. 59–75.

But there were others lower down the social hierarchy whose occupations and skills could be turned to medical use. The village blacksmith would have had the strength to reduce dislocations in the manner portrayed in the illustrations to Apollonius' *Commentary on Joints*, while, in Phaedrus' famous poem, it was the skill of the cobbler with needle and bradawl that took him away from his last to carry out a little surgery.[30] Remedies of humble peasants and craftsmen were taken and recorded by physicians. Even the learned Galen reproduced without comment recipes taken, often at second or third hand, from a Bithynian barber, Euschemus the eunuch, Flavius the boxer, and Orion the groom.[31]

This great variety of evidence for the participation in medicine by men (and women) of all classes throughout the ancient world proves beyond any doubt that medical knowledge was by no means confined to those who called themselves doctors. The learning of the so-called supporters of medicine (*philiatroi*) was frequently more than theoretical. The line between a Cornelius Celsus and a practising physician was a very narrow one, and had at least as much to do with an individual's perception of his own role and position in society as with his competence in book-knowledge or practical experience. Failure to appreciate this fact has resulted in much barren argument among modern scholars seeking to discover traces of a medical profession, and in a general bewilderment at the range of healers calling themselves doctors. The wide gulf between M. Modius Asiaticus, champion of the Methodist sect in early imperial Smyrna, and Fadianus Bubbal, a doctor from Morocco around A.D. 250, is evident from their memorials.[32] The Greek is beautifully carved, with an extremely elegant bust of a man of fashion, the African rustic in its lettering, and somewhat alarming in its crude display of brandished knife and cleaver. Yet both men were called by the same word, 'physician'.

This accessibility of medical knowledge was not without advantages to the patient. It enabled some members of the community to pass

[30] Phaedrus, I.14. Cf. the story in Eunapius, *Vit. Phil.*, p. 386 Wright, of the barmaid cum midwife.
[31] XIII.104, 204, 294, and 260 K.
[32] G. Richter, *Portraits of the Greeks*, vol. III (London, 1965), p. 282, fig. 2021; P. Gauckler, *Le Musée de Cherchel* (Paris, 1895), pl. III, n. 2. Much of the surprise may simply result from the translation of the Latin and Greek terms as 'physician' with its modern connotations. 'Healer' would carry different meanings and would easily allow a broad range of styles and statuses among those it denoted.

judgement with reasonable certainty on the abilities of those who claimed to possess healing powers. Galen assumed that, when a choice of doctor was available, the illness itself was not too pressing and no personal recommendation by a friend was to hand, an educated patient would submit the aspiring physician to a lengthy series of detailed and searching questions on all aspects of his art.[33] We may choose to dismiss this as a typically Galenic exaggeration, yet in many communities it was precisely men of Galen's own social class, the wealthy and respectable members of the local council, who had the task of selecting, investigating and appointing the town physician. Historians have argued at length about the duties and obligations of these civic doctors, yet all are agreed on one crucial point.[34] The appointment, which often brought with it such obvious privileges as a front seat at the local games or a rent-free surgery at the town's main crossroads, served at least to legitimate visibly the doctor's own claims to competence and to display in public his acceptability. Yet, unless a doctor happened to be a council member, it was a choice made entirely by laymen. It was a judgement by the future consumer, not by a technical peer. But it was not made entirely out of inexperience and ignorance.

The councillors were charged to review all appointments regularly, perhaps even annually, and they were empowered to sack any doctor found deficient in morality or learning. The facts that they could occasionally be fooled by a doctor's flashy instruments, poetic quotations and flamboyant rhetoric, that we have no definite evidence for any sacking of a civic physician, that increasingly it was members of local medical families who were appointed, or that a doctor might be unjustly stigmatised for a failure not of his own making, should not blind us to one important point. This method of selection, by those who were most likely to be able to know and follow the doctor's activities in practice, was, in the absence of anything resembling a system of medical licensing, a sensible and perhaps effective procedure. In the face-to-face society of the small towns of antiquity, where, in Galen's words, everyone knew each other's parentage, education and way of life, a check on performance was simple, and the provision by satisfied town councils of testimonials to the virtues of a departing

---

[33] Galen's tract 'On the examination of the physician' is being edited by Dr A. Z. Iskandar; see also A. Dietrich, *Medicinalia Arabica* (Göttingen, 1966), pp. 190–5.

[34] L. Cohn-Haft, *The Public Physicians of Ancient Greece* (Northampton, Mass., 1956); and my articles, 'Archiatri' and 'Continuity'.

doctor would have made the initial problem of selection occasionally easier.[35]

The evidence of honorary decrees and formal commemorations of departed physicians reveals that the layman's assumptions about the good doctor were almost identical to those of the physicians. The language of epigraphic testimonials differs but little from that of the Hippocratic treatises on medical decorum. The civic physician was a man of piety, philanthropy and consummate skill; he poured out his energy and compassion on all who sought his help; and he united within himself learning (*episteme*) and experience (*peira*).[36] There was general agreement also on his ideal intellectual pedigree. The importance of Cos as a medical centre in the Greek world of the fourth and third centuries B.C. is confirmed by the number of surviving requests from the small towns of the Aegean basin asking for a suitable Coan doctor to come and reside among them.[37] The later pre-eminence of Alexandria is likewise no happy fiction put about by its 'old boys'. It was a geographer who called it 'the foundation of health for all men', and a sober historian who declared that merely to have studied there was recommendation enough for any doctor.[38] This testimony can be confirmed by a story from an impeccable source, none other than St Augustine. According to him, an elderly lawyer from Carthage, by the name of Innocentius, had long been a sufferer from a fistula of the rectum. A first operation failed, and he dismissed with anger and contempt both his personal physician and a reputable local surgeon when they proposed to try again. It was only when a famous doctor from Alexandria arrived and recommended the identical operation that Innocentius was persuaded to submit himself again to the knife. But even as he was being prepared for the operation, a miracle occurred; the prayers of his friends were answered, and medical intervention was made unnecessary. The reputation of Alexandria was eclipsed only by the power of God.[39]

Only in one respect do the expectations of the layman differ from

35 Galen, XIV.624 K.
36 *Inscr. graec.*, XII.5.719; *Inscr. graec. ad res Rom. pertinentes*, III.534; IV.1087; *Mon. Asiae Minoris Ant.*, VI.114. See now D. Gourevitch, *Le triangle hippocratique dans le monde gréco-romain: le malade, sa maladie et son médecin* (Rome, 1984), pp. 414–37.
37 S. M. Sherwin-White, *Ancient Cos* (Göttingen, 1978), pp. 263–74.
38 Anon., *Expositio totius mundi*, p. 37; Ammianus Marcellinus, *Hist.*, XXII.16.18.
39 Augustine, *Civ. Dei*, XXII.8; cf. Theodoret, *Epp.* 114, 115, and the evidence cited by me at 'Ammianus and Alexandria', *Clio Medica*, VII (1972), 165–76.

those of the doctor, and even here the divergence may be more superficial than real. It is clear that to the man in the street the doctor's healing power resided as much in his words as in his actions. Cicero praised Dr Asclepiades for his eloquence as well as his therapies, and later legend magnified his achievements still more. He could awaken the apparently dead by a mere declaration. Where other doctors took the pulse, palpated the chest and grimly pronounced impending doom, the great physician had only to say the word and the patient recovered.[40] Five hundred years later, in the 370s, the same miraculous powers were credited to Magnus of Nisibis, professor of medicine at Alexandria. If the writings that go under his name are genuine, he seems to have been an uninspired synthesiser of Galen, an indifferent poet and, to judge from the correspondence of Libanius, an odious personality. But his reputation as a medical man was enormous.[41] The city of Alexandria built a special lecture hall for him; pupils flocked to hear him from many miles away; and an epigrammatist could depict him descending to Hades to bring back the dead. The secret of his success is revealed by his contemporary biographer, Eunapius. In his opinion, Magnus was generally thought less able as a healer than as an orator; he could convince patients that they were cured or were still in need of his assistance purely by his command of eloquence and logic. In more than one sense, Magnus was an iatrosophist.[42]

Rhetoric, the ability to speak well, was thus seen by patients as a guide to medical competence. Doctors might bemoan the fact that the good speaker could outwit the good but somewhat tongue-tied practitioner, and they might offer helpful advice to the would-be physician: he should avoid flowery poetic quotations (the sign of a mis-spent education), violent argument (which would damage the

40 Apuleius, *Flor.* 19; for Asclepiades' rhetorical skills, see E. D. Rawson, 'The life and death of Asclepiades of Bithynia', *Classical Quarterly*, n.s., XXXIII (1982), esp. 362–7. The story about Asclepiades goes back via Pliny, *Hist. nat.*, VII.124; XXVI.15, and Celsus, *De med.*, II.6.15, perhaps to Varro, but the motif is much earlier. There are close parallels in Christian texts, e.g. Luke 7: 11–17 and Acts 9: 36–41. The emphasis on the healer's actual words can also be seen in the preservation by Mark of some Aramaic words used by Christ in his healing miracles, Mark 5: 41 and 7: 34.
41 Philostorgius, *Hist.*, VIII.10; Libanius, *Epp.*, 843, 1208, 1358; *Anth. Pal.*, XI.281. On his poetry, *Anth. Pal.*, XVI.270, and cf. M. L. West, 'Magnus and Marcellinus: unnoticed acrostics in the Cyranides', *Classical Quarterly*, n.s., XXXII (1982), 480–1.
42 Eunapius, *Vit. phil.*, pp. 530–2 Wright. The term is applied to him by a later writer, Palladius, *Anth. Pal.*, XI.281, and may not be his contemporary title.

prestige of the art of medicine) and inappropriate language.[43] According to Galen's pompous banalities, he should adapt his tone and even vocabulary to suit each individual patient; he should be able to communicate with the intellectual as well as with the illiterate.[44]

But any idea that the pursuit of eloquence was ever followed unwillingly by doctors is a gross exaggeration. On the contrary, in a society where public discussion and debate were common and where education and culture set a high premium on rhetoric, doctors seem gladly to have used their skills as orators. Lectures on medicine in the public gymnasia, open confrontations at the bedside, challenge matches and debates at street corners, these were the very stuff of medical life. The travelling physician, the 'crowd-puller', attracted attention by the torrent of words pouring from him, or even by the volume of his voice.[45] More elegant productions do not disguise the effects of rhetoric. Tracts such as *On Breaths* or *On the Ensoulment of the Foetus* are closer to declamations than to scientific theses, while Galen's success owed much to his ability to tell a good story and to refute his opponents by the vigour of his arguments, not to mention the sheer number of his words.[46] Rhetoric and showmanship, if carried to excess, were deprecated by all parties, yet it is clear that they were what attracted audiences and drew the crowds, and that they were necessary weapons in the battle against disease. The doctor needed them, and used them gladly in his attempt to gain the patient's confidence, for without that confidence, the victory was won only with difficulty. The stronger the patient's belief in the physician, the greater the chance of cure, and no doctor would neglect in this the power of the word.[47]

My argument has been so far that medicine in classical antiquity was an open science. The doctor performed in public; his surgery was as

43 [Hippocrates], *De nat. hom.*, 1; *Praecepta*, 12–13.
44 Galen, XVII B.145–8 K., with the excellent discussion of K. Deichgräber, *Medicus gratiosus* (Mainz, 1970), pp. 33–41.
45 On lectures, cf. L. and J. Robert, 'Bulletin épigraphique', *Revue des études grecques*, LXXI (1958), n. 336; on challenge matches, Galen, II.642 K.; on quacks and crowd-pullers, F. Kudlien, 'Schaustellerei und Heilmittelvertrieb in der Antike', *Gesnerus*, XL (1983), 91–8.
46 [Hippocrates], *De flat.*, II.226–52 Jones (cf. also 221–2); K. Kalbfleisch, 'Die neuplatonische fälschlich dem Galenos zugeschriebene Schrift Ad Gaurum quomodo animetur foetus', *Abhandlungen der Akademie der Wissenschaften zu Berlin, Philologisch-historische Klasse* (1895); on Galen's own abilities as a narrator, see my 'Style and context in the *Methodus Medendi*', forthcoming in the proceedings of the 1982 Galen conference, Kiel.
47 L. Edelstein, *Ancient Medicine* (Baltimore, 1967), pp. 65–86.

much a meeting-place for gossip as a medical sanctuary;[48] and his theoretical principles, as well as many of his techniques, were familiar to many of the community in which he served. Medicine, in short, formed part of general culture, and doctors showed little reluctance to recommend their subject as a worthwhile intellectual pursuit for young and old alike. The idea of medicine as a holy art, whose secrets were to be kept within a close circle, was far from being shared by all physicians. The boundary between the self-acknowledged doctor and the educated layman was very narrow. The distance that separated a Galen from a Cornelius Celsus or a Seneca is far less than that between a modern cardiologist and the average G.P.

There were, of course, good and bad physicians. The ancient sources catalogue with relish the crimes of quacks, charlatans, magi and incompetent healers of every description; sex, alcohol and bungled operations figure as much in them as in the *News of the World*. Galen's view of his competitors is so lurid that one is surprised to find any member of the Roman aristocracy living to middle age, let alone surviving treatment by hands other than Galen's. But such stories are universal, and can tell us little about attitudes towards medicine and medical men. Nor should we be surprised to find great divergencies of income and status between practitioners. A doctor to the emperor is clearly a cut above an ex-slave doctor at Assisi, even though he too might be wealthy; and the social situation of a doctor from a family long resident in a town in Asia Minor is different from that of a Greek immigrant to Italy.[49] A doctor with claims to descend from the gods or with generations of local magistracies in his family was a suitable relative for a provincial governor; a travelling physician, like Lucius Clodius of Ancona, 'always on the road, and hurrying to get to the next fair', was a figure as much to be suspected as welcomed.[50]

---

[48] *Ibid.*, pp. 87–92; G. Harig, 'Zum Problem "Krankenhaus" in der Antike', *Klio*, LIII (1971), 182–5. Cf. also the comments of Polybius, *Hist.*, XII.25d.6, on the crowds that gathered around a rhetorical physician.

[49] *Inscr. lat. sel.* 5369, 7812, a wealthy freedman. See also V. Nutton, 'The medical profession in the Roman Empire, from Augustus to Justinian' (University of Cambridge Ph.D. thesis, 1970), pp. 67–86. Not that an immigrant doctor's family could not equally within a few generations become accepted among the local gentry, e.g. *Corp. Inscr. Lat.*, IX.1655, 1971 and *Notizie degli Scavi*, 1913, 311 (on a Greek family at Beneventum), or that a travelling physician in the East was less respectable than a resident civic doctor.

[50] Contrast *Inscr. graec. ad res rom. pert.*, III.693 and *Mon. Asiae Min. Ant.*, VI.373, for example, with Cicero, *Pro Cluentio*, 14.40. C. Stertinius Xenophon, doctor to the emperor Claudius, claimed descent from both Asclepius and Heracles, see A. Maiuri, *Nuova Silloge epigrafica di Rodi e Cos* (Florence, 1925), n. 461.

Yet even the best-connected or the wealthiest of physicians might not be thought to come from the right social bracket. In a society such as the Roman Empire, where landed wealth and the ability to enjoy a life of ease and honour (*otium cum dignitate* in Cicero's phrase) were the marks of a true aristocrat, any connection with medicine was to some extent demeaning, even if it only involved having to take exercise in a gymnasium under the supervision of a trainer.[51] Even the two authors whose opinions about doctors and medicine have been thought to be highly favourable, Cicero and Seneca, display the understandable prejudice of the senatorial order. Seneca's eulogy of his own physician, whose constant and devoted attentions to his millionaire patient turned him from a hireling into a friend, reveals by its saccharined eloquence the generally low expectations with which he approached his physicians.[52]

The evidence of Cicero is somewhat more complex. His public pronouncements on his own physicians are indeed laudatory. He recommends Dr Asclapo of Patras as a man of kindness, learning and fidelity, while the death of Dr Alexio causes him immense grief. As for Dr Glycon, none other than the noble Brutus could praise him as a 'modest and frugal man, whom no thought of self-advantage could drive to crime'. These paragons were practising something more than a mere craft; they exercised an *ars liberalis* or an *ars honesta*, an art worthy of a gentleman.[53] Yet a closer examination of these texts reveals a very different story. Cicero's praise of medicine, if indeed it is his own and not, as Peter Brunt has suggested, lifted bodily from a work by a Greek philosopher, is subtly and damningly qualified.[54] Medicine is a nobler art, but only by comparison with the work of tax-collectors, small traders, carpenters, cooks and dancers: it ranks below oratory, politics and large-scale farming, and is suitable only for men of an appropriate social class (*eis quorum ordini convenit*).[55] Nor are Cicero's individual physicians all that they might seem. His commendatory letter of Asclapo is distinctly cool by comparison with others

---

[51] Seneca, *Ep.*, 15.2., cf. 15.4.

[52] *Idem, De Benef.*, VI.15.4.

[53] Cicero, *Ad fam.*, XIII.20; *Ad Att.*, XV.1–3; *Ad Brut.*, I.6; *De off.*, I.151.

[54] P. A. Brunt, 'Aspects of the social thought of Dio Chrysostom and of the Stoics', *Proceedings of the Cambridge Philosophical Society*, n.s., xix (1973), 26–34.

[55] Cicero, *De off.*, I.150–1. On the problem of medicine as a 'liberal art' in Roman law, see K. H. Below, *Der Arzt im römischen Recht* (Munich, 1953), pp. 57–81; J. Visky, 'Osservazioni sulle Artes Liberales', in *Synteleia: scritti in memoria di V. Arangio-Ruiz* (Naples, 1964), pp. 1068–74.

that he wrote; and his own experience with Asclapo in Greece had revealed him to be lacking in effort and attentiveness.[56] Nor should the fame and eloquence of Brutus blind us to the fact that his letter was intended to secure Cicero's help in freeing Glycon from gaol, where he had been confined on suspicion of murdering his patron.

If Cicero and Seneca, for all their supposedly enlightened and liberal views, refused to recognise the physician as one of themselves, one can understand how a later historian could regard the attempt by the son of an imperial physician to become emperor as the culminating proof of the decadence of society. When in A.D. 219 Gellius Maximus, a legionary commander in Syria, raised his standard against the emperor Elagabalus, Cassius Dio commented tartly: 'Things have come to a pretty pass when the son of a doctor can aim at empire.'[57]

Such prejudice on the part of the landed aristocracy would be unremarkable, were it not for the reverence of medical historians for the medical profession and their desire to set the ancient physician on the highest social plane. They have, on the whole, neglected the fact that the *iatroi* and *medici* were but one of many specialists who claimed to cure disease. The services they provided could be compared with those of the herb-cutters, druggists, midwives, gymnastic trainers, diviners, exorcists and priests of both private and public shrines.[58] Medicine, as practised by a Galen or a Hippocrates, had to compete, or at least to coexist, with other forms of healing. Of the arguments of its opponents only dim echoes can now be heard. It was alleged that medicine was merely a development of gymnastics, and that certain conditions, for example, war-wounds and the stone, should best be left to specialists to treat, while the tract *The Art* is a rejoinder by a layman to the criticisms of those who have 'vilified the arts in order to show off their own learning'.[59] The last two of their objections, that patients

56 Cicero, *Ad fam.*, XVI.4.
57 Cassius Dio, *Hist.*, LXXX.7.1. Cf. V. Nutton, 'L. Gellius Maximus, physician and procurator', *Classical Quarterly*, n.s., XXI (1971), 262–72.
58 Lloyd, *Magic*, pp. 38–9. It should also be noted that there might be disputes within the physicians over the propriety of using remedies of a particular type, and the bias of the surviving sources leads modern historians to take Galen or Rufus as typical. Hence remedies rejected by Galen or Scribonius, but accepted by Pamphilus, Xenocrates and Alexander of Tralles, are condemned as magic and superstition. Perceptions of what was suitable for a doctor to use might differ from doctor to doctor, and one should be wary of accepting Galen's standpoint as the most obvious or as the usual. His own long training, wealthy background in a large and affluent city, and intellectualism were by no means typical of his fellow physicians.
59 Anon. Londin., IX; p. 48 Jones; [Hippocrates], *Medicus*, 14; *Iusiur*, 5, with Edelstein's comments, *Ancient Medicine*, pp. 26–31; *Ars*, 1, 4–8.

die even after medical treatment and that doctors themselves recognise some cases as hopeless, are easily rebutted, but the first two, that patients often recover without medical help and that cures are due to luck or fate, demand closer consideration. It should be stated at the outset that we have no way of knowing how far these arguments were spread, although they can be traced over the centuries and are not without influence today. At the same time, these problems – which may be roughly interpreted as 'Are doctors necessary?' and 'Is medicine necessary?' – take on a subtly different aspect as a result first of Rome's conquest of the Greek world and its gradual hellenisation, and secondly of the spread of Christianity in the Roman world. Objections which, to the author of *The Art*, contributed to the same end, the refusal to admit that there was a specific art of medicine, became separated, and were put forward for different reasons and with different results, as the rest of this paper will show.

For the early defender of medicine, a man skilled in the art was necessary both to enable the healing process to continue and to give the patient confidence to resist his disease. But need he be a doctor? A patient might recover through doing or eating something, unwittingly, which counteracted his disease. He might be his own physician without knowing it. The doctor, then, possessed greater knowledge than the patient, but, as we have already seen, such knowledge was by no means difficult to obtain or to put into practice. Hippocratic medicine, which in general preferred diet to drugs, and drugs to surgery, was little more than good nursing – and is not to be despised for that; its precepts were not hard to follow, and many of its allopathic cures could be easily deduced from first principles.[60] If nature's way was obvious, then following her guidance need not be difficult. Unless the secrets of the art were to be kept for the few – and the author of *The Art* rejects that opinion – then it was possible for anyone to be his own physician.[61] The art of medicine may be

---

[60] Edelstein, *Ancient Medicine*, pp. 87–110; I. M. Lonie, 'A structural pattern in Greek dietetics and the early history of Greek medicine', *Medical History*, XXI (1977), 235–60.

[61] [Hippocrates], *Ars*, 8–9. The authors of the *Oath* and the *Law* prefer to restrict a knowledge of medicine to 'those who have been initiated into the mysteries of knowledge', *Lex*, 5, but, as Lloyd has argued, *Magic*, pp. 246–67, much of the peculiar character of Greek, as opposed to Babylonian or Egyptian, medicine derives from its openness and, at times, public accountability. Neither in Greece nor in Rome does an acquaintance with medical ideas appear to be confined to a particular social class (although the illiterate and the rural peasant were obviously less advantaged than a literate town-dweller), nor, except at a very superficial level, is the choice of remedy determined

necessary, but the intervention of physicians, it is implied, is not always
so.

This argument against doctors was given an added twist when, from
the fourth or third century B.C. onwards, the Romans came into
contact with Greek medicine. What survives of early Roman medicine
suggests a reliance on a relatively small number of local plants and
herbs, in which the power to heal resided in the plants themselves or
in the chants and charms with which, from time to time, they were
administered. Remedies were handed down within the household, and
could be applied to man or beast by a family patriarch or the humblest
cowherd. It was an egalitarian medicine, appropriate to the ideal
Roman farm, wherein the humble cabbage could cure everything from
gout to deafness and from insomnia to cancerous sores. It was a
medicine without doctors, and, for that reason, inexpensive.[62]

But Rome's growing contact with the Greek world, as well as the
steady drift away from the fields to the city of Rome itself, was already
changing this domestic medicine even before the elder Cato, in his
book *On Agriculture* and in an open letter to his son, both written
between 175 and 160 B.C., took up the challenge on behalf of traditional
medicine. His own experiences in Greece and in provincial Italy had
convinced him that the medicine of the Roman patriarchs was far
superior to anything that the Greeks could offer. Their physicians, he
believed, were far more likely to corrupt and destroy even than love
poetry. As he told his son, they had sworn an oath to kill all barbarians
by their medicine; they charged fees merely to allay the suspicions of
their victims; and they were inclined to insult the Romans as barbarians
or worse.[63] This is strong stuff, and yet far from lacking evidence in
its favour. The failure of the first Greek surgeon to come to Rome
as a civic physician, Archagathus the Peloponnesian in 219 B.C., was
already notorious. Within a short time of being welcomed with a
public surgery and citizen rights, Archagathus was being derided as
'executioner' and returning home to the obscurity from which he had
come.[64] But Cato was no simple educator or medical publicist: he was

entirely by social class. The ingredients might be different for a rich and for
a poor patient, but the *type* of remedy, pill, ointment, potion and so on, often
was not.

[62] W. H. S. Jones, 'Ancient Roman folk medicine', *Journal of the History of
Medicine*, XII (1957), 459–72; U. Capitani, 'Celso, Scribonio Largo, Plinio il
Vecchio', *Maia*, n.s. II (1972), 120–40.

[63] Pliny, *Hist. nat.*, XXIX.7.14.

[64] *Ibid.*, 6.12–13. The correct interpretation of this story was first given by
Cohn-Haft, *Public Physicians*, p. 48, n. 18. Pliny's opinion that he was the first

a politician, with a strong populist and nationalist line, as well as an orator with more than a gift for colourful hyperbole. As Professor Astin puts it, 'although the underlying conviction was doubtless that Greek medicine was hazardous, it found expression not as a rational assessment but with the emotional twists and illogical conjunctions of unmistakable prejudice. A number of prejudices associated with the Greeks, including that against Greek doctors, impinged upon and reinforced each other.'[65]

Prejudiced or not, Cato's denunciation became famous. It provoked Plutarch 250 years later to defend his fellow Greeks by implying that Cato had mixed up a Hippocratic oath with a misunderstood version of the story whereby Hippocrates refused to lend his services to Artaxerxes, king of Persia, on the grounds that he would never help the enemies of Greece.[66] By contrast the elder Pliny, writing his *Natural History* in the early 70s, felt no need to excuse or defend his predecessor. The words of Cato, now viewed as a sage, a moralist and the incarnation of true Roman virtue, fitted perfectly with his own sentiments of a gradual decline of Rome under the corrupting influence of Greece; and the rhetoric of the earlier writer challenged him to emulation. The result was the most sustained, influential and potentially devastating attack on doctors and their medicine ever mounted. Even today the vigour of Pliny's prose and the salacious magnificence of his examples still compel admiration, if not assent.

For Pliny, medicine, as generally practised in the Rome of Nero and the Flavians, is wholesale murder, and unpunished at that. Its victims go eagerly to their deaths, seduced by wishful thinking and a belief in things Greek. A medical book not in Greek has no prestige at all, and the less the patient understands, the more he praises his attendant. There is a constant confusion of doctrine; the man in the street is blown along by each blast of a new fancy, now for cold baths, now for hot, now for luxury foods, now for fasting. Drugs have become more and more complicated, and are easily falsified. Poisons are substituted for remedies willy-nilly, and to trust in a drug-dealer is akin to suicide. Doctors are continually quarrelsome, always vicious and never without

doctor to come to Rome is more often interpreted literally or to mean that he was the first 'scientifically trained' physician, so G. Baader, 'Der ärztliche Stand in der römischen Republik', *Acta Conventus XI 'Eirene', 1968* (Warsaw, 1971), p. 9; J. H. Phillips, 'The emergence of the Greek medical profession in the Roman Republic', *Transactions and Studies of the College of Physicians of Philadelphia*, ser. 5.2 (1980), 269.

[65] A. E. Astin, *Cato the Censor* (Oxford, 1978), pp. 170–3.
[66] Plutarch, *Cato Maior*, 23.3–4.

money. They buy popularity with the lives of their patients, from whom they also extract huge sums to spend on villas, estates, and occasional public benefactions. They use medicine as a way to political influence, and do not scruple to take advantage of their positions to commit adultery even with imperial princesses. Pliny's sole consolation is that native Roman citizens have not taken up the practice of medicine in large numbers, despite the lure of immense wealth, and the existence of such exemplars as the wealthy Antonius Castor, pottering around his little herb garden, hale and hearty in his hundredth year, offers Pliny hope for the future. His aim in his encyclopaedia is threefold: to warn his fellow-citizens, to encourage them to go out and hunt for herbs and simples themselves, and to offer a collection of remedies that will enable the Roman reader to treat himself, just like old Cato.[67]

It is not the intention here to determine whether or not Pliny succeeded in any part of his campaign, and it makes no difference whether he is shown to be exaggerating wildly or accurately reporting the actual situation.[68] What is significant is that Pliny is articulating an attitude towards doctors that makes its appearance otherwise only in the writers of satire or humorous epigram. He may well be wrong, but he is at least expecting to find some response, especially by playing also upon the well-worn theme of moral decay and anti-Greek sentiment. In an age when all the doctors to the emperor came from the Greek East or from Marseilles, that little Athens beyond the Alps; when ninety-three per cent of doctors recorded over three centuries on inscriptions from Rome and Italy bear non-Roman, and usually Greek, names; when only fifteen of the almost 180 doctors named thereon in the first century A.D. can be shown beyond any doubt to come from citizen families, it is hardly surprising that there should be some adverse comment at the invasion of eager foreigners.[69] Yet one should be careful not to take Pliny's evidence as having universal significance or to assume that he is attacking medicine in general. He stands for self-treatment, tested remedies and a commendable distrust of cant, not for the wholesale abandonment of medicine and medical theory.

That even this extreme view found some supporters is already clear

[67] Pliny, *Hist. nat.*, XXIX.1–8.28.
[68] I have discussed this problem at length in a paper 'The perils of patriotism: Pliny and Roman medicine' delivered at an international conference on Pliny in London in December 1983, and forthcoming in the proceedings of the conference.
[69] Nutton, 'The medical profession', pp. 258, 262–3.

from the comments of the author of *The Art*, and Cicero records a similar belief among the Stoics in the overriding power of fate, without in any way assenting to it or indicating that it was widespread.[70] But it is only with Judaism, and, still more, with Christianity, that one finds passive acceptance of disease and suffering enjoined upon the true believer because they are part of God's judgement. The Book of Job is not a Greek tragedy, while the discussion in Anastasius of Sinai over the correct interpretation of Jeremiah 21.9–10, which apparently recommends flight as the best way of avoiding a plague sent as punishment from God, cannot be transferred to a pagan setting.[71] The enquirers at the oracle at Claros during the great plague of the late 160s were clear what they wanted from Apollo. They wished to know when the pestilence would end, and what steps they might take to avoid or mitigate it;[72] a man who, when given the opportunity to escape, chose from moral scruples to stay, would have been seen as a fool, not a saint. By contrast, the Christian preacher Tertullian delighted exuberantly in famine and plague as God's cure for overcrowding, while, somewhat calmer, St Cyprian advised his African flock to welcome the plague of A.D. 252 as proof of God's love and mercy: 'Why should we be afraid? It is God's will, and we should welcome it with gladness. For by it, the unbelievers are sent swifter to Hell, and the just attain even more speedily their everlasting refreshment.'[73] Such an attitude would have drawn forth derision from a non-Christian audience, who rarely shared such certainty of a future life of happiness for the true believer. Their minds were set on more earthly things: self-preservation and flight.

That the advent and spread of Christianity introduced new tensions into the relationship between religion and medicine is only too obvious, although the loss of many pagan religious documents may have helped to exaggerate the difference. Paganism had its religious healers in its priests, exorcists and diviners; it had its healing centres

---

[70] Cicero, *De fato*, 13. This opinion could shade into a belief in astrology that was far from unacceptable to many doctors, e.g. *Inscr. graec.*, XIV.809; K. Deichgräber, 'Ausgewähltes aus der medizinischen Literatur der Antike: I', *Philologus*, CI (1957), 135–47; W. and H. G. Gundel, *Astrologoumena* (Wiesbaden, 1966).

[71] Anastasius Sin., *Quaestiones*, 114; *Patr. graec.* 89.765–6.

[72] J. N. Wiseman, *Studies in the Antiquities of Stobi* (Belgrade, 1973), pp. 143–83; L. Robert, *A travers l'Asie Mineure* (Paris, Athens, 1980), pp. 402–8; the whole section on Alexander the false prophet, pp. 392–421, is of relevance. Cf. also *Pap. Oxyrrh.* 3078.

[73] Tertullian, *De anima*, 30; Cyprian, *De mort.* 9.

in the shrines of Asclepius, Sarapis, Apollo or of local gods like Amphiaraus or Nodens; it had its religious therapies in incubation, expiation, sacrifice. In theory at least, any disease might have a religious cause and be healed by religious means, and some, in particular plague, mental disorders, epilepsy and chronic conditions, were regularly so treated. Yet in all this there is a striking collaboration between priest and doctor, and a remarkable lack of polemic between the two. Boundaries might be delimited, but there was not total annexation. Only one sect of doctors, the Methodists, utterly rejected the possibility of divine healing, for although their gods existed, they were too far removed from this world to be able to effect anything.[74] But the average doctor accepted that the gods might heal where he could not: to acknowledge his own limitations was a sign of strength, not of weakness. Many went far beyond this in their support for divine healing. The doctor Asclepiacus acted as one of the interpreters at the shrine of Asclepius at Pergamum; an elderly physician was one of the leading contenders for the succession to Alexander of Abonuteichos as priest of his shrine; and Galen, himself a devotee of Asclepius, did not think it at all odd to cure himself, and even his patients, by remedies vouchsafed to him by the god in a dream.[75] This devotion could be expressed in buildings as well as in creeds. Caius Stertinius Xenophon, doctor to the emperor Claudius, largely rebuilt at his own expense the famous Asclepieion of Cos, and showed no embarrassment at referring to his direct descent from two healing deities, Asclepius and Heracles.[76] A century or so later, in the highlands of central Turkey, Menodorus, doctor and priest of Asclepius, joined with his son in providing a vaulted annexe, two columns and a new roof for their local shrine.[77] Conversely, in Edelstein's words, the god learned medicine. Many of the therapies ordered by the god at the Asclepieion of Epidaurus differed only slightly from those of the physicians; there was no religious objection to doctors as priests and interpreters; and even Aelius Aristeides, who shocked his medical attendants by obeying the

---

[74] Edelstein, *Ancient Medicine*, pp. 205–46, remains fundamental; see also F. Kudlien, 'Der Arzt des Körpers und der Arzt der Seele', *Clio Medica*, III (1968), 1–20.

[75] Aristeides, *Or.*, 48.25; Lucian, *Alexander*, 60; F. Kudlien, 'Galen's religious belief', in V. Nutton (ed.), *Galen: Problems and Prospects* (London, 1981), pp. 117–30.

[76] R. Herzog, 'Nikias und Xenophon von Kos', *Historische Zeitschrift*, CV (1922), 189–247; for his divine descent, see *ibid.*, p. 218, n. 3.

[77] *Inscr. graec. ad res Rom. pert.*, IV.520.

orders of Asclepius and plunging into winter torrents, never stopped asking their advice, as well as that of the god, or rejected them entirely as useless.[78] Inscriptions recording divine cures may mention the failure of physicians, but in sadness rather than anger, and the invocation of Euandridas to mighty Heracles 'who hast favoured me, unlike the physicians' is rare in its explicit dislike of doctors.[79]

This easy coexistence may have been assisted by the general absence of any linkage between disease and sin. At the Asclepieia the patient made a bargain for the future, not a repentance of the past: Euandridas expected Heracles to help him because of his erection of a sacred fountain. If, as in the famous plague that begins Homer's *Iliad*, disease was the result of divine wrath, its cause was more often a ritual offence against the god than any moral transgression. The several texts from upland Lydia (West Turkey) that record divine punishments on those who failed to fulfil their vows or foolishly cut down a sacred oak are unusual in their explicitness. The sinners were visited with blindness, 'all manner of misfortunes', a stroke, even madness, which only the open confession of their misdemeanours and acknowledgement of the power of the divinity could cure. Here is illness as a divine punishment, but for a specific cult offence, not a moral failing. Furthermore, upland Lydia was well off the beaten track, and likely to preserve longer traces of older beliefs, and the rarity of similar pagan records elsewhere shows up the changes brought about by Christianity.[80]

Nor is there much trace among Greek and Roman religion of the crowds of demons which infested the world of the Bible. The Roman personifications of disease, such as Dea Febris, and their very rare Greek equivalents,[81] do not resemble the malignant demons that attacked the madmen of the New Testament. What in Christian authors appears as a nightmare demon, the *incubus*, is in our earliest Greek source merely a metaphor.[82] Individual illness is thus less caught up in the eternal

---

[78] E. and L. Edelstein, *Asclepius* (Baltimore, 1945); for Aristeides, note his relations with Satyrus, Galen's teacher, *Or.* 49.8–10, and Theodotus, *Or.*, 47.13, 55–6; 48.34; 50.21, 38, 42; 51.57.

[79] *Inscr. graec.*, V.1.1119. Cf. also O. Weinreich, *Antike Heilungswunder* (Giessen, 1909), pp. 195–7.

[80] *Tituli Asiae Minoris*, V.509, 541, 586, 598; cf. also A. D. Nock, *Essays on Religion and the Ancient World* (Oxford, 1972), vol. 1, pp. 65–7, and F. Kudlien, 'Beichte und Heilung', *Medizin-historisches Journal*, XIII (1978), 1–14.

[81] K. Deichgräber, 'Parabasenverse aus Thesmophoriazusen II des Aristophanes bein Galen', *Sitzungsber. Akad. Wiss. Berlin, Kl. Spr., Lit., Kunst* (1956), 35f.

[82] *Ibid.*, p. 38.

struggle between the mysterious forces of good and evil; bodily infirmity is explicable on physical, not moral grounds. In these circumstances, religion and medicine coexist, even co-operate.

By contrast, from its inception Christianity offered itself as a direct competitor to secular healing. It took over the Jewish conception of a theocratic universe, in which God alone was a source of strength, and in which illness was the result of man's failure to keep his covenant with God, and extended it in two ways. In Christ, God incarnate, it had the saviour on earth, the great physician, whose help was available to all believers, and at no monetary cost. The woman with the issue of blood had spent all her savings on doctors and drugs, yet she was not cured by them, but by merely touching the hem of Christ's robe.[83] Secondly, the healing powers of Christ were also given to his followers, who could thereby cast out devils, heal the sick and even bring the dead to life again, by the Christian healing by faith, prayer, unction and confession. The healing miracles of Christ, his apostles and saints were paraded as proof of the unmistakable efficacy and truth of the Christian message, and a formal place within this religion was allotted to the healers and exorcists. The early apologists of Christianity laid stress on the effectiveness of Christian cures, and their message of hope to the sick was a major factor in the eventual triumph of Christianity over other cults.[84]

The existence of a specifically Christian method of healing and of an explanation of disease as the result of sin exacerbated a tension already visible in Jewish tradition. The apparently favourable advice

---

[83] Mark 5: 26. The literature on Christian healing is vast, and not always helpful. See, for example, C. F. D. Moule, *Miracles* (London, 1965); *Die Wurderbegriff im Neuer Testament* (Darmstadt, 1980); K. Hauck, 'Gott als Arzt', in C. Meier and U. Ruberg (eds.), *Text und Bild* (Wiesbaden, 1980), pp. 19–62 (for artistic evidence); F. Kudlien, 'Gesundheit', in T. Klauser *et al.* (eds.), *Reallexikon für Antike und Christentum*, vol. 10 (Stuttgart, 1978), pp. 936–43; D. W. Amundsen, 'Medicine and faith in early Christianity', *Bulletin of the History of Medicine*, LVI (1982), 326–50, is far too bland. Many Christian texts stress that Christ's healing is *free* to all believers, cf. e.g. H. Schipperges, 'Zur Tradition des "Christus medicus" im frühen Christentum und in der älteren Heilkunde', *Christianische Arzt*, XI (1965), 12–20; P. Maas, *Kleine Schriften* (Munich, 1973), pp. 308–9; Robert Murray, *Symbols of Church and Kingdom* (Cambridge, 1975), pp. 199–203.

[84] First emphasised strongly by A. Harnack, 'Medicinisches aus der ältesten Kirchengeschichte', *Texte und Untersuchungen zur Geschichte der altchristlichen Literatur*, VIII.4 (1892), 37–152. See also G. W. H. Lampe, in Moule, *Miracles*, pp. 165–78, 205–18; A. D. Nock, *Essays*, vol. 1, pp. 308–30; and R. MacMullen, *Paganism in the Roman Empire* (New Haven and London, 1981), pp. 50, 168–9.

of Jesus ben Sirach to 'honour the physician with the honour due unto him, for the uses which ye may have of him; for the Lord hath created him' was there balanced by the cautionary tale of King Asa, who was condemned because, in his serious disease of the feet, 'he sought not to the Lord, but to the physicians'.[85] The Gospel narratives reveal similar ambiguities. Although doctors are not condemned, their failures are made obvious; although Christ never explicitly proclaims sin as the direct cause of suffering, his disciples, on at least one occasion, were convinced that an illness had its origin in sin, not a physical change; although faith, repentance and moral purity were necessary in order to receive healing, nowhere is it stated that physical illness resulted from their absence.[86] The injunction of St Paul to Timothy to take a little wine for his stomach's sake is countered by the Epistle of James, which enjoins on the sick only the true Christian healing.[87]

This obvious tension within the very earliest writings of Christianity over the place of secular healing within a Christian society did not disappear in time. True, Clement of Alexandria and his follower Origen at the end of the second century proclaimed that the existence of medicine was highly laudable: it was a gift from God, who did not wish men to be bereft of help in time of illness.[88] Such a compromise between medicine and religion was accepted by most Christian writers,

[85] Eccl. 38: 1–15, with the comments of S. Noorda, 'Illness and sin, forgiving and healing: the connection of medical treatment and religious beliefs in Ben Sira 38: 1–15', in M. J. Vermaseren (ed.), *Studies in Hellenistic Religions* (Leyden, 1979), pp. 215–24. Asa, 2 Chron. 16: 12, with the discussion of later Jewish commentary in J. Preuss, *Biblical and Talmudic Medicine* (New York and London, 1978), pp. 22–4. I doubt the suggestion of J. Fink that the puzzling 'anatomical' scene from the Via Latina catacomb represents the death of Asa, 'Die römische Katakombe an der Via Latina', *Antike Welt*, vii (1976), 3–14. The Jewish historian Josephus, *Ant.*, VIII.2.5, claimed that Solomon's wisdom extended to medicine, in which he was a master of all chants and exorcisms.

[86] The Jewish scriptures made a link, occasionally, between sin and disease (so Preuss, *Biblical Medicine*, pp. 22–3), and it is clear from John 9: 1–4 that the Apostles were convinced that the cause of a man's blindness lay in his or his parents' sin. But Jesus expressly refuses to answer their question on this point, and although he heals by forgiving sins, e.g. Mark 2: 5, 9–11, and reminds a cured paralytic that he should sin no more or he might suffer something worse, John 5: 14, the purification is a preparation for healing, not an acknowledgement of the cause of disease, cf. Nock, *Essays*, vol. 1, p. 373; Kudlien, 'Beichte', p. 11.

[87] I Tim. 5: 23; James 5: 13–16.

[88] Clement, *Strom.*, 6.17; Origen, *Contra Cels.*, 3.12. See also H. J. Frings, *Medizin und Arzt bei den griechischen Kirchenvätern bis Chrysostomos* (Bonn, 1959), pp. 8–17; Amundsen, 'Medicine and faith', *passim*.

particularly by St Basil and St John Chrysostom. But the alternative view never lacked supporters, although few were as violent as Tatian (fl. A.D. 160), who saw a belief in drugs as apostasy from God and as faith in evil matter, and who explained secular cures on the grounds that all that had happened was that the demons who were the true cause of disease had decided, for the time being, voluntarily to end their sport and had flown away.[89] Others, including even Origen, could argue that the medicine of the physicians was suitable for the average Christian; but for those of higher capabilities, like Macarius' Egyptian monks, prayer and faith alone sufficed.[90] The crypto-paganism of many of the later professors of medicine at Alexandria only added to Christian suspicion of secular physicians, while the Lives of the Saints frequently pointed to the expensive failures of the physicians by comparison with the sure healing, available at no cost, from the hands of a Cosmas and Damian, or an Artemius.[91] This strain of Christianity continually reappears throughout the centuries, in St Bernard of Clairvaux, the mediaeval Waldensians, or St Bernardino, and it comes as no surprise to find that the controversy was reopened by the Wittenberg reformers in the sixteenth century.[92] The extremist

[89] Tatian, *Or. ad Graec.*, 16–18. *Pace* Amundsen, I am still inclined to see in the Christian texts before A.D. 300 a more obvious hesitation about secular medicine than in later texts, although I agree that the compromise view of Clement was probably by far the most usual. I would connect this suspicion, however, not with a feeling of anti-Hellenism, later reduced by a greater knowledge of the Greek classics, but with the position of Christianity as a cult that offered physical and spiritual healing. The suspicion of providers of healing, particularly pagan magi, exorcists and the like, is clear from the *Didache* and the *Apostolic Constitutions*, and from the bitter rivalry between Asclepius cult (and the like) and Christianity. The destruction of the great healing shrine of Sarapis is famous, but it should be noted also that the sack of the Asclepieion at Pergamum was so thorough that scarcely any trace has been found of cult offerings, statues or other reproductions of the Pergamene Asclepius on the site itself or in the city.

[90] Macarius, *Hom.* 48.3–6; cf. 51: p. 19 Marriott, and the rule of St Macarius, *Patr. graec.* 34.982 (cf. that of St Basil, *Patr. graec.* 31.1046); Arnobius, *Adv. gent.*, 1.48; 3.23 (but his hostility was also sharpened by the continuing paganism of many intellectuals, *ibid.*, 2.5); Origen, *Contra Cels.*, 8.60. One can find many other examples, e.g. Diadochos of Photike, *De scient. spirit.*, 53–5; Nicetas of Remesiana (?), *Patr. lat.*, 52.866.

[91] For a general survey, see my essay, 'From Galen to Alexander: aspects of medicine and medical practice in Late Antiquity', forthcoming in J. Scarborough (ed.), *Byzantine Medicine* (Washington, 1984); on lives of the saints, P. Horden, 'Saints and doctors in the early Byzantine Empire: the case of Theodore of Sykeon', in W. J. Sheils (ed.), *The Church and Healing* (Studies in Church History XIX, Oxford, 1982), pp. 1–13, is an excellent introduction.

[92] For Bernard, see C. H. Talbot, *Medicine in Mediaeval England* (London, 1967), p. 180; on the Waldensians, P. Biller, '*Curate infirmos*: the medieval

Carlstadt preached, to Luther's disgust, against the use of secular medicines by any true Christian, while Melanchthon's *Encomium of Medicine* defended the traditional compromise against those who sought to deny the value of medicine or its place in a divinely created universe.[93]

Melanchthon's oration is a Christian transmutation of an old theme, and is unusual precisely in its refusal to rely on classical pagan texts in defence of contemporary medicine. Other authors, such as Poggio, Erasmus and Cardano, reeled off the opinions of Cicero, Seneca and Galen in praise of medicine, and thought that they had thereby silenced the snobbish complaints of orators or philosophers.[94] But they were unable to eliminate the influence of Pliny. Editions and commentaries on him poured from the presses; the lectures on him by Johannes Lange at Leipzig in 1516 attracted a remarkably large and talented audience; and, perhaps even more significant, his writings were pillaged to provide the basis for all Renaissance encyclopaedias and handbooks of learning.[95] Through works like Ravisius Textor's *Officina* and Theodore Zwinger's *Theatrum humanae vitae*, Pliny's prejudices were transmitted

Waldensian practice of medicine', in Sheils, *The Church and Healing*, pp. 55–77; San Bernardino, cited by R. J. Palmer, 'The church, leprosy and plague', in Sheils, *The Church and Healing*, p. 86. It should perhaps also be stated that, while such injunctions are found most often when medical aid is either absent (as in Nicetas' Dacia) or largely unhelpful (as in plague), their acceptance does not easily fit into categories of either social class or intellectual ability.

93 M. Luther, *Tischreden* (Weimar, 1912), vol. 1, n. 360, which gives the variant versions of Luther's comments. The shorter German text is translated by T. G. Tapper, *Luther's Works*, vol. 54 (Philadelphia, 1967), pp. 53–4. P. Melanchthon, *Encomium medicinae*, perhaps written in 1529. This was often reprinted, and was made accessible in the next century by being reprinted by J. van Beverwyck, *Medicinae encomium* (Rotterdam, 1644), pp. 129–40. See also W. Maurer, *Der junge Melanchthon*, vol. 1 (Göttingen, 1967), pp. 162–6, 238f.

94 Poggio, see L. Thorndike, *Science and Thought in the Fifteenth century* (New York, 1928), pp. 28–41; Erasmus, *Encomium medicinae*, ed. J. Domanski, *Erasmi opera omnia*, I.4 (Amsterdam, 1973), pp. 146–60. It was written in or before 1499 (*ibid.*, pp. 147–9), probably for Ghysbert Hessels, civic physician at St Omer, although it was not published until 1518 at Louvain; cf. also J. C. Margolin, 'Erasme et la médecine', *Respublica Litterarum*, II (1979), 187–203, esp. 199f.; H. Cardanus, *Medicinae encomium*, in *Opuscula quaedam* (Basle, 1559), but written in the 1540s. The encomia of Erasmus and Cardano were both reprinted by Beverwyck, *Medicinae encomium*, pp. 82–105, 106–27.

95 C. G. Nauert, 'Caius Plinius Secundus', in F. E. Cranz and P. O. Kristeller (eds.), *Catalogus translationum et commentariorum*, vol. IV (1980), pp. 297–422; on Lange, N. Reusner, Preface to J. Lange, *Epistolae medicinales* (Hannover, 1589), which suggests that, *pace* Nauert, p. 313, the study of Pliny was already in fashion in Germany before the Lutheran transformation at Wittenberg.

to an ever-widening circle. The notoriety of the surgeon Archagathus increased markedly: his unhappy career at Rome was described or alluded to in almost every book on surgery, even if its author could not spell his Greek name correctly.[96] None defended him against Pliny's imputations, but merely added to his alleged incompetence by an assertion of the obvious superiority of modern surgery. Pliny's strictures against Greek physicians were repeated by respectable doctors, surgeons and city councillors from Saxony to South America, as they strove to check the lesser practitioners, the barbers, wisewomen and urine-diagnosticians.[97] His praise of practical Roman herbalism was enshrined in the statute of the new University of Frankfurt-an-der-Oder and welcomed by the Paracelsians.[98] Above all, his dislike of medicine inspired Michel de Montaigne to create, in calmer prose, perhaps the most devastating attack on medicine written by a layman.

Montaigne knew the physicians of contemporary France, and was not impressed. Their diagnoses and remedies seemed to him to lack the certainty he found among the surgeons; their drugs were expensive and ineffective concoctions; their theories were mere rhetoric; and their bedside manners were tyrannical in the extreme. They needed to be controlled equally as much as the mountebanks, quacks and imposters who travelled the roads of France.[99] Montaigne's opinion was not derived entirely from the pages of Pliny, for it was based on a broad acquaintance with medical therapies and ideas. Handbooks of medicine for the layman, from both antiquity and later,[100] were easily accessible to him, and carried often the same message. Medical

---

96 So F. le Fevre, *Les trois premiers livres de la chirurgie d'Hippocrate* (Paris, 1555), sig. c.1, who calls him Archibutus.

97 J. Lange, *Epistolae*, I.pf.; II.47; J. T. Lanning, *Pedro della Torre* (Baton Rouge, 1974), p. 7.

98 K. Pielmeyer, *Statuten der deutschen medizinischen Fakultäten im Mittelalter* (Bonn, 1977), p. 57; Petrus Severinus, *Idea medicinae philosophicae* (Basle, 1571), pp. 4, 15, 110, 142.

99 Montaigne, *Essais*, II.37.

100 To give but four ancient examples, Galen's shorter *Method of Healing* was expressly written for a non-medical audience; Rufus of Ephesus' major work (alas, now surviving only in fragments) was entitled 'The layman', while the late Latin handbooks of Marcellus Empiricus and Theodore Priscian are aimed at the non-medical man. For fifteenth century England, see F. M. Getz, 'Gilbertus Anglicus anglicized', *Medical History*, xxvi (1982), 436–42, and for sixteenth century England, P. A. Slack, 'Mirrors of health and treasures of poor men', in C. Webster (ed.), *Health, Medicine and Mortality in the Sixteenth Century* (Cambridge, 1981), pp. 239–43. Similar long lists could be drawn up for the Continent.

treatment should be the treatment of the individual and his idiosyncrasies, and, in such circumstances, who better to know his temperament, his habits, and any deviations from his natural state than the patient himself? The basic doctrines of humoralism, as we have seen, were by no means hard to understand, certainly for a Montaigne, and they offered every man the opportunity to be his own Galen. The warnings of Pliny merely confirmed the advantages of self-medication.

When Montaigne, a chronic sufferer from the stone, made his journey round the spas of Switzerland and Italy in 1580–1, he astonished the doctors of Plombières, Baden and Bagni di Lucca by disregarding their advice and prescribing his own course of treatment. It is obvious from their comments that the strangeness of his behaviour did not lie in his decision to look after his own health himself, and, indeed, he could claim support for this even from other doctors.[101] His oddity consisted in carrying out his plan at a spa, a health centre presided over by physicians and visited by patients eager to receive treatment at their hands. For a Frenchman to travel so far and then to treat himself was carrying the layman's approach to medicine far beyond what custom and propriety allowed. Montaigne's crime was not self-help, but exaggeration.

I am grateful to Faye Getz, Ghada Karmi and Roy Porter for their comments and suggestions.

[101] Montaigne, *Journal de voyage*, ed. Thibaudet and Rat, pp. 1122, 1139, 1287–8. For Montaigne and medicine, see F. Batisse, *Montaigne et la médecine* (Paris, 1962), somewhat superficial on medical theory, but good on the place of spas; and the articles by V. Nutton and M. Brunyate, in K. Cameron (ed.), *Montaigne and his Age* (Exeter, 1981), pp. 15–38, 163–72.

3

Puritan perceptions of illness in seventeenth century England

ANDREW WEAR

Introduction

Not many historians so far have examined Puritan attitudes to physical illness. A lot of the contextual spadework, however, has already been done by social, cultural, political, religious and demographic historians.[1] They provide the larger picture in which to place the subject and they also help to illuminate related issues (for instance, the spiritualisation of life, providence, the different shades of Puritanism, the material conditions of society, etc.). Moreover, thanatology has recently become popular.[2] As death was often the expected consequence of illness in the seventeenth century, people's attitudes to it had a close relationship to their perceptions of illness.

Attitudes to illness itself have been studied by Keith Thomas and

[1] See for instance: William Haller, *The Rise of Puritanism* (New York, 1938; my edition Harper Torchbook, 1957); Perry Miller, *The New England Mind: The Seventeenth Century* (Cambridge, Mass., 1967; 1st edn. 1939); C. Hill, *Society and Puritanism in Pre-Revolutionary England* (London, 1964) (hereinafter *Society*); Owen Watkins, *The Puritan Experience* (London, 1972); Lawrence Stone, *The Family, Sex and Marriage in England 1500–1800* (London, 1979); George Yule, *Puritans in Politics* (Appleford, 1981); E. A. Wrigley and R. S. Schofield, *The Population History of England 1541–1871* (London, 1981); Keith Wrightson, *English Society 1580–1680* (London, 1982); Peter Laslett, *The World We Have Lost – Further Explored* (London, 1983) (hereinafter *Lost World*). This is a small sample; the list is huge.

[2] For example: Philippe Ariès, *The Hour of our Death* (London, 1983); Michel Vovelle, *La mort et l'Occident de 1300 à nos jours* (Paris, 1983); David E. Stannard, *The Puritan Way of Death* (New York, 1977) (hereinafter *Death*); John McManners, *Death and the Enlightenment* (Oxford, 1981); Gordon E. Geddes, *Welcome Joy. Death in Puritan New England* (Studies in American History and Culture No. 28, Ann Arbor, 1981); C. Gittings, *Death, Burial and the Individual in Early Modern England* (London, 1984).

Alan Macfarlane.[3] Both bring out the importance of providence as a means by which Puritans made sense of illness. Thomas also provides an influential and important overview of cultural change in seventeenth century England that shows magic declining with a trend towards secularisation after the Restoration. It may be, as Jonathan Barry points out in this volume, that secularisation was not as rapid or as clear-cut as some historians, following Thomas, have imagined.[4] Also, more specifically, the case for providentialism may have been over-emphasised, and in this essay I shall spell out in detail the nature of the eclectic use of physical and religious explanations of illness.

Psychological illness in the seventeenth century has received some recent attention. Michael MacDonald has produced a brilliant study of the practice and the patients of Richard Napier, an astrological physician working at the beginning of the seventeenth century.[5] Napier's case notes cover thousands of patients, throwing light on medical practice and on the types of events and situations that produced psychological disorders in a wide range of people. However, MacDonald's work is of limited use for this essay. Mainstream Puritans did not approve of astrological medicine, and they certainly would not have conjured the Archangel Raphael as Napier sometimes did.[6] Furthermore, MacDonald is concerned with psychological rather than physical illness. Also, if the perceptions of the *patient* are to be the focus of study, it is not clear whether Napier's case notes can be safely used, for it is possible that patients' conversations were 'made sense of' by Napier.

Historical work on mental illness, however, does act as a point of reference for this essay's concern with physical illness. Elsewhere, MacDonald and others have described Puritan, Anglican and Non-conformist attitudes to mental illness in the pre- and post-Restoration period.[7] The Puritans should have been interested in the workings of

---

[3] Keith Thomas, *Religion and the Decline of Magic* (London, 1971) (hereinafter *Religion*); Alan Macfarlane, *The Family Life of Ralph Josselin* (Cambridge, 1970) (hereinafter *Josselin*).

[4] See below, note 9.

[5] Michael MacDonald, *Mystical Bedlam* (Cambridge, 1981).

[6] *Ibid.*, p. 210.

[7] As well as *Mystical Bedlam* see also MacDonald's, 'Religion, social change and psychological healing in England 1600–1800' in W. J. Sheils (ed.), *The Church and Healing* (Oxford, 1982), pp. 101–25; Thomas, *Religion*; D. P. Walker, *Unclean Spirits: Possession and Exorcism in France and England in the Late Sixteenth and Early Seventeenth Centuries* (Philadelphia, 1981); Roy Porter, 'The rage of party: a glorious revolution in English psychiatry?', *Medical History*, xxvii (1983), 35–50; H. D. Rack, 'Doctors, demons and early

the mind was natural, given Calvin's 'institutionalisation' of the believer's inner anxiety and his injunction to know and to be displeased with ourselves[8] (a recipe for guilt-laden self-analysis). Puritans put much effort into understanding mental processes, and it is no accident that the first chapter of Haller's *The Rise of Puritanism* is entitled 'Physicians of the Soul'. With the Restoration and the consequent dislike for 'enthusiasm'[9] in religion (already apparent in the 1650s and earlier in Robert Burton)[10] the healing role of religion in mental illness declined, though Nonconformists continued the practice of religious healing.

Can the history of physical illness be interpreted in the same way? Christopher Hill wrote of the 'spiritualisation of the household' to describe how the minutiae of family life came under the influence of religion.[11] Were the body and its illnesses spiritualised also? Certainly the body's perceived closeness to the soul would have made it a likely candidate. This essay will show, however, that among mainstream Puritans the spiritualisation of illness was only partially accomplished. More tentatively, the essay supports the view that post-1660s Anglicans moved to a more secular, rational view of illness, though Barry's paper warns us against easy generalisations.

Methodist healing', in W. J. Sheils (ed.), *The Church and Healing* (Oxford, 1982), pp. 137–52.

[8] Paul Delany, *British Autobiography in the Seventeenth Century* (London, 1969) (hereinafter *British Autobiography*), pp. 34–5, citing Calvin's *Institutes*, I, 1, 1 and II, v, 19.

[9] An important work for the reaction to enthusiasm is M. C. Jacob, *The Newtonians and the English Revolution* (Hassocks, Sussex, 1976); Michael Heyd has a good article on enthusiasm, pointing out the nature of the opposition to it: 'The reaction to enthusiasm in the seventeenth century: towards an integrative approach', *Journal of Modern History*, LIII (1981), 258–80. See also Porter, 'The rage of party' and MacDonald, *Mystical Bedlam* and 'Religion, social change and psychological healing'. Christopher Hill finds the reaction to enthusiasm significant; see his *Some Intellectual Consequences of the English Revolution* (London, 1980), pp. 62–7. However, historians could be putting too much explanatory power on enthusiasm. Jacob's idea that the scientific laws of the later seventeenth century are the result of religious and political positions taken on enthusiasm relies too much on the imaginative use of analogies. Moreover, the social historian – unless a historian of elites and of professional society – must be unhappy at the limited extent of pro- and anti-enthusiasm ideas.

[10] MacDonald in his 'Religion, social change and psychological healing', p. 104, gives the impression (no doubt inadvertently) that Robert Burton associated religious melancholy mainly with strict Puritans ('giddy precisians'); sectarians did figure in his argument but, overall, the vast majority of Burton's examples and descriptions came from Catholic or pagan history.

[11] Hill, *Society*, pp. 443–81.

I take 'Puritan' to mean the 'godly' sort of people who up to the
1640s tended to conform and who were not openly hostile to the
establishment though they wished for further reformation.[12] Moderate
Puritans like William Perkins, Richard Greenham and William Gouge
have been seen as shaping the mainstream of Puritan thought.[13] I have
looked at their views and related them to the perceptions of illness of
a generally later group of diarists and autobiographers who shared the
same moderate views (after 1640 many would be Presbyterians). As
they disliked Sectarians, Baptists, Ranters and Quakers as much as
Papists, I have not discussed the more 'enthusiastic' healing miracles
of the sects nor the material on religious healing in George Fox's
Journal. Also left to one side are the radical Puritan reformers who, as
Charles Webster shows, were concerned with changing the relationships between religion and medicine,[14] as they were more interested
in institutional relationships than with how an individual should
approach illness and death.

Finally, some comments are needed on the material that I am using.
How individuals perceived illness can be discovered by looking at

[12] The definition of 'Puritan' and 'Puritanism' has produced a huge literature.
   See for example: Haller, *Rise of Puritanism*, pp. 18–20; Charles and Katherine
   George, *The Protestant Mind of the English Reformation* (Princeton, 1961);
   Michael G. Finlayson, *Historians, Puritanism and the English Revolution: The
   Religious Factor in English Politics Before and After the Interregnum* (Toronto,
   1984) – the last two deny the existence of Puritanism; John F. H. New,
   Anglican and Puritan, The Basis of their Opposition (London, 1964); C. Hill,
   Society, pp. 13–29 gives a social as well as religious definition; J. Sears McGee,
   *The Godly Man in Stuart England: Anglicans, Puritans and the Two Tables,
   1620–1670* (New Haven, 1976); William Lamont, *Godly Rule: Politics and
   Religion 1603–1660*, pp. 25, 93–7 (hereinafter *Godly Rule*); Peter Lake, *Moderate
   Puritans and the Elizabethan Church* (Cambridge, 1982), pp. 11–14. My own
   description has been influenced most by Haller, and the following: Claire
   Cross, *Church and People 1450–1660* (London, 1976); G. Yule, *Puritans in
   Politics* (Appleford, 1981), pp. 72–105; Basil Hall, 'Puritanism: the problem
   of definition', in G. J. Cumming (ed.), *Studies in Church History* (London,
   1965), vol. 2, pp. 283–96. Hall writes 'before 1642 the "serious" people in
   the Church of England who desired some modification in Church government
   were called Puritans: after 1640 party names came increasingly into use, of
   Presbyterian, Independent and Baptist'; he goes on to point out that
   Presbyterians such as Baxter did not think of themselves as Puritans, who they
   associated with the time before 1640.

[13] Haller, *Rise of Puritanism*, pp. 49–82; H. C. Porter, *Reformation and Reaction
   in Tudor Cambridge* (Cambridge, 1959), pp. 216–26 (hereinafter *Reformation*);
   Lamont, *Godly Rule*, p. 42; Yule, *Puritans in Politics*, pp. 75–7.

[14] Charles Webster, *The Great Instauration* (London, 1975), pp. 245–323 (hereinafter *Instauration*).

diaries, autobiographies, 'lives' and letters. In seventeenth century England diary writing flourished. The cosmos of the Puritan diary centred on the individual and his or her personal communion with God, though Puritans were also intensely interested in the wider world. The Puritan was encouraged to keep a reckoning and judgement of his actions. John Dod wrote:

If we keep an assises at home in our own soules, and find ourselves guilty, and contemn ourselves, then shall not we be judged of the Lord: but because we deal very partially in our own matters, therefore is the Lord driven to help us, by laying his correcting hand some way or other on us.[15]

The diary became the vehicle for this confessional assessment, and seventeenth century England saw a great expansion in diary writing.[16] Isaac Ambrose wrote that the diarist 'observes something of God to his soul, and of his soul to God'.[17] John Fuller in his introduction to John Beadle's *The Journal or Diary of a Thankful Christian* used an accounting or trading metaphor:

A Christian that would be exact hath more need, and may reap much more good by such a journal as this. We are all but stewards, factors here, and must give a strict account in that great day to the high Lord of all our ways and of all his ways towards us.[18]

The Puritan diary, then, was written with an eye towards God. By noting 'God's ways towards us' as well as 'our ways', the diarist was constantly trying to discover evidence of the hand of God as it touched his life.

It is no surprise, therefore, that Puritan diarists should emphasise God's providence. Was a Puritan diary merely a formalism, a literary artefact written for religious reasons and bearing little relation to 'real life'? Although the diaries have to be used with caution, the writing of the diaries was part of the real life of the authors, and they contain enough width of daily experience to give us confidence that what was

---

[15] John Dod and Robert Cleaver, *Seven Godlie and Fruitful Sermons* (London, 1614), p. 44 (hereinafter *Seven Sermons*). The first six sermons are by Dod.
[16] On diaries see Watkins, *Puritan Experience*, which analyses Puritan perceptions through diaries and autobiographies. Haller, *Rise of Puritanism*, p. 38; Macfarlane, *Josselin*, pp. 3–11 who regrets the small use made of diaries by historians, though see now Linda Pollock, *Forgotten Children* (Cambridge, 1983).
[17] Isaac Ambrose, *Prima, The First Things in Reference to the Middle and Last Things* (London, 1674), p. 118. Cited by William Sachse in his edn of *The Diary of Roger Lowe* (London, 1938), p. 2 (hereinafter *Diary*).
[18] Quoted by Delany, *British Autobiography*, p. 64.

put down to God's providence was not merely a circumscribed part of the author's life. Yet it has to be remembered that this highly providentialist vision was relatively short-lived and limited mainly to Puritans, and many diaries were written by Puritan ministers who would naturally think in this way. In other words, although the religious ethos of Puritan diaries was for their authors normal and not artificial, for the historian, who puts them into an overall context, they may appear to have the aura of artificiality associated with any genre of writing.

The religious background

Religion had always been closely associated with illness, and Puritan interest in healing and illness was nothing new. Similarities between Catholic and Protestant views will often occur in this essay. However, there were differences. Protestants did not make Church processions, or offer prayers to saints or to their relics when seeking cure from community-wide or individual illness.[19] Calvin's emphasis on God and the Bible moved people away from the pantheon of minor Christian divinities. The structure, nevertheless, remained the same: communal and individual prayer was still offered to relieve physical ills.

More specifically, Puritans had a different view from Roman Catholics of the role of religion at the sick-bed. In Puritan eyes, the age of miracles had long since past, and in their attack on the superstitions of the Roman Church Puritans stated that the Catholic sacraments had merely a symbolic meaning without any real or material power. This meant that the Church could no longer heal. William Perkins, perhaps the outstanding Puritan writer at the turn of the century,[20] wrote that the Catholic rite of anointing the sick was an ineffectual imitation of that of the primitive Church:

The fifth of James is commonly alleged to this purpose, but the anointing there mentioned is not of the sa: :c kind with this greasy sacrament of the Papists. For that anointing of the body was a ceremony used by the Apostles and others, when they put in practise this miraculous gift of healing, which gift is now ceased. Secondly, that anointing had a promise that the party should recover his health, but this popish anointing hath no such promise,

[19] See for instance R. Palmer, 'The Church, leprosy and plague in early modern Europe', in Sheils (ed.), *The Church and Healing*, pp. 79–100, and C. Cipolla, *Faith, Reason and the Plague* (Brighton, 1979).

[20] Haller, *Rise of Puritanism*, p. 91; Yule, *Puritans in Politics*, pp. 75–6. For modern accounts of Perkins' life see Haller, *Rise of Puritanism*, pp. 64–5; W. Perkins, *The Works of William Perkins*, ed. I. Breward (London, 1970), pp. 3–131.

because for the most part the persons thus anointed die afterward without recovering; whereas those which were anointed in the primitive Church always recovered.[21]

The Reformation not only took the power of healing from the priest, it also took from him the power of judging and absolving men from sin (sickness and sin came together for 'by God's word...sickness comes ordinarily and usually from sin'[22]). All that was left for the reformed Church was, in Perkins' words, 'but a ministry of reconciliation',[23] where the minister tried to reconcile the sick-man to God.

The denial of the Church's God-like and miraculous power formed part of the 'disenchantment'[24] of the world and its consequent rationalism that gains momentum through the seventeenth century. Keith Thomas has charted this process, and, as with all pioneering efforts, his research can be modified. Although the rejection of the Church's role as an institution of divine power through which man's relations with God were mediated led to a direct and personal communion between the two, this does not mean that religion had ceased to be a third party. Puritans such as Richard Greenham, William Perkins and William Gouge emphasised the teaching role of the Church. At the same time, like any other didactic institution, religion needed authority. Through the century, many Puritans whether pre-1640 conformists, or later, Presbyterians or Congregationalists, believed in some level of organisation, and certainly in the specific calling of the ministry, and in the transcendent authority of the Bible to uphold them in their calling. How illness and death relate to the authority of the Church and to its teaching is discussed next.

Religion, illness and death

In the first half of the seventeenth century religion was a dominant system of thought.[25] Moreover, at the institutional level, Puritan

---

[21] William Perkins, *A Golden Chaine* (London, 1612), p. 501 (hereinafter *Chain*). The same passage in James was used by Baptists to justify their healing practices: see Thomas, *Religion*, p. 149.

[22] Perkins, *Chain*, p. 501.

[23] *Ibid.*, p. 500, citing II Corinthians 5: 18.

[24] See Heyd, 'The reaction to enthusiasm', p. 258. The word comes from 'Entzauberung' used by Max Weber in the essay 'Wissenschaft als Beruf'.

[25] Hill, *Society*, p. 32 writes, 'In the sixteenth and seventeenth centuries the Church had a monopoly of thought control and opinion forming. It controlled education; it censored books.'

ministers such as William Gouge[26] exuded a self-confident belief in
their power to govern all aspects of men's minds. This belief in the
right of a minister to control and influence behaviour had its mirror-
image on the political stage from the Elizabethan to the Civil War
period, where religion was a major influence. The power of religion
also showed itself on a more local and intimate level, with consistory
courts, and later Presbyterian and Congregational officials, punishing
breaches of personal morality; and paralleling this policing was the
belief held by clergymen that they had the right and duty to give
advice ('practical divinity') on how individuals should live their
lives.[27] This included guidance on how to be ill and how to die, and
how to look after the sick.

Advice books set down the hierarchical relations and reciprocal
duties between rulers and subjects, husbands and wives, parents and
children, masters and servants, and it was in such a context that Puritan
ministers stressed that looking after a sick wife, husband, child or
servant was one of the duties of each member of a family.[28]

There were other more theological or theoretical reasons for the
Church's interest in giving advice about health and sickness apart from
the attempt at social education and control. At the level of the
individual rather than of society, religious writers saw the body as
God's workmanship: Robert Horne called it the Temple of God which

26   See especially William Gouge, *Of Domesticall Duties* (London, 1622) (herein-
     after *Duties*). On Gouge see Haller, *Rise of Puritanism*, pp. 67–9; Porter,
     Reformation, pp. 222–3.
27   Haller, *Rise of Puritanism*, pp. 24–6; Porter, *Reformation*, p. 222, 'For Perkins,
     as for Aristotle, the family was a natural institution, "the seminary of all other
     societies", though "the only rule of ordering the family is the written word
     of God". By this rule he laid down the essentials of domestic justice: with
     particular chapters on the duties of husband and wife and son, and on to the
     relation of master and servant. This tradition of practical divinity was
     continued in William Gouge's...*Of Domesticall Duties*'; Hill, *Society*,
     pp. 443–81.
28   Whether the sick were, in fact, looked after by their families is a difficult
     question to answer. Despite the small nuclear family of seventeenth century
     England where grown-up children left parents to form separate family units,
     it seems that few people lived in institutions and that widowers and widows
     rarely lived separately (7 and 14 per cent respectively in one study: Laslett,
     Lost World, pp. 295–6). Not surprisingly, no diarist that I have read, admits
     to having deserted a family member who was ill or dying (with the
     characteristic exception of Pepys who, when his servant Susan fell ill with
     an undiagnosed illness that might have been plague, sent her away to her
     mother: Samuel Pepys, *The Diary of Samuel Pepys*, ed. Robert Latham and
     William Matthews (11 vols., London, 1970–83), vol. 7, pp. 115–22 (hereinafter
     Diary); the illness proved to be an ague).

had to be kept pure and clean;[29] John Sym argued that failure to look after one's body was an indirect form of suicide.[30] The body had an appointed and natural span of life and it was man's duty to survive that span; Gouge, therefore, condemned 'the practise of gluttons, drunkards, unchaste and voluptuous persons, who to satisfy their corrupt humours, impair their health, pull diseases upon them and shorten their days'.[31] Perkins made it clear that the body could not be divorced from the soul, the secular from the divine, and he stated that the hold of God extended to this life and to our bodies:

Whereas our bodies are God's workmanship, we must glorify him in our bodies, and all the actions of body and soul, our eating and drinking, our living and dying, must be referred to his glory: yea we must not hurt or abuse our body, but present them as holy and living sacrifices unto God.[32]

A further reason for placing the body within the ambit of religion was that body and soul were taught to be intimately connected. The body was the instrument of the soul; if the body was impaired the soul could not express itself in this world:

the body of man is the organ or instrument whereby the soul works organically: and therefore, he that kills his own body destroys all those works, that the soul was to work in it, and which it cannot do without it.[33]

How far people took note of religious advice to look after their own health is unknown. Certainly the interest that religiously orientated diarists such as Ralph Josselin, Henry Newcome and Oliver Heywood had in their health can be explained not only in providential terms (illness or health being a mark of God's providence) but as a sign that they were heeding the advice to look after their bodies. That religious writers expected to be able to affect health practices is indicated by the sometimes quite detailed guidance that they gave on matters such as wet-nursing,[34] or on a husband's duty to satisfy his pregnant wife's 'longing', the want of which could result in her death or that of the child or both.[35]

There were other ways in which the Church and ministers entered

[29] Robert Horne, *Life and Death, Foure Sermons* (London, 1613), p. 25 (hereinafter *Life*). Horne was citing I Corinthians 6: 15, 19.
[30] John Sym, *Lifes Preservative Against Self-killing* (London, 1637), pp. 109–10 (hereinafter *Self-killing*).
[31] Gouge, *Duties*, p. 85.
[32] Perkins, *Chain*, p. 153.   [33] Sym, *Self-killing*, p. 81.
[34] See Thomas Becon, *The Catechism*, ed. J. Ayre for the Parker Society (Cambridge, 1844), pp. 347–8.   [35] Gouge, *Duties*, p. 399.

the world of illness and also of death, and at this point I want to concentrate on the latter. The death-bed scene constantly recurs in diaries, 'lives' and autobiographies. The similarity between its various enactments points to the fact that dying was a learnt procedure, part of the ceremonial of life. When dying one had to show evidence of piety (hence prayers and quotations from the Bible), a repentance of sin, and most importantly the mind had to be prepared to accept death, which was shown by exclamations of eagerness to enter Heaven. For example, John Angier described the death-bed scene of his wife:

they called me up, she being very ill, she then said Lord receive my spirit, into thy hand I commit my spirit, for thou hast redeemed it, come Lord Jesus, come quickly, make no tarrying he doth not yet come, will he not make hast?[36]

There was a whole genre of religious writing in the seventeenth century teaching people how to die (stemming from the medieval *ars moriendi*, the art of dying) and stressing the transitory nature of life. The period of one's life was secretly determined by God and known to him alone; any illness could presage death – thus Robert Yarrow called sickness 'the messenger of death'.[37] Robert Horne wrote 'I know not when I shall die, and therefore every day shall be as my dying day'.[38] Life had, therefore, to be a constant preparation for death. Puritans poured scorn on the Roman Catholic belief in death-bed repentances;[39] Horne wrote that they were a 'charm and a sorcery',[40] and that 'late repentance is seldom, or never true repentance'. Instead one needed to be in a constant state of repentance.[41]

Ariès has written that the move away from the death-bed scene to a constant preparation for death was a product of humanist writers and of the 'reformist elite of the Catholic and Protestant Churches',[42] with the consequence that 'death has become the pretext for a metaphysical

[36] Oliver Heywood, *Autobiography, Diaries* etc., ed. J. Horsfall Turner (4 vols., Brighouse and Bingley, 1882–5), vol. 1, p. 73 (hereinafter *Diaries*). See note 2 above on the literature on the history of death.
[37] Robert Yarrow, *Soveraigne Comforts for a Troubled Conscience* (London, 1634), p. 406 (hereinafter *Comforts*).
[38] Horne, *Life*, p. 116 and Stannard, *Death*, p. 77 quotes Cotton Mather, 'A prudent man will die daily'.
[39] On French death-bed repentance see McManners, *Death and the Enlightenment*, pp. 191–233. Although Catholics advised against too great a reliance on death-bed conversions, they nevertheless were seen to work, for 'a man's disposition in his dying moments decided his eternal destiny' (pp. 193–4).
[40] Horne, *Life*, p. 116.   [41] *Ibid.*, p. 69.
[42] Ariès, *The Hour of our Death*, p. 303.

meditation on the fragility of life that is intended to keep us from giving in to life's illusions. Death is no more than a means of living well'.[43] Ariès' view has to be modified in two respects. From the personal records of seventeenth century Puritans it is clear that there still remained an intensity around the death-bed. The formalised pattern of dying with its set speeches was a sign that Puritan society still retained death as one of the crises of life to be celebrated with ritualised behaviour learnt for the occasion. Moreover, in religious terms, the time of dying was that of most danger since this was when Satan's temptation was greatest.[44] Secondly, the life-long meditation upon death not only led one to pursue a better life, but also had another function: it integrated life with death and therefore enhanced the authority of the Church on the mundane level. Death, as religious writers had never tired of telling, was the gate-way to the world of the spirit and the destroyer of the social world and its hierarchy.[45] It was the leveller that struck down rich and poor alike:

Fearfull death, of all miseries the last and the most terrible...how quickly and suddenly stealest thou upon us? how secret are thy paths and ways? how universal is thy signiory and dominion? The mighty cannot escape thee, the strong lose their strength before thee, the rich with their money shall not corrupt thee. Thou art the hammer that always striketh: thou art the sword that never blunteth...[46]

[43] *Ibid.*, p. 301.
[44] Yarrow, *Comforts*, p. 393: 'He is not ignorant to take opportunity fittest for his purpose. And therefore now (above all other his desired times) he will devise and sound into the bottom of all his subtilties: to intrap, and so to make conquest of the Christian soules, knowing that this is the last combat that he is like to make with such a one...Assure thyself therefore that he will prepare the best he can stretch every limb in this final conflict.' Also Horne, *Life*, p. 71: 'there is business and work enough in the mind and external man of deaths condemned prisoner to resist and prepare against the extremity of that combat, which (because it is the last of the day) is like to be the sharpest'.
[45] Stannard, *Death*, pp. 16–17.
[46] Thomas Hastler, *An Antidote against the Plague* (London, 1625), pp. 35–6 (hereinafter *Antidote*). The theme of 'fearful' death seems to have been a Puritan one. Death was the 'king of Terrors', and Puritans combined their fear of death with the traditional view of death as a welcome release: Stannard, *Death*, pp. 78–99; Vovelle, *La mort et l'Occident*, p. 300. Jeremy Taylor's *Holy Living and Dying* shows many similarities with traditional and Puritan thought – 'that we should always look for death, every day knocking at the grave' (ch. 11, sect. 1) – but it differs from Puritan attitudes in not putting great emphasis on the death-bed scene itself, and on presenting a positive image of death: 'It is so harmless a thing, that no good man was ever thought the more miserable for dying, but much the happier' (ch. 3, sect. vii). Given the Puritans' belief in predestination such a view was logically impossible for them to hold, though in practice they sometimes did.

The constant meditation upon death diminished the reality of the secular world and allowed the Church's area of greatest expertise and legitimacy – knowledge of the world after death – to permeate the world of life. Puritans like Isaac Ambrose expressed the traditional merging of death into life:

We live and yet whilst we speak this word, perhaps we die. Is this a land of the living or a region of the dead? We that suck the air to kindle this little spark, where is our standing but at 'the gates of death'? Psalm 9.13. Where is our walk but 'in the shadow of death' Luke 1.19. 'What is our mansion-house but the body of death'? Romans 7.24.[47]

The systematic reminder of death found in advice books, sermons and books on the art of dying might well be interpreted (possibly cynically) as bolstering the indispensability (*qua* source of knowledge about death) and power of the Church in this world. It also served as the background for the Puritan writers' mingling together of religion and medicine which I discuss below.

The Church's emphasis on death gained plausibility because it reflected physical reality. Death and funerals were frequent experiences in seventeenth century society.[48] Moreover, seventeenth century England was a time of increasing mortality; the expectation of life fluctuated wildly because of epidemics, but declined overall through the century until by 1681 it had fallen by about ten years.[49] But whether people actually thought of death all the time is debatable. Although this was the baroque era with the skull as its remembrancer of death,[50] there were, not surprisingly, many people who show in their diaries and letters that they did not go around meditating on death

[47] Isaac Ambrose, *Ultima, The Last Things in Reference to the First and Middle Things* (London, 1650), p. 5 (hereinafter *Ultima*).

[48] Though the conclusion of some historians that other people's deaths were expected to occur at all ages and not just in old age has to be treated with some caution, see for such an instance: Stone, *The Family, Sex and Marriage in England 1500–1800*, pp. 54–66. Hervé LeBras shows, however, that in the France of the 1750s there was a high expectation that young children would have living parents and grandparents. Thus, the experience of death in the immediate family was not as high as a high mortality rate would suggest. H. LeBras, 'Living forbears in stable populations', in K. W. Wachter with E. A. Hammond and P. Laslett (eds.), *Statistical Studies of Historical Social Culture* (New York, 1978), pp. 163–88.

[49] E. A. Wrigley and R. S. Schofield, *The Population History of England 1541–1871*, pp. 413–14.

[50] Cotton Mather wrote 'Let us look upon everything as a sort of Death's Head set before us, with a *Memento mortis* written upon it'. Quoted in Stannard, *Death*, pp. 77–8.

all the time.[51] It is the exceptions, men like the mystic Francis Rous, who took to heart the injunction constantly to reflect on death.[52] Indeed, religious writers often complained that death, despite its experienced closeness, was far from the minds of people.[53] In other words, normative writings can affect the morality of a culture but not always thoughts and behaviour.

Turning now to religion and illness, it is clear that for both religious writers and laymen there was a close connection between religion and medicine. The links that produced this were various, and included the general intertwining of death and life. The union of those 'amorous twins',[54] the body and soul, had traditionally allowed the language of medicine to be applied to both. Richard Greenham wrote:

If a man troubled in conscience come to a minister it may be he will look all to the soul and nothing to the body: if he come to a physician, he only considereth of the body and neglecteth the soul. For my part, I would never have the physician's council severed, nor the minister's labour neglected: because the soul and body dwelling together, it is convenient, that as the soul should be cured by the word, by prayer, by fasting, by threatening or by comforting: so the body also should be brought into some temperature [health] by physic, by purging, by diet, by restoring, by music, and by such means; providing always that it be done so in fear of God.[55]

The use of medical language to describe the healing of the soul was widespread. Puritan theologians constantly used medical metaphors. Perkins wrote that a sinner was frequently compared in the Scriptures to a sick man: 'And therefore the curing of the disease fitly resembleth

[51] It is difficult to prove a negative, but see the diary of Adam Eyre, or even the more devout diaries of Henry Newcome and Roger Lowe. Oliver Heywood expressed his pleasure that his father started to think of God a few months before his death, and did not leave the preparation for death until the last moment: Heywood, *Diaries*, vol. 1, pp. 30 and 85.

[52] 'For myself, I have taken out many lessons of dying and I pray God I may so perfectly learn the art of it, that I may make good that heavenly sentence; that not only to live but to die choist is gain: and that by believing in Him, I may never die, which is his own promise.' Francis Rous, Bodleian Lib., Tanner MS. 62/2 fo. 530.

[53] McManners, *Death and the Enlightenment*, pp. 223–7 discusses the difficult problem of knowing who read books on dying, and whether they were acted upon. He concludes the literate minority did so only when absolutely necessary. The illiterate mass would have to rely on oral instruction by the curé.

[54] Hastler, *Antidote*, p. 36.

[55] Richard Greenham, *The Words of the Reverend and Faithful Servant of Jesus Christ*, 4th edn. (London, 1605), p. 159. On Greenham see Haller, *Rise of Puritanism*, pp. 26–8; Porter, *Reformation*, pp. 216–18.

the curing of sin', a sinner stands 'in need of Christ, the good physician of his soul'.[56] Dod wrote that the offences of God's children could be healed only by the medicine of the precious blood of the Lamb of God.[57] Religious writers used the medical metaphor as a way of moving from the more to the less familiar. Ambrose explicated Hebrews 1: 3, 'When he had by himself purged our sins', by using medical terminology:

See here the manner of the cure: there is a Physician he, (the patient *himself*) [i.e. Christ as physician and patient], the physic administered 'When he had purged' the ill humours evacuated, 'when he had purged our sins'.[58]

The figure of Christ the physician, the healer of the body as well as the soul also served to link this world with the next, medicine with religion. In 1665 during the plague the Anglican Richard Kingston wrote, in a vein common also to Puritans, that Christ by his death became not only 'physician of the dead',[59] but also of the living:

Other physicians, either out of hope of gain or to buoy up their credits and repute in this world, promise those cures which they can never perform: but here is one whose word is his deed, that archetypal verity, who having the issues of life and death in his hand, when he promises life cannot be guilty of a lie...[60]

Christ, of course, had healed the sick in body, and his example gave the church an entrée into the world of medicine. Kingston cited St Matthew's Gospel and Jesus curing the halt, the lame and the blind, and he declared:

the learned physicians are but shadows of this sun of righteousness, when he appears with healing on his wings. Have we the plague spots upon us? If God will be our physician their very redness shall serve for a blush to confess their impotency when he bids them vanish. Does a fever burn us, or a dropsy drown us? One word of his mouth will prove a julip to cool our veins, and a sluice to let out that lake of humours which would engulf us.[61]

The double face of physical and spiritual healing (cure of bodies, cure of souls) showed itself in the very words health and salvation. The Latin word *salus* was taken to mean not only health but also salvation, and health itself could mean salvation. The early English protestant

[56] Perkins, *Chain*, p. 365, citing Luke 4: 18 and Matthew 9: 11–12.
[57] Dod and Cleaver, *Seven Sermons*, p. 4.
[58] Ambrose, *Ultima*, p. 156.
[59] Richard Kingston, *Pillulae Pestilentiales: Or a Spiritual Receipt for Cure of the Plague* (London, 1665), p. 102.
[60] *Ibid.*, p. 103.   [61] *Ibid.*, pp. 105–6.

Thomas Becon had written:

God's word worketh marvellously unto the health of them that believe. And therefore in the word of God it is called the word of health, or salvation; as it is written: 'Ye men and brethren the children of the generation of Abraham...the word of this health was sent unto you.'[62]

The merging of the two worlds of life and death, of body and soul, and the dual and interchangeable senses of Christ the physician, medicine and health, probably helped the sick to move easily from medicine to religion and vice versa, and reflects the fact that there was more than one mode of healing available in the seventeenth century.

The utterances (or belief-system or ideology, as the reader's historical bent directs) of religious writers who indicate a duality or ambiguity between religion and medicine reflected the world of practice. Many ministers, such as Richard Baxter, acted as physicians; and even if they did not, they often quoted medical writers, as did Perkins and Ambrose; or like Ralph Josselin and Oliver Heywood had a developed knowledge of medical terms; or might be friendly with the town's medical men while their wives acted as sources of medical expertise especially at births, as was the case with Henry Newcome at Manchester.

Socially, clergymen and physicians belonged to the same stratum of society – at the lower end of the class of gentlemen, above 'the men which do not rule'.[63] In terms of career choice, medicine and religion could appear equal possibilities.[64] The general proximity of physician and clergyman was reflected by their personal contact at the sick-bed. Given the close intellectual, social and practical links between religion and medicine, it is not surprising that religious and medical explanations should come close together. In fact, as Charles Webster has noted, Puritan reformers argued that all clergymen should routinely act as doctors and provide a medical service;[65] clearly the close connections existing between religion and medicine already noted served as a background for such ideas.

Relations between the clergy and physicians were not always

---

[62] Thomas Becon, *Prayers and Other Pieces*, ed. J. Ayre for the Parker Society (Cambridge, 1844), p. 490.

[63] Laslett, *Lost World*, pp. 35–8.

[64] See *The Diary and Letter Book of the Rev. Thomas Brockbank 1671–1709*, ed. R. Trappes-Lomax (Chetham Soc., N.S., LXXXIX, 1930), p. 64 (hereinafter *Diary*), where Brockbank's father set out the choice of medicine or religion as equal possibilities.

[65] Webster, *Instauration*, pp. 259 and 289.

amicable, for proximity breeds rivalry: ministers objected to doctors dominating the sick-bed,[66] and the Puritan reformers put their schemes forward because they disliked the monopoly of the physicians.[67] On the other hand, physicians such as van Foreest, Cotta and Primerose attempted to establish a monopoly for orthodox, university-trained physicians and attacked ministers together with empirics and wise-women as dangerous to patients.[68] The attacks of the two groups upon each other is further evidence of their closeness.

To sum up: illness and death formed part of the teaching of the Church and were so emphasised that they were seen to permeate the whole of life. This moved people to be good throughout life rather than merely at their death-bed, and enhanced the authority of the Church in the world of life. At the same time, the extension of death into life,[69] and the parallel but more specific merging of religious and medical language were both signs of, and justifications for, the involvement of religion with the process of healing. This section of my essay should, therefore, help to explain why there were religious explanations of illness, and although it can be used as background for the well-known providential view of illness, it should also indicate that there was more to religion and illness than providence.

The individual and God's providence

One of the ways many Puritans spiritualised illness was to see it as God-given; it was a rod, and God was a father correcting (in the sense of guiding and admonishing as well as punishing) his children. The remedy for the Christian was to discover the reason for the correction. In Nehemiah Wallington's manuscript collection of Puritan letters, Paul Bayne's 'Letter of Comfort and Instruction in Affliction' advised:

---

66 Perkins, *Chain*, p. 502.
67 Webster, *Instauration*, pp. 250–64.
68 Petrus Forestus, *De Incerto, Fallacii, Urinarum judicio...* (Leyden, 1589), trans. as *The Arraignement of Urines... Translated by James Hart* (London, 1623); John Cotta, *A Short Discoverie of the Unobserved Dangers of several sorts of Ignorant and Unconsiderate Practises of Physicke in England...* (London, 1623); James Primerose, *De Vulgi in Medicina Erroribus Libri Quatuor...* (London, 1638), trans. as *Popular Errors...* (London, 1651).
69 John Carey, *John Donne: Life, Mind and Art* (London, 1981), p. 202 points to Donne's terror of, yet impatience for, the Last Judgement. Donne's way of managing his fear of death is 'to treat death as a form of life, or to vivify it by giving it an active role in poems which are passionately concerned with living'. Although religious writers put death into life they also often saw events after death as a continuation of life.

First you must labour to apprehend God as a father correcting you by these infirmities. Secondly you must labour to find the cause why and to what purpose God doth follow you in such a kind.[70]

When in 1625 Wallington's wife was ill, his brother-in-law, Livewell Rampagne, wrote: 'I wrote doubtfully because I know not how it hath pleased God to dispose of my sister, who was then under his correcting hand.'[71] Rampagne made no reference to medicine, or to the natural course of the illness, but his attitude was not so much fatalistic as expectant of a higher power. Although Puritans stressed that the age of miracles was over, nevertheless in matters of providence, and illness was one such, God remained an active God, working amongst people. Although His purposes might be unknown, His presence was not.

As Keith Thomas and Alan Macfarlane have written,[72] illness was often seen in providential terms and it was included in the set of happenings or accidents such as fire, falling from horses and the occurrences of social life such as poverty which could be explained by God's providence. As illness, therefore, was one of the methods by which God showed 'his ways towards us', it was a subject to be noted by Puritan diarists along with the other happenings that indicated God's providence.

In this view of illness, guilt and a sense of sin (the natural allies and accompaniments of religion) were of course prominent. Health, a good night's sleep or recovery from illness were noted as a sign of God's favour, but the onset of illness stirred up anxiety, self-doubt and guilt. As Thomas has pointed out the illness of others could be perceived as a correction of oneself.[73] When Henry Newcome's child became ill, he blamed himself for having gone out the night before when, as he recorded at the time, at a private gathering for readings and prayers 'we had a pretty lively close of ye day'. So the next day he wrote:

Was sad this day. Could not sleep at night because of the child's illness. Surely my neglect of what I might have gotten last night, and needlessly going out as I did hath caused this sad affliction and withdrawment from my soul.[74]

---

[70] N. Wallington, *Letters on Religious Topics*, Brit. Lib., Sloane MS. 922, fo. 66r (hereinafter *Letters*).

[71] *Ibid.*, fo. 71r.

[72] Thomas, *Religion*, pp. 90–132; Macfarlane, *Josselin*, pp. 163–82.

[73] Thomas, *Religion*, p. 96.

[74] *The Diary of the Rev. Henry Newcome*, ed. Thomas Heywood (Chetham Soc., xviii, 1849), p. 107 (hereinafter *Diary*).

When his wife had a 'very sick night', Newcombe wrote 'I would
humbly see the rod and him that hath appointed it and beg a good
use of it'.[75]

Illness of others in a family could be perceived less as a punishment
and more as a warning and a sign to alter one's life. The effect was
the same: to change behaviour, and to act as a barometer to one's
conscience. Newcome wrote at different times: 'Ye Lord awaken me
to seriousness by my wife's illness'; 'My wife was ill this night, and
so it occasioned me to be a little more serious. Such need have I of
some load and ballast to keep my heart from carnality and security';
'I have cause to be awakened and to draw nearer to God, my wife
being so ill of a cold as she is.'[76]

The lack of institutional mediation between God and man helped
to internalise this sense of guilt and anxiety, but its root cause was the
ever-present doubt as to whether the individual was one of the elect.
Newcome, describing a colleague's sermon on the spirit, wrote:

Despite of ye spirit is ye soule's apoplexy. Deprives of all life, motion, sense
at once. Alas I doubt somet: I have a stroke of ye palsy on my soul taken
all one side that I am defective in all I do and sadly partial: *But if I could
be satisfied in this point that I am God's childe*, answer to all other objections
would fall in of itself [my italics; note also use of medical metaphor].[77]

All his character faults, misfortunes, illnesses would be as nothing if
Newcome could have known definitely that he was one of the elect.[78]
But as he could not, the everyday occurrences of life took on
significance and acted as indicators of God's decision. Illness, therefore,
became one of the signs of what God had in store. Puritan theologians
were aware of the possible dangers of such an approach, and cautioned
that a life of illness and misfortune did not mean that one was not one
of the elect.[79]

However, this was a period, like all others, when there existed a
plurality of explanations for illness, and people moved easily between
them. Thus belief in God's providence did not prevent Newcome
from having recourse to medicine when someone was ill. Equally,
when ill himself he went to the doctor. During April–May 1662

[75] *Ibid.*, p. 28.   [76] *Ibid.*, pp. 19, 137, 153.

[77] *Ibid.*, pp. 85–6.

[78] Certain signs might indicate if one was amongst the elect but there was no
certainty: Miller, *The New England Mind*, pp. 50–3, also Stannard, *Death*,
pp. 72–5, 83–5.

[79] Perkins, *Chain*, p. 492: 'And by the outward condition of any man, either
in life or death, we are not to judge of his estate before God'.

Newcome became ill, he was bled and he took a rosemary posset to make him sweat; and after going to the apothecary, Thomas Minshull, he wrote: 'After supper I was a little at Mr Minshull's. I am it seems for ye jaundice.' The next day he wrote: 'Read my chapter and after duties, taking [blank] for ye jaundice, went a walking.'[80] The medical expert seems here in Newcome's mind to be deciding his bodily fate (of course the illness could be seen to originate from God) and Newcome immediately acted on the diagnosis by taking medicine. Having a religious view of illness did not exclude recourse to the physician and his remedies, and this was in keeping with the religious injunction to look after one's body; however, once in the hands of the doctors, the religious dimension to illness was forgotten for the time being.

It is clear that the providential view of illness, as well as stirring guilt, which Puritans probably welcomed as part of their spiritual life, also gave a rationale for why someone was ill. For instance, in Paul Bayne's letter 'against the passionate lamenting of the death of a brother', the images of God the punisher and God the healer came together – linked by the image of medicine as painful – and helped to make illness understandable:

God is wise who when he giveth us physic, doth put all the outward comforts we affect far from us. Lest his chastisements should work less kindly and with the purpose to us dear sister the physic must make us sick that doth us any good.[81]

The providential model of illness not only explained sickness, but also allowed recourse to a traditional practice: prayer. Prayer, a promise of repentance or some other religious activity, could be offered up to God in return for a cure. Wallington wrote of one such vow:

and I remember that in the year 1624 I was sick of a fever that I had little hope of life and then I turned my face to the wall (like Hezekiah) and prayed and promised unto God that if he would spare me a little longer O then I would frequent his house more than ever I have done and I would become a new man in the reformation of my life. And now God hath heard my prayers (as he did Hezekiah) in adding near fifteen years to my life.[82]

Richard Baxter wrote scathingly that 'sick-bed promises are usually soon forgotten',[83] but prayer and pleading to God to prevent and cure

---

[80] Newcome, *Diary*, p. 80.
[81] Wallington, *Letters*, fo. 62r.   [82] *Ibid.*, fo. 118v.
[83] Richard Baxter, *Reliquiae Baxterianae* (London, 1696), p. 90 (hereinafter *Reliquae*).

illness was usual. Wallington wrote of others 'that were better than I who on their death-bed did so entreat the Lord to spare them and try them a little longer but the Lord would not hear to grant them their desire'.[84]

Prayers could be said in private but they were often part of communal healing. Puritan groups frequently had their own special days of humiliation, days set aside to assuage God's wrath where by prayer and fasting the community would plead with God that an individual's illness should be taken away or, in the case of an epidemic, that his people as a whole should be spared. Providence, therefore, although it affected individuals, could lead to a group response, and this should be borne in mind as a counter-balance to the picture of introversion and isolated individuality often painted of Puritans and their providential view of life.[85]

In the hands of Keith Thomas and others the providential view of illness has been paraded (and rightly so) as a historical wonder and curiosity. Some questions could now be put: What was the function of providence for religion? Did it retain the faithful by satisfying a need for explaining inexplicable events such as the onset of illness and by providing a method for recovery? The vengeance of God was seen to be inexorable, the case of plague often being taken to demonstrate the implacable efficacy of God's arrows of retribution,[86] but how much did this image of a powerful God depend on the failure of medicine, and to what extent was it used as a means of eliciting belief in God – the material success of the spiritual over the worldly, religion over

---

[84] Wallington, *Letters*, fo. 118v.

[85] Miller, *The New England Mind*, pp. 297–8; Haller, *Rise of Puritanism*, pp. 36–7, 90–1; Delany, *British Autobiography*, p. 56; Stannard, *Death*, p. 41 quotes Max Weber's 'unprecedented inner loneliness' of the Puritan.

[86] See William Gouge, *Gods Three Arrowes, Plague, Famine, Sword in Three Treatises* (London, 1631), p. 14 (hereinafter *Arrows*): '*Prepare to meet thy God O England*. This beginning of the plague is a real demonstration of a greater plague yet to come...The lion hath roared, who will not fear? The Lord God hath spoken, who can but prophecy?' Also pp. 65–6: 'Extraordinary it is, because the immediate hand of God in sending it, in increasing it, in lessening it, in taking it away, is more conspicuously discerned than in other judgements.' Hastler, *Antidote*, pp. 39–40: 'our sins have provoked *Bellatorum fortem*, the mighty warrior, the Lord of Hosts, the righteous judge, to whet his sword and bend his bow and made them ready to prepare the instruments of death, and arrows to destroy us: our customary sins have forced out the Lord's decree, and have brought forth three deadly weapons; his Sword and Famine hover over us...and we are already beset...with a conflict of many diseases; the Angel is darting the right aiming arrows of the Lord's wrath at every man's door: God's deadly tokens: the only marks of his displeasure'.

medicine? Such functional questions could be leavened by a psychological interpretation (always suspect in some historians' eyes). Apart from the well-worn approach that focusses on the figure of authority conjured up by God the chastiser and on the tremulous Puritan anxiously waiting for the next thunderbolt (Josselin's 'my dear angry Lord'),[87] another path could lead to the fear of illness and death and its channelling into a providential context. By focussing upon their putative sins rather than upon illness, Puritans could take away some of the anxiety that they felt about the latter – a form of conversion hysteria in reverse!

Finally, what of the duration and popularity of the providential view of illness? It was popular in the early to mid seventeenth century and amongst Puritans. Devout Anglicans such as John Evelyn and Lady Elizabeth Delaval also believed in providence and God's afflictions.[88] Many Anglicans, however, especially after the Restoration, tended not to refer to providence so much. Laud, who in his simultaneous belief in and denial of dreams, and in his astrological interests, was typical of the first half of the seventeenth century, nevertheless did not mention providence when noting his illnesses in his diary.[89] The attitude of the Anglican martyr was generally followed by later members of the Church in the more secular and less 'enthusiastic' Restoration period. For instance, the correspondents of the Hatton family, most of whom were conformists, writing in the later seventeenth century, used medical terminology when discussing illness and hardly mentioned God.[90] The early eighteenth century Yorkshire diaries of John Hobson

---

[87] Macfarlane, *Josselin*, p. 173; Delany, *British Autobiography*, p. 60 writes of 'the Calvinist image of man cowering before a wrathful God'.

[88] See, for example, Evelyn's account of the death of his son Richard where he commented 'The L. Jesus sanctify this and all other my afflictions: Amen', and when his youngest son died immediately after he wrote 'The afflicting hand of God being still upon us': *The Diary of John Evelyn*, ed. E. S. de Beer (6 vols., Oxford, 1955), vol. 3, pp. 210–11. Also *The Meditations of Lady Elizabeth Delaval*, ed. Douglas G. Greene (Surtees Soc., CXC, 1978 for 1975), p. 77: 'Pain seldom seizes us but physicians can tell what evil is the cause of it from whence our distempers proceed, and what are the most proper remedies (or at least they make us believe so), and by those remedies one may be cured, perhaps suddenly too; but if not me, who it may be God will punish longer making me smart under his rod, even till I humble kiss it, by suffering willingly, yet some other person in pain's might find ease by the physician's skill.'

[89] William Laud, *The Autobiography of Dr William Laud* (Oxford, 1839); this prints the diary.

[90] *Correspondence of the Family of Hatton, Being Chiefly Letters Addressed to Christopher First Viscount Hatton A.D. 1601–1704*, ed. E. Maunde Thompson (2 vols., Camden Soc., N.S., XXII, 1878).

and James Fretwell also described illness in medico-naturalistic terms.[91] The Reverend Giles Moore, rector of Horstead Keynes in Sussex from 1655 to 1679, was a strong supporter of the Restoration settlement. When in London he bought 'rolls on the burning of London, God's terrible voice in the City'. He noted that as his brother died 'he sent forth with great earnestness four or five most divine prayers'.[92] Yet these were mere echoes of godliness. When he, or his maid, was ill, references to prescriptions and physicians predominate, and amongst the many details of his brother's illness the only reference to God was the one given above. God the healer seems to have receded into the background. A similar picture emerges from the diary of the Reverend Thomas Brockbank.[93] Of course, Anglicans did not ignore God, and thanks were often given to God for recovery after illness, for example by Pepys after his operation for the stone. However, after 1660 it was generally only Nonconformists – now an identifiable and limited part of the population – who seemed to view the occurrences of life in spiritualised and providential terms.

Even within Puritan ranks a providential view of illness was by no means universal. A Puritan might believe in providence but not see it working in illness. Richard Rogers, the Puritan lecturer and evangelist writing at the end of the sixteenth century, did not use the providential model in his diary when noting his illnesses.[94] However, clergymen *were* more likely to take a providential view of illness in their diaries. Oliver Heywood, Henry Newcome and Richard Baxter, who were by no means extreme Nonconformists and were close to Anglicanism in other respects, nevertheless contrast sharply with Anglican clergy in their constant recourse to providence. On the other hand, Puritan laymen less intensely devout than Roger Lowe or Joseph Lister were less constant in their reliance on providential explanations. It is almost as though the providential model of illness depended upon one's religious training and devotion. The young Simonds D'Ewes, when studying law in London between 1622 and 1624, showed himself in his diary to be a reasonably devout Puritan layman, but did not see illness as a punishment coming from God. Another layman, Thomas

---

[91] *Yorkshire Diaries and Autobiographies* (Surtees Soc. LXV, 1875) (hereinafter *Yorkshire Diaries*).

[92] 'Extracts from the Journal and Account Book of the Rev. Giles Moore', *Sussex Archaeological Collections*, 1, pp. 101, 109.

[93] Brockbank, *Diary*.

[94] M. M. Knappen (ed.), *Two Elizabethan Puritan Diaries* (Chicago and London, 1933) (hereinafter Rogers, *Diary*).

Dudley, the deputy governor of New England, could see God's hand in the diseases affecting his colony, yet he was able to distance himself from the providential view and, almost like a modern sociologist, see behind the systems of medical and religious explanations. On the causes of the widespread deaths in the colony in 1630–1 Dudley wrote in a Hippocratic vein:

The natural causes seem to be in the want of warm lodging and good diet to which Englishmen are habituated at home, and in the sudden increase of heat which they endure that are landed here in summer, the salt meats at sea having prepared their bodies thereto...

He also mentioned

the poorer sort, whose houses and bedding kept them not sufficiently warm, nor their diet sufficiently in heart. Other causes God may have, as our faithful minister Mr Wilsonne (lately handling that point) showed unto us, which I forbear to mention, leaving this matter to the further dispute of physicians and divines.[95]

It is difficult to tell whether being a layman, having a cosmopolitan range of experience (Dudley had been page to the Earl of Northampton, clerk to a judge and steward to the Earl of Lincoln) or living in the metropolis (as did D'Ewes) produced a greater detachment from a providential way of thinking. Detailed research linking place in society, domicile and personal experience to religious attitudes may elucidate the issue, but I suspect that, as in all periods, there will be frequent contradictory findings, especially as the period up to 1660 was a time of great confusion as regards the religious identity of the gentry (for instance, Dudley's superior was the wealthier John Winthrop who was a consistent believer in providence).

Moreover, much of the evidence has an inherent bias. As one of the purposes of writing a diary was to express the communion between the individual and God, it is almost inevitable that a diarist would favour a providential view. The fact that a Puritan diarist like the parliamentary Captain Adam Eyre[96] did not constantly look for the hand of God in daily life, or like D'Ewes hardly mentioned it, shows that not all Puritan diaries were written as a reckoning of God's ways to man and vice versa. No doubt the rising consciousness of the 'middling' sort of people expressed in politics, commerce and religion found an outlet in diary writing. But, for those imbued with the

[95] Everett Emerson (ed.), *Letters from New England* (Amherst, 1976), p. 76 (hereinafter *New England*).   [96] See *Yorkshire Diaries*.

providential view of things, namely clergymen and devout laymen, the perception of illness as God's correction was habitual. However, together with or underlying the providential view of illness are found more widespread ideas about illness, which are discussed later in the essay.

The plurality of models of illness

Religion held no monopoly in explaining illness. Even thorough-going Puritans often used medical or physically based explanations. This is not surprising given the intellectual and social proximity of religion and medicine discussed earlier. However, from mediaeval times there had been a third way of understanding illness. Magic and folk-wisdom still permeated the English countryside in the seventeenth century.[97] This was oral knowledge and so generally hidden from us, often only surfacing in some disapproving mention in court record, letter or diary. In other words, we know of popular magic only through literary sources, and they almost always disapprove, unless they take an explicitly magical or Paracelsian approach. The magical tradition, however, lies outside the scope of this essay. My focus rests upon religious and naturalistic (medical) explanations, for these were the ones employed both by religious writers and by Puritan diarists.

Although, as we shall see, medical and religious explanations could at times be used by Puritans without relation to each other, there was a standard perceived relationship between the two. In the minds of Puritans, medicine, like other aspects of life, was integrated with religion. For instance, medical remedies were seen as a gift of God, put on earth for men's use. Perkins wrote:

In the preserving of life, two things must be considered: the means, and the right use of means. The means is good and wholesome physic, which, though it be despised of many as a thing unprofitable and needless, yet must it be esteemed as an ordinance and blessing of God.[98]

Perkins added that the medicines had to be authorised 'by the word of God and prayer'.[99] They had to be 'lawful and good' and 'by prayer we must entreat the Lord for a blessing upon them, in restoring of health, if it be the good will of God. 1 Tim. 4.3'. In this way Puritans (and Anglicans like Robert Burton)[100] placed medicine within the

97 See Thomas, *Religion*.   98 Perkins, *Chain*, p. 505.
99 *Ibid.*, p. 506.
100 Robert Burton, *The Anatomy of Melancholy*, ed. Floyd Dell and Paul Jordan-Smith (New York, 1938), pp. 384–6, 389–91 (part 2, sect. 1, member 2 and 4).

bounds of religion, for the word of God (the Bible) defined what was acceptable medicine, and a remedy worked on a specific occasion only because of prayer (which thus gave religion priority over medicine) and God's blessing.

In Perkins' eyes what was allowed by God's word was essentially the medicine of orthodox Galenic physicians. He condemned uroscopy, astrology and enchanters who, he wrote, were in fact witches and wizards though they might be called cunning men and women. Perkins' advice on the choice of physician could be found in many Galenic text-books (in a scholium he cited the attack on uroscopists by Lange and Foreest who were both Galenists). Moreover, the physician should be of 'good conscience and good religion', a sentiment echoed by John Sym who likewise attacked empirics and required physicians to be 'conscionable for religion and piety that God may bless their labours the better'.[101] The requirements that the medicine used should be lawful was understandable given the existence of magical remedies – Perkins condemned the use of spells and charms which 'are all vain and superstitious: because neither by creation, nor by any ordinance of God's word have they any power to cure a bodily disease'.[102]

The attack on empirics shows how moderate Puritan clergymen were closely in tune with their fellow professionals, the Galenic physicians, and had a similar interest in attacking competitors, especially of the oral or 'little' tradition. (It would be an interesting test of Charles Webster's link between Puritanism and Paracelsianism[103] to examine the attitude of moderate Puritan theologians and diarists to Paracelsian medicine.)

The definition of medicine as God-given 'means' not only placed religion on top of medicine, but also had implications for the sick person. The need to gain God's blessings upon 'means' by prayer was an expression of obedience to God. By praying and showing his willingness to accept God's control over medicine the individual avoided the possibility that God might take the use of means as an expression of rebellion, as a method of escaping punishment. In this way the possible conflict between religion and medicine could be avoided, and Puritan diarists and autobiographers – men like Ralph

---

[101] Sym, *Self-killing*, p. 15.
[102] Perkins, *Chain*, p. 506. Burton, *Anatomy of Melancholy*, p. 382 also condemned magic ('sorcerers are too common: cunning men, wizards, and white-witches as they call them, in every village'), but unlike Perkins he accepted astrology (p. 390).   [103] Webster, *Instauration*, pp. 273–82.

Josselin, Henry Newcome, Joseph Lister and Richard Baxter – took special care to note that the success of a remedy was due to God's blessing.[104] The Puritan Lady Brilliana Harley wrote to her son in 1640:

Edward Pinner hath been very sick. I sent to Doctor Wright to him, who hath been here the most part of this week, and hath given him physic which hath done him (by the blessing of God) upon that means, much good.[105]

Was there any conflict between providential, God-controlled means of medicine, and a naturalistic medicine in which a remedy would work whether God's blessing was given or not? Certainly, Puritan writers were aware of the possibility that people could rely too much upon means and not enough upon God, and that they could sin by thinking that medicine worked without God's blessing – that is, that it worked naturalistically. John Sym wrote:

In taking of physic we are always to observe these subsequent cautions. First, that we *dote not* upon, nor *trust*, or *ascribe too much* to physical means; but that we carefully look and pray to *God* for a blessing by the warrantable *use* of them. For, it is *God* that both directs the *physicians* judgement and conscionable practise about a *patient*, and also puts virtue into, and gives healthful operation to the medicines.[106]

Sym also argued that a man might indirectly kill himself when he 'doth not depend upon God, for a blessing upon means, who by his over-riding providence directs the course and blesses the means'. The possibilities were that men would 'slavishly enthrall' themselves to means and so exclude God or 'perplex themselves if they cannot have them [means], or that the success answers not their expectation: because the Lord disposes things so, as he also may effect his work and will, often by crossing ours'.[107] The God of the early seventeenth century was not yet the giver of immutable laws to be discovered by reason and by the scientist, as was thought in the late seventeenth and eighteenth centuries. For Puritans who believed in providence, all things were subject to the secret will of God, and reason could not discover his plan, though a minister, as in the case of plague, might interpret his actions.[108] However, there was some uniformity in the working of

[104] Miller, *The New England Mind*, p. 234 writes that the idea of means 'prevented believers from being lured into the heresy of natural autonomy'.
[105] *Letters of the Lady Brilliana Harley*, ed. Thomas Taylor Lewis (Camden Soc. LVIII, 1853), p. 91.
[106] Sym, *Self-killing*, pp. 14–15.   [107] *Ibid.*, p. 92.
[108] Gouge, *Three Arrows*, p. 13 gave ministers a privileged position as interpreters of God's word (the Scriptures) who could discern what particular sins had brought on the plague.

nature. God, after all, could achieve his ends through natural means, in other words he used the natural (God-given) tendency of a remedy to behave in a particular way. Perkins, for instance, wrote of how a life-span was measured by a predetermined amount of 'radical moisture' in the body.[109] God's determination of a person's existence was thus achieved by natural means. The acceptance of the workings of nature and, more especially, the exhortation not to depend too much on means show that Puritan writers implicitly recognised the existence of naturalistic explanations which might be divorced from providence. And their teaching can be seen as an attempt to exclude the latter possibility from people's minds.

Ralph Josselin, who is discussed in detail elsewhere in this volume by Lucinda McCray Beier, illustrates in his diary how providential and naturalistic explanations of illness could be interchanged – sometimes connected in his mind, sometimes not. The two do not seem to come into overt conflict; after all, even today recourse both to prayer and to doctors often takes place without any inner stress.

Josselin had a sore and suppurating navel between 1648 and 1650. His attitude was that God could heal it directly or could do so indirectly by blessing 'the remedies applied'.[110] When the remedies did not work he 'applied nothing to it hoping in god it will do well'.[111] Here God worked directly rather than through means. Sometimes, providential and naturalistic explanations were placed side by side. At one time Josselin saw his sore navel as God's way of minding him of his folly, but at the same time he wrote that his going outside and taking cold may have been a precipitating factor, and he also added: 'And I observe that I swett very much too or three nights before it was sorish.'[112] Josselin's attempt to make sense on a natural level of his illness by looking for precipitating causes is independent of his ideas of what caused God to make him ill (though Josselin, being a good Puritan minister, would have probably used the standard link between divine ends and means and replied that God worked by indirect means, by cold, to achieve his correction). However, it is clear that Josselin's anxiety was not limited to the divine level, for he was anxious about the natural possibilities threatened by his sore navel, writing: 'heard of one that after 2 years illness was killed with a rawness in his navel, but god shall heal me of this infirmity, and I shall praise him'.[113] Here,

---

[109] Perkins, *Chain*, p. 506.
[110] *The Diary of Ralph Josselin*, ed. Alan Macfarlane (Oxford, 1976), p. 141 (hereinafter *Diary*).   [111] *Ibid.*, p. 147.
[112] *Ibid.*, p. 157.   [113] *Ibid.*, p. 159.

Josselin was setting the divine against the natural. Again, when noting cases of smallpox he wrote that God's providential will could allay the natural, contagious nature of smallpox: 'he can preserve my family or me when others ill';[114] and he prayed 'the lord stand betwixt the whole and sick, and suffer his rod to proceed no farther if it be his will'.[115]

There were times for Josselin, however, when naturalistic and providential explanations of illness coincided. He employed medical metaphors for religious purposes and carried them through their origins in physical illness:

This day I had a little pose and roughness of rheume in my throat, my god will ordain all for my good...my desires are with David that god would purge and wash me thoroughly from my sin, oh let not the humour have no settling stay behind if it be thy pleasure.[116]

Here Josselin slid from the medical to the religious and perhaps back again. He moved from a description of his body to wish God to purge and wash him of sin, then he asked that the humour (of sin? of phlegm?) have 'no settling stay behind': the language could apply just as well to his chest or throat as to his soul. In a sense we are seeing the homely medical metaphor of Dod and Cleaver, Perkins and Ambrose put powerfully into practice; for it draws religion into medicine by borrowing medicine's language, but also appropriates medicine for religion by showing that there is a supreme, providential physician who cures both body and soul. Perhaps it was such language and such metaphors which allowed the possible tensions between religious and naturalistic (medical) explanations of disease to remain hidden from view. Certainly if God was a physician and worked like one then the potential conflict could be evaded, and Josselin did at times picture God like this: 'the lord is pleased to give me some mixtures and rubs in my condicions that my heart may upon every thing look up to him'.[117]

Turning to naturalistic ideas of illness, it is clear that Puritans often thought of the natural causes of illness in two ways. There was knowledge, possibly derived from professional medicine but certainly current in society, involving humoral ideas and specific disease conditions such as 'ague', 'rheum', 'gout', 'fit', 'palsy', etc. Secondly, and more generally, there was an ability to make sense of an illness

---

114 *Ibid.*, p. 154.
116 *Ibid.*, p. 204.

115 *Ibid.*, p. 158.
117 *Ibid.*, p. 206.

by referring to some precipitating event, often described in terms of wet, cold, dry and warm. This latter type of knowledge seems to have been widespread and to have transcended differences of domicile, religion and status. D'Ewes, for instance, wrote 'being somewhat thin clothed I got there a most fierce and bitter cold';[118] Josselin, as we have seen, felt that going outside and taking cold might have produced his sore navel; whilst the poor Puritan servant Roger Lowe wrote 'I went to Leigh and was ill wet'.[119] Thomas Dudley reported 'there died Mrs Shelton, the wife of the other minister there, who, about eighteen or twenty days before, handling cold things in a sharp morning, put herself into a most violent fit of the wind colic and vomiting, she at length fell into a fever and so died'.[120] Pepys also tried to make sense of his illnesses in this way: 'this day under great apprehensions of getting an ague from my putting on a suit that hath lain without ayring a great while, and I pray to God it do not do me hurt'.[121]

This way of thinking, relying upon a qualitative (hot, cold, dry, wet) view of things, had analogies with the more complex and technical system of orthodox medicine, which in its practice was also qualitative despite the advent of Paracelsian and then mechanical ideas which tended to change its theoretical structure. It may be that an anthropological analysis, as MacDonald has suggested,[122] instead of, or as well as, a social history approach will give insight into what seems to have been a common resource in literate society (and most probably in non-literate ones as well). Anthropologists have studied hot–cold/dry–wet systems of ideas in various societies. The need of sick people to find for themselves a precipitating cause for an illness is something that we find today,[123] and a psychological as well as an anthropological perspective may be helpful in understanding it. For this type of explanation, depending as it does on the sick person's actual

[118] *The Diary of Sir Simonds D'Ewes (1622–1624)*, ed. Elizabeth Bourcier (Paris, 1974), p. 124 (hereinafter *Diary*).

[119] William L. Sachse (ed.), *The Diary of Roger Lowe of Ashton-in-Makerfield, Lancashire 1663–74* (London, 1938).

[120] Emerson, *New England*, p. 82.

[121] Pepys, *Diary*, vol. 6, p. 32.

[122] Michael MacDonald, 'Anthropological perspectives on the history of science and medicine', in P. Corsi and P. Weindling (eds.), *Information Sources in the History of Science and Medicine* (London, 1983), pp. 61–80.

[123] As I write, newspapers report the death of a girl whose parents believed that the piercing of her ears was responsible, despite doctors' statements to the contrary.

experience and his own verbalisation of it, which is usually different from the complex and probably alienating reasoning of the medical profession, has the function of giving personal understanding of, and hence a measure of personal control over, illness.

The vocabulary of illness

The vocabulary used to express knowledge of illness varied greatly. Richard Rogers gave few descriptions of his own illnesses and hardly any of other people's. When visiting the sick he recorded no details of the illnesses that they suffered from; what we have is the laconic: 'One of these days I visited a goodly sick woman with comfort.'[124] Apart from mentioning a cough and cold,[125] Rogers did not have a developed vocabulary for illnesses (at least in his diary), though as one of the early 'physicians of the soul' he did for his psyche and its troubles, for his great interest was 'seeing myself':

And I had this med[itation] one morn[ing] that, comparing this course in which I view my life continually with the former wherein I did it by fits and thus was oft unsettled, out of order, and then either not seeing myself, though I had been less unwatchfull [*sic*] walked in great danger by every occasion or, seeing it, could not easily recover myself, and so went unfit, many hours and sometimes days, for my calling, sometimes dumpish and too heavy, sometimes loose and many fruits following, as no study but unprof[itableness].[126]

Clearly Rogers' emphasis was on his mind not on his body, and the adjectives 'unsettled' and 'out of order', 'unfit', 'dumpish', 'too heavy', 'loose' all testify to the fact that he had developed a rich and variegated vocabulary of fine distinctions to describe the state of his mind. Napier's patients also seemed to have the same wealth of vocabulary for their mental states,[127] so this fullness of language may not have been limited to Puritans; certainly as Haller points out it is found in the literature of the time.[128] Whether Rogers had the same full vocabulary for physical illness but did not put it in his diary is impossible to tell.

In the diary of Roger Lowe the vocabulary both for his mental and for his physical states was very limited. As his is almost a unique diary,

---

124 Rogers, *Diary*, p. 70. On Rogers see his editor's introduction and Haller, *Rise of Puritanism*, pp. 35–45.
125 *Ibid.*, p. 83.   126 *Ibid.*, p. 70.
127 On the vocabulary of psychological states see MacDonald, *Mystical Bedlam*, p. 243.
128 Haller, *Rise of Puritanism*, pp. 31–3.

from a poor but literate servant, it is worth looking at it in a little detail. 'Sad' was one of Lowe's major descriptive terms for mental trouble and 'sick' for physical. He often put the two together, expressing the typical union of body and mind: 'Tuesday, I was sadly sick and had a very sick night, but the Lord restored me in the other morning.'[129]

Lowe, however, gave a little detail of his own and others' physical illnesses. Obvious, visible ailments were noted, Lowe at different times recording that 'A tedious stitch took in my back, so I was unable to stay shop, and held me very sore till noon, and then the Lord helped me'; 'I was in an afflicted state in my body by reasons of cold'; 'and so we parted and were ill wet'.[130] However, more serious complaints were vague, in a sense unknowable, for affliction and recovery belonged to God. From March to May 1666 Lowe suffered from some illness which was probably serious but which he did not identify, apart from his references to God's affliction and mercy; the physical descriptive terms used were 'ill', 'pains', 'well'.[131]

When describing the illnesses of others Lowe noted some obvious ailments and well-known conditions. He mentioned toothache (often specifically noted by diarists), accidental poisoning by arsenic, 'a hurt by a fall off a horse', 'neck broken in riding', 'dropsy', 'falling sickness', 'troubled with sores'. However, he was usually less specific when describing illness.

At first sight this is surprising, for his acquaintance with illness and death was far greater than that of a modern lay person. Although not a minister, he visited the sick regularly (as Puritans were enjoined to do); he was present at death-beds and he attended many funerals. Judging from other diaries such as William Bulkeley's[132] and Adam Eyre's, this was not unusual for a lay person in the seventeenth century. Lowe certainly gained some knowledge of illness and death from his exposure to the sick. (Accounts of death-bed scenes not only portrayed the piety of the dying, but also described their symptoms and thus expressed medical knowledge, and being read became sources of knowledge.) Lowe thought that he knew the signs of approaching death:

This evening old Izibell and John Hasleden and I went to Gawther's and were merry when we parted. We went all together into old John Jenkins', we

---

[129] Lowe, *Diary*, p. 56. [130] *Ibid.*, pp. 22, 75, 86. [131] *Ibid.*, pp. 99–101.
[132] *The Diary of Bulkeley of Dronwy, Anglesey 1630–1636*, ed. H. Owen (Anglesey Antiquarian Society, 1937), pp. 27–172.

thought he would have died this night. When I was with him he shook me by the hand and I conferred with him. After a while I parted. [In fact he did not die that night.][133]

On another occasion Lowe wrote: 'I went into old William Hasleden's in Ashton, his wife was sick and I read in the *Practice of Pietie*, and as I was reading she gave up the ghost.'[134] However, despite his familiarity with the sick, Lowe had little vocabulary to describe different diseases or perhaps had no interest in having one. He went to a large number of funerals, but gave no cause of death, and on his visits to the sick, with few exceptions he seemed uninterested in recording what particular illness was involved. Lowe was interested in medicine only in so far as it related to religion. So he recorded a religious rhyme for staunching blood;[135] and a visit to 'one George Clare, who lay sick' provided a religious motif: 'I went into church yard to look at graves, as is my common custom, and there stayed a while admiring the common frailty of mankind: how silently now they were lying in dust.'[136]

For Lowe the sick were sick, and no explanation or diagnosis of their condition was required; but the sick, even if strangers, could act as the focus of social activity and be the recipients of religious comfort. We should thus remember that the sick were not only perceived in 'medical' terms but also in religious and social terms.

It may also be the case that Lowe's knowledge of medical terminology was slight. Certainly men like Newcome, Josselin, Heywood who were ministers and in daily contact with sickness, and who sometimes read medical authors, used a wider vocabulary. And Richard Baxter, who had a consuming interest in his own illness as well as being a minister and a medical practitioner, came close in his autobiography to emulating the language found in medical text-books (whether contact with physicians produced an acquaintance with medical terminology, or whether it was a shared resource of a particular section of society needs further research). However, it is possible that these men were the exceptions and that many people were specific only about accidents (broken legs etc.), obvious ailments (toothaches, colds, joint pains) and a few well-known illnesses (dropsy, ague, etc.), with the large majority of cases being labelled 'sick'. In other words, for some people knowledge of illness as shown by a differentiated terminology may have been slight. Or, it may be the

[133] Lowe, *Diary*, pp. 42–3.   [134] *Ibid.*, p. 109.
[135] *Ibid.*, pp. 76–7.   [136] *Ibid.*, p. 57.

case that there was a difference between the first and second half of the century. The diaries of Robert Bulkeley, Adam Eyre and the reports of the early American colonists tend to support the view that in the earlier part of the century less medical terminology was used, while the diaries after 1660 are richer in the vocabulary of illness. A comparison of the diary of Laud and the autobiography of Baxter, the former written in the first half of the century and the latter in the second half, also shows this difference. However, generalisations are dangerous; Baxter was *so* interested in his health that his knowledge would probably have been as great had he been living at the beginning of the century.

To conclude the more general part of this essay: it should now be apparent that physical illness was only partly 'spiritualised', that there was a guarded note of acceptance by Puritan writers of physical medicine and that, given the wide diversity of knowledge and vocabulary amongst different people, generalisations are most difficult.

So far I have discussed problems and approaches; the people involved have not really shown their faces. The English historian in taking the thematic approach has tended to use snippets of evidence to support a particular point; this means that a person's overall 'life trajectory' or experience as shown in a diary or autobiography is lost in the attempt to describe particular problems and to produce generalisations. This is especially unfortunate in such a personal matter as attitudes to illness. By looking in some detail at the autobiographies of Joseph Lister and Richard Baxter I hope to remedy the defect.

The autobiographies of Joseph Lister and Richard Baxter

A Puritan autobiography, as opposed to a diary, highlighted significant events and episodes in the author's life.[137] Rather than a day by day account of illness we are presented in the autobiographies of Lister and Baxter with a selection of significant illnesses; and health and illness are treated in a more considered if distanced fashion, being remembered after a period of years.

Joseph Lister (1627–1709) was an apprentice, and a servant, who finally became reasonably well off after the death of his wife's uncle who left land worth £20 a year. Although not a minister himself, Lister sent his sons into the ministry. His autobiography is full of examples of God's providence, whether it was saving him from accidents or

---

[137] On Puritan autobiographies see Delany, *British Autobiography*, and Watkins, *Puritan Experience*.

illness; however, the autobiography is not a mere recital of pious paradigms but, like Lowe's diary, also a lively and almost innocent account of social life (his reasons for not marrying his master's daughter spring to mind).

Lister's first brush with divine providence came when he fell off a horse and 'I was taken up for dead...O how near was I to death at this time! and had I died then, surely I had gone down to the pit'.[138]

Another example of God's providence occurred when, as an adult, he was at Hartlepool and he was caught by the tide. Lister put his trust in God:

Then I cried unto the Lord, who can do everything; and I thought, though I be in the sea, I am not in the whale's belly; and if I was, yet God could demand deliverance for me; so I depended upon his ability to save me...yet God enabled the horse to grapple with the flood.[139]

Here Lister's horse as well as God could help him, but in most accidents it was God alone who could be a protector. In illness, however, medicine and doctors could be of use as well as God. This brings us back to the problem of the perception of illness as naturalistic and/or divine. After his ordeal, Lister came home wet and fell ill (he saw illness in functional terms: he could not rise, food was disagreeable and appetite and sleep departed from him). His reaction was to send his urine to a physician who, without knowing of the episode with the tide, could form no judgement except that 'the person had been under some sad overpowering fear'. Rather than wait upon providence Lister acted. He was dissatisfied with his physician:

I fell into a violent fever, in which, after I had laid some weeks in great extremity and the doctor ordering me nothing but some easy cordial things, I desired him to give me a bill, for I purposed employing another man; for though I was not against cordials for relieving and strengthening nature, yet I thought it very proper to have some working physic that might be likely to weaken and remove the distemper, which he was not willing to give me.[140]

There are some points to note here. Lister was a free agent, who like Josselin and anyone else who could afford it, could decide on his own treatment. We in the age of the National Health Service have forgotten how easy it is to change a doctor if the patient is paying. However, Lister like Josselin had his own opinion of medical matters, and the

---

[138] Joseph Lister, *The Autobiography of J. L....*, ed. T. Wright (London, 1842), p. 4.
[139] *Ibid.*, p. 42.   [140] *Ibid.*, p. 43.

plastic, qualitative language of seventeenth century medicine – 'working physic...weaken and remove the distemper' – was far easier for lay people to use than that of modern medicine. Lister could not only sack his doctor, but he was also much more able to make a decision on the rationale of his treatment and could do so whilst using the language of the physicians. One might also say that by helping himself, Lister was not waiting upon God's providence, for, as Perkins wrote, the Christian had the duty actively to look after the health of his body. Lister got a new doctor:

a good man, I believe, and they said a young convert...He first let me blood, and then gave me what he thought proper, and *God so blessed his prescriptions*, that I did soon recover. [my italics][141]

Even if it appears illogical to us that God should work through one doctor and not the other, it was not to a Nonconformist, for every moment was subject to God's providence. Providence worked not uniformly but at each moment of time, and in the face of providence consistency was a meaningless concept – and the doctor being a convert may have helped.

Yet the difference between blind acceptance of providence as in the case of accidents and an ability to act to evade illness was still there. Although Lister recovered, he fell ill again, not because of providence but because he walked into the garden and was 'much worse than before'. In this case Lister's actions did not bring healing but disease. Nevertheless, his explanation was a naturalistic rather than a providential one. The point, however, is that Lister was able to use both explanations without feeling any tension between them. Providence in a sense encompassed the natural, for it could work through natural means. Certainly, after being close to death both from drowning and illness, Lister saw providence behind all his recent experiences. He got back to Bradford among his Christian friends who:

assisted me in returning a thanks-offering to the Lord for his past mercies, for I had been under a series of gracious and merciful providences for a long time past.[142]

Lister's attitude to death was not one of anxiety. Like Josselin he was sure that he would go to heaven. He wrote of his relapse: 'I now lay long in a languishing condition, expecting nothing but death; and being easy, and well satisfied about my future state, was borne

---

[141] *Ibid.*, p. 43.   [142] *Ibid.*, p. 45.

90   *Andrew Wear*

comfortably.'[143] This serenity may have been unusual, for the Puritan's belief in his predestination ensured that no worldly event such as a death-bed confession or repentance could change God's unknown decision as to his fate after death. Hence, anxiety should in theory have continued up to the moment of death. But the older tradition of dying well to which Puritans still subscribed emphasised that the dying person should achieve a state of peace and reconciliation with God.[144]

For both Catholics and Puritans the approach of death was usually something that was known to the ill person. The religious preparation for death would be enough to ensure this.[145] Lister perceived the intimation of death in terms of execution (a recurring image in diaries). After his wife's death, he was attacked by a 'violent fever' so that:

for a week or ten days I was, in the judgement of almost all spectators, a gone man; and I had received the sentence of death in my own apprehension, and yet, at last, even to a wonder, God was pleased to rebuke the distemper, and raise me up again. Bless the Lord, O my soul and all that is within me praise his holy name![146]

Illness and death were spectacles in which the spectators and the patient could make their own judgement; the medical expert did not have a monopoly on prognostication. At the same time, God was the ultimate judge, giving his sentence of death through bodily intimation to the patient. Whatever the theologians might have said and a Puritan expected after death, loss of life was still a punishment (an execution).

Richard Baxter (1615–91), the Puritan divine, also discussed his health and illnesses in his autobiography.[147] Baxter left the materials for an autobiography which were published after his death as *Reliquiae Baxterianae* (1696). In it are accounts of his involvement in religion and politics as well as intimate details of his personal life. Health and illness were given places of great importance. Baxter saw himself as suffering pain and illness continually through his life. He perceived these illnesses as being sent by God, but his interest in providence was, on this subject, at times only nominal in relation to the large amount of detail about

---

143 *Ibid.*, p. 44.
144 Stannard, *Death*, pp. 69, 78–9, 88, describes the conflicts of the two views.
145 Puritan theologians stressed that physicians should tell the patient if the prognosis was bad and call a minister. In France a physician was required by law to advise the patient to call in a confessor on the second day of a serious illness: McManners, *Death and the Enlightenment*, p. 244.
146 Lister, *Autobiography*, p. 57.
147 On Baxter see G. F. Nuttall, *Richard Baxter* (London, 1965); Delany, *British Autobiography*, pp. 72–6; Watkins, *Puritan Experience*, pp. 121–43.

his ailments. It was his illnesses *per se* that interested Baxter, their symptoms, causes, treatments and his sufferings under them. In short, Baxter was morbidly obsessed with his ailments, but as I do not want to label Baxter with what his doctors tagged him with, this will be my last pejorative comment about Baxter's interest in his own health.

The reasons that Baxter gave for writing about his health varied. At the beginning of the book Baxter stressed the importance of his body for understanding his soul:

And because the case of my body had a great operation upon my soul, and the history of it is somewhat necessary to the right understanding of the rest, and yet it is not a matter worthy to be oft mentioned, I shall here give you a brief account of the most of my afflictions of that kind, reserving the mention of some particular *deliverances* to the proper place. [my italics: Baxter was indicating the formal structure of a Puritan autobiography][148]

The same note of apology is present later when Baxter gave another reason for talking about his health. Students and physicians might learn something and other men's health might benefit, so 'I must here digress, to mention the state of my vile body, not otherwise worthy the notice of the world'.[149] Whatever the ostensible reasons for writing about his health, its place in his autobiography is clearly justified for he must have spent many hours both suffering from, and thinking about, his illnesses. Not only did he treat himself (which was quite usual) but, like other ministers, he became a medical practitioner.

Baxter opened his case history by describing his general constitution ('sound...but very thin and lean and weak and especially of a great debility of the nerves').[150] The structure of his narration was totally secular and 'medical'. He listed his childhood illnesses and how he had caught a chronic catarrh and cold which he was afraid had turned into a consumption. From this point on we have a catalogue of treatments, and Baxter's explanations of why they failed. His account would have provided Molière with good material for his satire on medicine, but for Baxter the treatments did not fail because they were *useless*, but because they were not *appropriate* – the physicians had neither properly diagnosed the illness and its causes, nor correctly assessed what treatment would supply the required qualities to counteract the illness. At first, Baxter ate garlic, 'but this put an acrimony into my blood, which naturally was acrimonious'. Baxter then sought advice:

[148] Baxter, *Reliquiae*, p. 9.
[149] *Ibid.*, part III, p. 173.   [150] *Ibid.*, part 1, p. 9.

After this the spitting of blood increased my fears. After that Sir Henry Herbert advised me to take the flower of brimstone, which I continued till I had taken seven ounces; which took off most of the remainder of my cough; but increased the acrimony of my blood.[151]

Then Baxter consulted an 'unskilful physician' who persuaded him that he had a hectic fever:

and to cure that I took much milk from the cow, and other pituitous cooling things, and constantly anointed my stomach and reins [kidneys] with refrigerating oils of violets and roses; and was utterly restrained from my usual exercise! By this time I had an extream chilliness without, and yet a strange scurf on my tongue, with a constant desire of stretching, that I thought I would almost have endured the rack; and an incredible flatulency at the stomach, and a bleeding at the nose.[152]

Clearly Baxter did not agree with his doctors. It would be tedious to recount the diagnoses, the treatments, and the reasons for their failure. Baxter wrote he had 'at several times the advice of no less than six and thirty physicians, by whose order I us'd drugs without number almost, which God thought not fit to make successful for a cure'[153] (who was to blame – God or the doctors?). A number of epistemological and social issues are involved here.

Baxter felt that his knowledge was equal to the physicians'. It was not of a different kind from theirs, but Baxter thought that he could apply it better than the doctors. He believed that his illnesses stemmed 'from latent stones in my reins, occasioned by unsuitable diet in my youth'.[154] He had observed that his catarrh and cough had come on after eating raw apples, pears and plums (note the search for a precipitating cause), and he was confirmed in his opinion that diet was at the root of his troubles when Sir Theodore Mayerne (physician to James I) advised him to eat apples 'which of all things in the world had ever been my most deadly enemies', with the result that:

Having taken cold with riding thin clothed in the snow, and having but two days eaten apples before meat, as he persuaded me, I fell into such a bleeding as continued six days, with some fits of intermission; so that about a gallon of blood that we noted was lost, and what more I know not.[155]

In the end, perhaps because he felt he knew better, Baxter 'at last forsook the doctors for the most part except when the urgency of a symptom or pain constrained me to seek some present ease'.[156]

[151] *Ibid.*, part 1, p. 9.
[153] *Ibid.*, part 1, p. 10.
[155] *Ibid.*, part 1, pp. 9–10.
[152] *Ibid.*, part 1, p. 9.
[154] *Ibid.*, part 1, p. 10.
[156] *Ibid.*, part 1, p. 10.

It was not epistemological freedom that was the crucial issue; Baxter never really successfully exercised such freedom. He never escaped from doctors; he was always asking their opinion despite his rejection of them. The reasons for this attraction are difficult to grasp (perhaps Baxter partly accepted physicians' claims that only they should make humoral interpretations of illness). Moreover freedom to diagnose and treat his illness was not the crucial factor in making him reject the physicians; it was a particular action of the doctors that mattered.

Baxter was variously diagnosed as suffering from a hectic fever, from scurvy and then came the blow: 'divers eminent physicians agreed that my disease was the hypochondriack melancholy'.[157] This was a diagnosis that Baxter did not want (it was one that was to recur), for it labelled him as mad, or possessed, or at least highly fanciful. Robert Burton wrote of windy or hypochondriack melancholy that physicians found it very difficult to locate the part affected. Signs of the illness included the tendency of the patient to exaggerate symptoms and to change physicians very often.[158] This particular category of melancholy was less associated with the extreme forms of madness, but it did fit Baxter and the label deprived him of the reality of his symptoms. He denied the diagnosis:

And yet two wonderful mercies I have had from God that I was never overwhelm'd with real melancholy. My distemper never went to so far as to possess me with any inordinate fancies, or damp me with sinking sadness, although the physicians call'd it the hypochondriack melancholy.[159]

Baxter had been willing to suffer for two years debilitating treatments for scurvy, but 'hypochondriack melancholy' was too much for him; although he was attracted to doctors and sought their expertise, their rejection of his symptoms and pains made him withdraw from them for a while. Interestingly, Baxter's denial of the doctors' diagnosis was based upon God's providence – 'mercies'. The strategy of using God's authority to counter that of the physicians was to recur.

Baxter came back to the question of 'hypochondriack melancholy' when he described how later on in life his kidneys started to trouble him. He first discussed his general state of health:

---

[157] *Ibid.*, part 1, p. 10.
[158] Burton, *Anatomy of Melancholy*, pp. 350–2, 392–3 (part 1, sect. 3, memb. 2, subsect. 2, and part 2, sect. 1, memb. 4, subsect. 2).
[159] Baxter, *Reliquie*, part 1, p. 10.

I have lain in above forty years constant weaknesses, and almost constant pains: My chief troubles were incredible inflations of stomach, bowels, back, sides, head, thighs as if I had been daily fill'd with wind...Thirty physicians (at least) all call'd it nothing but hypochondriack flatulency, and somewhat of a scorbutical malady: great bleeding at the nose also did emaciate me, and keep me in a scorbutickal atrophy.[160]

Baxter was fighting the doctors through the pages of the autobiography. This shows how much power they had in his eyes and how necessary a diagnostic label was for Baxter to legitimate his disease (unless the label was melancholy). Baxter wrote that 'I thought myself, that my disease was almost all from debility of the stomach, and extream acrimony of blood by some fault of the liver'.[161] Then in 1658 he suspected renal stones and

thought that one of my extream leanness might possibly feel it: I felt both my kidnies plainly indurate like stone: But never having had a nephritick fit, nor stone came from me in my life and knowing that if that which I felt was stone, the greatness prohibited all medicine that tended to a cure: I thought therefore that it was best for me to be ignorant what it was.[162]

Rather than thinking that he did not have kidney stones because he did not have colic Baxter took the gloomier view – the stones were so big that they could not be dislodged. After fifteen years his pains redoubled:

1673 it turned to terrible suffocations of my brain and lungs. So that if I slept I was suddenly and painfully awakened: The abatement of urine, and constant pain, which nature almost yielded to as victorious, renewed my suspicion of the stone, And my old exploration: and feeling my lean back, both the kidneys were greatlier indurate than before, that the membrane is sore to touch, as if nothing but stone were within them.[163]

The physicians replied that 'the stone cannot be felt with the hand!' Baxter asked for them to feel his back and they had to agree that the kidneys felt hard but with what 'they could not tell'. The reaction of the physicians was to tell Baxter that if both kidneys had such big stones then he would have been 'much worse, by vomiting and torment, and not able to preach, and go about'.[164] This argument between doctors and patient went on with Baxter relying on the

[160] *Ibid.*, part 3, p. 173.
[162] *Ibid.*, part 3, p. 173.
[164] *Ibid.*, part 3, p. 173.

[161] *Ibid.*, part 3, p. 173.
[163] *Ibid.*, part 3, p. 173.

authority of 'Skenkius[165] and many observators' that kidney stones could lie unsuspected. The debate had its spectators and the label of 'hypochondriack melancholy' could be hurtful when disseminated at large, and this indicates again the legitimating powers of the doctors:

> I became the common talk of the city, especially the women; as if I had been a melancholy humourist, that conceited my reins were petrified, when it was no such matter, but mere conceit. And so while I lay night and day in pain, my supposed melancholy (which I thank God, all my life hath been extraordinary free from) became, for a year, the pity or derision of the town.[166]

Baxter had the last word, stating that 'all physicians had been deceived', and as he perceived 'that all flatulency and pains came from the reins by stagnation, regurgitation and acrimony I cast off all of their medicine and diet'.[167] He decided to clean out his intestines twice a week with a mixture whose ingredients he gave. The result was that God eased his pains. The structure of the argument is important. Baxter gives his own diagnosis and aetiology, and applies an appropriate remedy (cleaning out the guts should get rid of stagnation and acrimony). Cause and remedy now make sense, and it is the success of the latter that justifies his belief that the doctors were deceived and his diagnosis was correct. Yet Baxter could not hide his anxiety, and his arguments were not totally convincing to himself; he gave a whole barrage of reasons why he was right, but could not shake off in his mind the authority of the doctors. He had to justify his illness. One of his arguments was that God had been merciful to him, despite his constant sufferings, for he had 'not one nephritick torment nor acrimony of urine (save one day of bloody urine) nor intolerable kind of pain. What greater bodily mercy can I have had?'[168] Baxter tried here to turn the doctors' arguments by recourse to God's providence. Again, as with Josselin, but in a different form, we have the divine being set up against the naturalistic and secular. Baxter also attacked the concept of hypochondria itself. Humoral medicine was enormously elastic and could explain most symptoms, and would *prima facie* not

---

[165] Skenkius may have been Johannes Schenck (1530–1598) who published a book of medical observations reprinted in the seventeenth century, or more probably his son Johann Georg Schenck who wrote on calculi.

[166] Baxter, *Reliquiae*, part 3, p. 173.

[167] *Ibid.*, part 3, p. 173.   [168] *Ibid.*, part 3, p. 174.

need to have recourse, if recourse it was, to hypochondria to hide
ignorance. But this is what Baxter thought was involved:

I have written this to mind physicians, to search deeper, when they use to
take up with the general hiding names of *hypochondriacks* and scorbuticks,
and to caution students.[169]

Baxter was willing to accept the framework of orthodox medicine
if not his place within it. Whether he was seen as 'deviant' by society
is difficult to judge, for Baxter's appeal to God's providence as
determining the nature of his illness – even if that providence produced
the topsy-turvy result of kidney stones without symptoms – was
sanctioned by Nonconformist tradition, though its force was being
challenged as Anglican rationalism came to the fore.

The extent of Baxter's 'deviancy' is also difficult to assess, for men
like Josselin were willing to treat themselves, the number of recipe
books of drugs was large, and despite the pretensions of the Royal
College of Physicians there was no set pharmacopoeia. So that when
Baxter made up his own drugs he was not, in the wider context, being
'deviant'. His actions would not have been interpreted in the way that
a rejection of orthodox medicine for herbalism would be today. Yet,
in his own mind, Baxter was being 'deviant': the doctors could not
be ignorant; they were in principle powerful and knowledgeable; he
had to justify his reaction against them. Part of his strategy was to place
his own alternative remedies within the framework of orthodox
medical theory, but then give them further validation by referring their
powers to God. When Baxter had a constantly running eye, his doctor
prescribed chalk to counteract the acidity of his stomach, but Baxter
wanted to try something of his own:

At last I had a conceit of my own that two plants which I had never made
trial of, would prove accommodate to my infirmity, *heath* and *sage*, as being
very drying and astringent without any acrimony: I boiled much of them
in my beer instead of hops, and drank no other: When I had used it a month
my eyes were cured, and all my tormenting tooth-aches and such other
maladies.[170]

Baxter found that it was the sage that was most effective and he
described its effect on different types of people. His choice of sage was
based on the same reasoning that his doctor had used, but God was
responsible for its nature and power – God the Physician ('This I
thought myself obliged to mention to the praise of my heavenly

169 *Ibid.*, part 3, p. 174.   170 *Ibid.*, part 1, p. 82.

physician, in thankfulness for these ten years ease; and to give some hint to others in my case').[171] Baxter used the idea of God the Physician and the belief that God blessed medicines to put God against the physicians: 'In a word, God hath made this herb do more for me (not for *cure* but for *ease*) than all the medicines that ever I used from all physicians in my life.'[172] Preferring his own medicine, Baxter appealed to another system – that of divine medicine. His separation of the divine and the naturalistic view of illness was more explicit than Josselin's, perhaps because of his love/hate relationship with orthodox medicine. The paradox with Baxter is that he did not believe exclusively and consistently in providential medicine. Far from it: although at times he used the divine physician against the human and also referred to instances of divine providence in relation to his illnesses, the tenor of Baxter's views on illness was frequently naturalistic. Immediately after his thanks to the 'heavenly Physician' Baxter added that the sage was diminishing in effectiveness because of constant use:

Though now, through age and constant use, this herb doth less with me than at the first; yet am I necessitated still to use it...After sixteen or seventeen years benefit it now faileth me, and I forsake it.[173]

Baxter moved from the providential to the naturalistic; he did not mention the possibility that sage no longer worked because God had withdrawn his blessing from it. In a sense, both medical theories and God's providence were bodies of knowledge (resources) that Baxter used when appropriate. He was not aware of it, but we are. Whether one should concentrate on Baxter's consciousness, or on a more distanced 'social', 'objective' view is a moot point.

Although Baxter made much use of orthodox medical categories, at times he also perceived illness in a predominantly religious sense. Like Lister, Baxter saw God as a judge handing out sentence and punishment. That Puritan relationship to God, more personal even than that of human beings with each other, was fully present in Baxter. On occasion he viewed his pain and illnesses not as medical entities but as the language that God used. After detailing his persecution for refusing to conform Baxter wrote:

But God was pleased quickly to put me past all fear of man...by laying on me more himself than man can do...day and night I groan and languish under God's just afflicting hand...As waves follow waves in the tempestuous seas,

[171] *Ibid.*, part 1, p. 83.
[172] *Ibid.*, part 1, pp. 82–3.   [173] *Ibid.*, part 1, p. 83.

so one pain and danger followed another, in this sinful miserable flesh: I die daily, yet remain alive: God in his great mercy, knowing my dulness in health and ease, doth make it much easier to repent and hate my sin and loath myself, and contemn the world, and submit to the sentence of death with willingness than otherwise it was ever like to have been. O how little is it that wrathful enemies can do against us, in comparison to what our sin, and the justice of God can do? And O how little is it that the best and kindest of friends can do, for a pained body, or a guilty sinful soul, in comparison of one gracious look or word from God. Woe be to him that hath no better help than man! And blessed is he whose help and hope is in the Lord.[174]

Here illness was put into a framework where the secular is excluded in favour of the divine. Illness is merely one of the providential instruments or signs of God, used as part of a communication with his own, which was far more intimate and effective than any human relationship. The afflictions of Lowe, Josselin and Newcombe were all part of this communion between God and man.

Yet, the language was notoriously ambiguous. Baxter himself pointed this out. At the time of the Great Plague, God's providence upon the whole community was variously interpreted according to particular interests:

Yet under all these Desolations the *wicked* are *hardened*, and cast all on the fanaticks: and the true dividing fanaticks and sectaries are not yet humbled for former miscarriages, but cast all on the *prelates* and imposers: And the ignorant vulgar are stupid, and know not what use to make of anything they feel: But thousands of the sober, faithful servants of the lord, are mourning in secret...From *London* it is spread through many counties, especially next London. Where few places, especially corporations are free: which makes me oft groan and wish, LONDON AND ALL THE CORPORATIONS OF *ENGLAND* WOULD REVIEW THE CORPORATION ACT AND THEIR OWN ACTS AND SPEEDILY REPENT.[175]

If it was easy to interpret the cause of plague to suit one's own prejudices, it was also convenient to have a nosebleed at a particular time. Much of Baxter's autobiography was a justification for his Nonconformist stance, though he was at pains to stress that he was against Charles I's execution and in favour of a monarchy. Baxter had been chaplain to the Parliamentary Army and when it seemed that it would move decisively against the King he tried to stop it. But providential nosebleed came in the way and excused him from taking any further action:

174 *Ibid.*, part 3, p. 192.   175 *Ibid.*, part 2, p. 448.

I came to our Major Swallow's quarters at Sir John Cook's house...in a cold
and snowy season, and the cold, together with other things coincident, set
my nose on bleeding. When I had bled about a quart or two, I opened four
veins, but, it did not good. I used divers of other remedies for several days
to little purpose; at last I gave myself a purge which stopt it. This so much
weakened me and altered my complexion, that my acquaintance who came
to visit me scarce knew me. Coming after so long weakness, and frequent
loss of blood before, it made the physicians conclude me deplorate after it
was stopped; supposing I would never escape a dropsy.

And thus God unavoidably prevented all the effect of my purposes in my
last and chiefest opposition to the Army; and took me off the very time when
my attempt should have begun...But the determination of God against it
was most observable: For the very time I was bleeding the Council of War
sate at Nottingham, where (as I have credibly heard) they first began to open
their purposes and act their part...And as I perceived it was the will of God
to permit them to go on, so I afterward found this great affliction was a mercy
on my self; likely to have had small success in the attempt, but to have lost
my life among them in my fury. And thus I was finally separated from the
Army.[176]

Thus high politics, providence, physicians and a nosebleed all came to
be mixed together.

There is much else in Baxter's autobiography to interest the
historian: his view that God made use of sickness to acquire converts,
his observation that the 'Religiouser sort' were protected from the
plague until they boasted of it, and his use of a Gold Bullet for 'a case
like mine' would all provide evidence of the multifaceted face of illness
in this period.[177]

P.S. In 1766 and up until 1830 the stone from Baxter's bladder was
in the British Museum at Montague House.[178]

This essay is part of a larger study of health and illness in seventeenth
century England. I would like to thank Roy Porter and George Yule
for their advice and help.

---

[176] *Ibid.*, part 1, pp. 58–9.
[177] *Ibid.*, part 1, p. 90; part 3, p. 1; part 1, p. 81.
[178] G. F. Nuttall, *Richard Baxter*, p. 42.

4

In sickness and in health: A seventeenth century
family's experience

LUCINDA McCRAY BEIER

The sufferer's experience of illness, although a relatively recent subject
of historical research, is not difficult to investigate. In all ages, people
have been fascinated by illness. Thus, diaries and autobiographies are
replete with descriptions of the disorders suffered by both writers and
their family members, friends and acquaintances. Seventeenth century
England was rich in such documents. However, historians who have
used these source materials have generally been interested in such
subjects as politics, religion, economics and family relationships,
leaving the great wealth of medical information they contain virtually
untapped.

The extent to which diaries reflect general experience is frequently
and deservedly questioned. The seventeenth century diarists whose
writings have survived were members of the middle and upper classes.
Furthermore, diarists and autobiographers are unusual in any age,
feeling a need most people never feel to commit thoughts and
experience to paper. Their attitudes and behaviour can be taken as
representative neither of general experience nor of the experience of
others at their social level.

Nonetheless, such records of unique, personal experience are
invaluable to the historian, providing as they literally do, a voice from
the grave which can make the past live as no other source can. And
the fact that the experiences they describe may not be representative
is, perhaps, insignificant, since each individual's experience is to a large
extent unique, whether or not he or she describes it in a diary. One
cannot quantify pain, fear, grief, confidence or comfort.

However, one can place suffering in its historical and cultural
context. An individual's experience of ill-health reflects a great deal
about contemporary living conditions and the methods society provided

to deal with illness. The investigation of one family's health and illness is therefore a valuable exercise, providing an example of the ailments suffered and feared and the choices of preventive measures and therapy made. This paper will describe the medical history of the Josselin family as related by the male head of that family, Reverend Ralph Josselin.

Josselin was born on 25 January 1616 and died in August 1683. His diary, preceded by a brief autobiography and annual notes, covers the period between autumn 1643 and July 1683.[1]

Josselin's diary is well known largely through the efforts of Alan Macfarlane, whose transcription of the diary itself is the source upon which this paper depends. Macfarlane's analysis of the diary, entitled *The Family Life of Ralph Josselin, A Seventeenth-Century Clergyman: An Essay in Historical Anthropology*, mentions the Josselins' illnesses in several places. However, Macfarlane is chiefly interested in Ralph Josselin's religious orientation to misfortune. Neither his discussion, nor those of other historians familiar with the Josselin diary such as Keith Thomas and Lawrence Stone, provides an investigation of the disorders the Josselins suffered and what they did about medical problems.[2] The present study attempts this investigation.

From late 1640 until his death, Ralph Josselin was the vicar of Earls Colne in Essex. In the course of his life there, he became a prosperous landowner, one of the ten wealthiest men in his village.[3] He and his wife, born Jane Constable, produced ten live-born children, five of whom were living at the time of Josselin's death. Although the Josselins were 'middle class' by any definition of that vague term, they socialised with upper class members of the community, including two gentry families, the Harlakendens and the Honeywoods. They kept one maid-servant to help with the housework, hired nurses for short periods surrounding childbirth, and, in later years, employed a man-servant.

Josselin's diary is an unusually good source of information about medical matters. He was interested enough in medicine and disease to

[1] *The Diary of Ralph Josselin, 1616–1683*, ed. A. Macfarlane (London, 1976), hereafter cited as *Diary*.
[2] A. Macfarlane, *The Family Life of Ralph Josselin, a Seventeenth-Century Clergyman: An Essay in Historical Anthropology* (Cambridge, 1970); K. Thomas, *Religion and the Decline of Magic* (Harmondsworth, 1973), pp. 83 and 117; L. Stone, *The Family, Sex and Marriage in England 1500–1800* (London, 1977), pp. 113, 210.
[3] Macfarlane, *Family Life*, p. 78.

have read at least two works on the subject.[4] In addition to his intellectual interest, he appears to have been unusually preoccupied with his own ailments, describing symptoms of both major and minor disorders in loving detail, always fearing the worst. Fortunately for the historian, he was also concerned about the ailments of his wife, children, servants, friends, neighbours and relations. Thus, the diary provides medical information about quite a large number of people, something which is not equally true about otherwise rich diaries of the period. The length of the Josselin diary is also an advantage. Josselin was very conscientious about making his entries. Thus we have a nearly daily record of the family's illnesses, accidents and childbearing during a period of approximately forty years. In referring to these disorders, Josselin's own terminology will be used, rather than anachronistic diagnoses of what the seventeenth century sufferer 'really' had. The health incidents Josselin described will be discussed within three major categories: the discomforts and dangers relating to childbearing, children's accidents and illnesses, and adult disorders, including Ralph Josselin's own.

Pregnancy and childbirth

Jane and Ralph Josselin took seriously the Biblical injunction to be fruitful and multiply. They married relatively young; Jane was just under and Ralph just over 20 years old. In their first twenty-two years of marriage Jane had at least fifteen pregnancies, producing ten live-born children and at least five miscarriages. She probably breast-fed all of her children.[5]

Both of the Josselins were delighted when Jane became pregnant some ten months after their wedding. Ralph's diary entry for July 1641 attests to their 'great joy and comfort' concerning her condition. He was not as communicative about the news of her subsequent pregnancies, although he was never happy about her miscarriages, regardless of the

---

[4] L. Lessius, *Hygiasticon, or the Right Course of Preserving Life and Health unto Extreme Old Age* (London, 1634) and D. Sennertus, *Institutionum Medicinae* (many Latin and English editions). See *Diary*, pp. 154, 181.

[5] Definite mention is made of Jane feeding her first, second, third and sixth babies. The weaning of all the children is noted. Since Josselin would probably have remarked upon the employment of wet-nurses (which he did not), and since conception of the next child usually followed a few months after the weaning of the preceding one, I think it can safely be assumed that Jane fed all of her children herself.

size of their family. On one occasion in June 1656, when four of the seven children which by then had been born to the Josselins were living, he wrote 'This morning my wife thought she miscarried, lord a miscarrying womb is a sad affliction'.[6]

Jane's feelings when anticipating yet another pregnancy were not recorded, but they certainly must have been mixed. She did not carry her babies easily. She was sick and uncomfortable throughout her pregnancies and dreaded her confinements for months before the baby was due. She suffered from nausea, faintness, weakness and pain in her back, false labour, after-pains, and pain in her breasts, in addition to sometimes long, usually painful, and always frightening deliveries.[7] Indeed, Ralph recognised his wife's unusually uncomfortable pregnancies, writing on 30 October 1653, 'My poor wife very ill, she breedeth with difficulty', and later in the same pregnancy, on 11 December, 'My wife very ill, and weakly in her childing'.[8] Surely Jane must have echoed his prayer at the beginning of that pregnancy: 'the lord bear up her head under the difficulties of her condition'.[9]

Nonetheless, Jane apparently accepted her obstetrical fate with equanimity and interest. She had, for example, a considerable degree of success in predicting the sex of her unborn children very early in her pregnancies. Ralph reported her predictions for five babies. The first four were accurate. The fifth guess she muddled by changing her mind. On 15 May 1657 she reported being pregnant with a girl; by 31 May she was sure she carried a boy. Mary was born 14 January 1658. Jane should have stood by her first hunch. Nonetheless, Ralph was right when, in recording her prediction of the sex of their third child, he wrote 'She useth not to be mistaken'.[10]

Jane's fears about her deliveries were understandable and, probably, very common. The hazards of childbirth in seventeenth century England were immense. Complications which today would be regarded as minor — such as an unusual presentation of the baby, or the mother's inability to expel the child once it was in the birth canal — were almost invariably fatal to both mother and child. Even normal deliveries were fraught with danger. Haemorrhages could not be stopped. Infections could be neither prevented nor cured. Neither midwives nor surgeons could do much to help the labouring women who came into their hands. Both could be responsible for causing a great deal of pain —

[6] *Diary*, p. 371.
[7] E.g. *ibid*., pp. 37, 50, 102, 108, 313.   [8] *Ibid*., pp. 313, 315.
[9] *Ibid*., p. 313.   [10] *Ibid*., p. 89.

the midwives with well-meant but ill-judged interference intended to speed up labour and delivery; the surgeons with their clumsy instruments used, mainly, to extract dead babies when all other means of delivering them had failed.[11]

Jane Josselin's fears had been shared and written about in the 1620s by a woman with the oddly coincidental name of Elizabeth Joceline. Elizabeth was so convinced that childbirth would kill her that 'when she first felt herself quick with child (as then travelling with death itself) she secretly took order for the buying of a new winding sheet'.[12] She wrote her book in order to provide religious instruction for her unborn child, doomed to grow up without a mother.

Like Elizabeth, Jane Josselin took her fears to God. On one occasion she prayed with neighbour women when she felt the child quicken.[13] On another, she and Ralph prayed together the night before her labour began, because Jane 'was oppressed with fears that she would not do well on this child'.[14] Jane feared her next delivery with particularly good reason. In the preceding year, 1646, two neighbour women had died in childbed, one after an excruciating labour lasting for two weeks.[15] Even years of fortunate experience did not lay Jane's fears to rest. When in August 1661 she thought she might be pregnant, Ralph wrote 'I see she apprehends a breeding again with fear, the blessing of a fruitful womb is by weakness of nature her fear'.[16]

For Jane and her contemporaries, childbirth was a social occasion. Indeed, the Church required that at least two or three 'honest women' in addition to the midwife be present to witness the birth for legal reasons.[17] When Jane was delivered of her third child at nearly midnight in November 1645, the midwife and 'almost all' of the women Ralph had summoned were present.[18] When her fourth child was born the midwife was not there, and she was attended by 'only'

[11] I avoid mentioning the notorious forceps of the Chamberlen family, since very few women had the benefit of this family monopoly. Compare Adrian Wilson's essay in this volume.

[12] *The Mother's Legacy to her Unborn Child* (London, 1894; reprint of 1632 edition), from 'The Approbation'.

[13] *Diary*, pp. 402–3.

[14] *Ibid.*, p. 50. See also p. 162.

[15] *Ibid.*, pp. 54, 64.   [16] *Ibid.*, p. 482.

[17] See e.g. J. Hitchcock, 'A sixteenth century midwife's licence', *Bulletin of the History of Medicine*, xli (1967), 75–6. These women witnessed the mother's conversation during labour and could report on statements made as to the paternity of the child. They could also protect the mother and the midwife from accusations of infanticide in cases of stillbirth.

[18] *Diary*, p. 50.

five neighbour women.[19] In her turn, Jane attended the confinements of her neighbours and her daughters.[20] In one case, Ralph reported that she saved the life of a labouring neighbour woman.[21]

Jane Josselin was fortunate in that all of her labours and deliveries appear to have been quite straightforward. This is not to say that they were easy. Ralph reported Jane's experience of 'sharp pains' or unusually long difficult labours during the births of their third, eighth, ninth and tenth children.[22] In two cases she gave birth without a midwife present.[23] Even when a midwife was there, her presence was not always regarded as an unmixed blessing. After the birth of her eighth child Jane criticised the midwife for not having done 'her part'. Not only was the labour unusually 'sharp', the baby appeared to be dead at birth. Josselin attributed its revival to the intervention of God.[24]

After the birth was over, the mother's health was a subject of special concern for a few weeks at least. Jane was again fortunate. She suffered from sore breasts after the birth of her first child.[25] When her fourth child died ten days after birth, she became 'weak and faint with the turning of her milk'.[26] Otherwise, there was no apparent cause for concern. Jane left her bed within three weeks, and left the house between one and two months after her deliveries.

Because Ralph Josselin was so conscientious about recording the details of the symptoms and illnesses of the members of his family, it is possible to compare Jane's health during her childbearing years (1642–63) and during the last twenty years of her marriage (1663–83). During their first twenty-two years of married life, Ralph reported 131 instances of Jane being unwell. Of these, seventy-three cases were clearly related to pregnancy and childbirth. On the other fifty-eight occasions a plethora of symptoms were recorded ranging from toothache, to ague, to being 'sickly with toiling over' an ailing child.[27] Some of these miscellaneous disorders may actually have arisen from gynaecological or obstetrical problems. For instance, in July 1656 Jane suffered from symptoms which she first diagnosed as the 'falling down of the mother' (prolapse of the uterus) and later, with relief, as piles.[28] This episode occurred a month after a miscarriage.[29]

Once Jane's reproductive years were over, she apparently became

[19] *Ibid.*, p. 111.
[20] E.g. *ibid.*, pp. 215, 570, 604, 615.
[21] *Ibid.*, p. 215.
[22] *Ibid.*, pp. 50, 415, 465, 502.
[23] *Ibid.*, pp. 111, 165.
[24] *Ibid.*, p. 415.
[25] *Ibid.*, p. 12.
[26] *Ibid.*, p. 115.
[27] E.g. *ibid.*, pp. 64, 189, 354, 429.
[28] *Ibid.*, pp. 374, 376.
[29] *Ibid.*, p. 371.

much healthier. In the last twenty years of their marriage, Ralph reported that Jane was unwell only seventeen times. This significant improvement might be explained in a number of ways. It is possible that for a short period of time Ralph lost interest in recording his family's symptoms. Certainly the years between 1665 and 1672 are remarkably poor in their references to illness. However, it is more likely that the Josselins were fairly healthy during those years. It is also possible that after November 1672, when Ralph was first troubled with the leg ailment which probably killed him, he ceased to mention any but the most dramatic illnesses of family members, concentrating, as the elderly and sick may be excused for doing, on his own problems.[30] However, this is also unlikely, for he did mention a cold Jane had in November 1680.[31] Indeed, Jane's health was of great concern to Ralph for purely selfish reasons. He frequently echoed the prayer he made when she was ill with a pregnancy in 1648: 'oh continue her a comfort to me and mine'.[32] Certainly the prospect of being left alone to care for a large house and family would have been grim indeed. Thus it seems that Jane's health did improve considerably once she finished childbearing. Certainly she outlived her husband and was apparently healthy at the time of his death.

Children's illnesses and accidents

In seventeenth century England, as in most developing societies, childhood was an especially dangerous period of life. The London Bills of Mortality included special categories for infants and 'chrisom' children, infancy seeming to be in itself a sufficient explanation of the cause of death.[33] Certain illnesses, such as ailments associated with teething and rickets, were peculiar to the first years of life. Other ailments, including the scab and worms, although they affected adults as well, were most common and dangerous in children.

Of the five Josselin children who died before their father, three were under the age of 8. One baby, the first Ralph, died at 10 days old. The second Ralph died at 13 months. Mary, the first-born, died aged 8 years and 1 month. Each of the three died under circumstances which would have been tragically familiar to Ralph Josselin's contemporaries.

The first baby Ralph died 'full of phlegm' with 'red mattery stuff' issuing from his mouth. No diagnosis of his illness was made. He was

---

[30] *Ibid.*, p. 566.   [31] *Ibid.*, p. 630.   [32] *Ibid.*, pp. 145, 150.
[33] John Graunt, 'Natural and political observations made upon the Bills of Mortality' (1662), in *The Earliest Classics* (Westmead, Hants., 1976).

very ill from the moment of his birth, and his parents did not expect him to live.[34] Although the second Ralph lived longer, his short life was tormented by continual illnesses, ranging from suspected rickets through skin and eye disorders to a condition his father described as being livergrown.[35] His death surprised no one. Mary, who died of worms, was exceptional, since she had had a relatively healthy childhood, and was ill for only a month before her death.[36]

Of course, childhood illnesses and accidents were not always fatal. Many of the Josselin children were ill when they were cutting teeth.[37] They suffered from numerous skin ailments, ranging from spots and pimples, to shingles, rashes on their scalps, the itch, and boils.[38] They were also subject to worms. The first Mary had worms when she was nearly 3 and John was 'full of worms' at age 4.[39] Ralph senior and several of the children had the rheum in the eyes and other eye ailments.[40] The second Ralph and Jane were supposed to have had rickets, which, in Jane's case, may have been associated with weaning.[41]

The children also suffered from ailments which today are commonly viewed as childhood diseases. In July 1649 one of Ralph's two sons (probably 5-year-old Thomas) developed 'great swellings' under both his ears – possibly mumps.[42] In March 1655/6 John, Jane and Ann developed 'colds nigh chincolds', Josselin describing their 'fierce and troublesome cough that is too hard for means that we can use'.[43] This may have been whooping cough. And two of the Josselin children and a maid had the measles.[44]

Although Josselin and his wife apparently escaped the ravages of smallpox, their children were not so fortunate. Thomas, John, Ann and Elizabeth each caught the disease as teenagers, while living in London.[45] Only 15-year-old Thomas, who contracted smallpox only two weeks after being sent to London as an apprentice, returned home to be nursed. The others remained in London, sending word of their condition home to their anxious parents. Despite the seriousness of the disease and the fear it inspired, these adolescents survived it without any permanent handicap worthy of remark.

Like their father, the Josselin children suffered from frequent colds and occasional bouts of ague. Colds were very common. On a number

[34] *Diary*, p. 114.
[35] *Ibid.*, pp. 184–205.
[36] *Ibid.*, pp. 198–203.
[37] E.g. *ibid.*, pp. 26, 80, 184, 272.
[38] *Ibid.*, pp. 48, 152, 274, 508.
[39] *Ibid.*, pp. 37, 338.
[40] E.g. *ibid.*, pp. 29, 64, 187, 190.
[41] *Ibid.*, pp. 97, 186.
[42] *Ibid.*, p. 172.
[43] *Ibid.*, p. 364.
[44] *Ibid.*, pp. 283, 428.
[45] *Ibid.*, pp. 447, 545, 546, 615.

of occasions the whole family suffered together.[46] Colds were usually regarded as unpleasant, but inevitable; worthy of comment, but not of fear. However, in children they were occasionally regarded as dangerous. When 3-year-old Mary suffered from a 'great cold' during which she 'strained and spit much blood', her parents sought help for her from a local gentlewoman, Lady Honeywood. Ralph was worried about her to the extent that he prayed that 'the lord will preserve her'.[47] Colds were even more dangerous to infants. When 10-month-old Thomas developed a cold in the night which seemed 'ready even to stop him up', Jane Josselin was so frightened 'that she was even at death's door'.[48]

Agues were generally regarded as more severe than colds. The intermitting hot and cold fits were very unpleasant and the disease was debilitating, often lasting for months. When she was only about 8 months old, Elizabeth picked up an ague which lasted from early February until mid-April.[49] Nonetheless, Ralph Josselin apparently feared the consequences of an ague only once, and that, perhaps understandably, was when he suffered from a bad case of it himself in February 1648.[50]

Living conditions gave rise to accidents involving the Josselins and their friends and neighbours. Like many another Puritan, Josselin regarded his family's brushes with disaster as marks of God's providence. Thus he wrote on 7 October 1644, 'I found god had graciously kept my daughter Mary who was struck with a Horse her apron rent off with his nails and her handkerchief rent and yet she had no hurt'.[51] Mary was 2 at the time. While adults also had accidents, children were most at risk because they were only beginning to learn how to deal with their environment.

Fire was particularly hazardous. The Josselin house had six hearths and presumably burned open fires in each of them. The family used candles for light. In all, the Josselin children either fell into fires or set their clothing alight six times without receiving any serious hurt.[52]

Then as now, children frequently fell and hurt themselves. The school stairs must have been particularly dangerous, since both Thomas and John fell down them, each without lasting damage.[53] In November

---

[46] E.g. *ibid.*, pp. 28, 337.

[47] *Ibid.*, pp. 40–1.

[48] *Ibid.*, p. 27.

[49] *Ibid.*, pp. 475–8.

[50] *Ibid.*, pp. 111–13.

[51] *Ibid.*, p. 24.

[52] *Ibid.*, pp. 113, 156, 433, 473, 545, 565.

[53] *Ibid.*, pp. 210, 330.

1653 2-year-old John broke a bone in his feet by falling at the street threshold.[54]

In addition, the children were injured by the adults looking after them. When the second Mary was 2 her arm was pulled out of joint 'by a snatch of our maid Alice'.[55] The Josselin children also endangered each other. In February 1648 2-year-old Jane 'dagged a pair of scissors in Thom: eyebrow', fortunately not much injuring him.[56] And in 1654 Jane, then nearly 9, dropped 2-month-old Ann into a bowl of milk. The baby was unhurt, but Jane swooned.[57] Equally, the children saved each other from harm. In December 1644 2-year-old Mary held 1-year-old Thomas out of the fire, crying until their father came to help. In order to survive, the children had to learn young the harsh rules of their environment.

Indeed, in view of the dangers which surrounded them, the Josselin children were remarkably fortunate in escaping both accidental injury and death from epidemic diseases. This good fortune certainly supported Ralph Josselin's belief in the special providence of God toward him and his.

Adult disorders

Although Ralph Josselin conscientiously reported the illnesses of his family, friends and neighbours, he was most interested in his own ailments. He was not a hypochondriac; his illnesses cannot be regarded as imaginary. However, he was unusually preoccupied with his symptoms, major and minor – so much so that his wife lost patience with him at one point. In January 1672 Josselin began to suffer from the pain, swelling and ulceration in his left leg which remained with him until his death over eleven years later. He wrote at that time, 'I am sensible I bear my infirmities about me, but my wife taxes me for great impatience. When I fear there is a provoking carelessness in her etc. and impatience too much, that bears nothing but expects I must bear all'.[58] The reader of the diary cannot help but sympathise with both Ralph and Jane. Certainly, Ralph spent most of his life handicapped by minor, annoying ailments. However, one imagines that his exhaustive (and exhausting) descriptions of his sensations found their way into breakfast-table conversation as well as into the pages of the diary.

Ralph noted the state of his health in both daily entries and weekly

[54] *Ibid.*, p. 314.   [55] *Ibid.*, p. 468.

[56] *Ibid.*, p. 113.   [57] *Ibid.*, p. 330.   [58] *Ibid.*, p. 566.

summaries, written on Sundays. In addition, he frequently made marginal notes which, as often as not, referred to an acute or chronic disorder.[59] Like his contemporaries, he was involved in determining the diagnoses and prognoses of his own illnesses, and helped decide the therapeutic 'means' to be used.

Josselin suffered from frequent long-lasting colds which he described in great detail. He mentioned colds in the throat, poses (the term he used to refer to head colds), rheumes, 'stuffing' and 'wheezing' (mainly at night), chest colds, 'stopping' in the chest, and aguish colds.[60] Out of some 317 mentions of his own illnesses, 114 referred to colds. He also gave full descriptions of the onset and various stages of his colds. For instance, he wrote in June 1646, 'I was now in taking of cold sensible of it most in my throat, a roughness and kind of soreness at the upper part next my mouth and especially on the left side'.[61] During another cold in December 1646, he wrote 'my cold begun to thicken, and to stuff and wheeze exceedingly'.[62] His conjectures about why he caught cold sound much like those we hear today. For instance, he believed came down with a pose and chest cold in October 1677 as a result of wearing thin stockings.[63]

Although Josselin very occasionally took medicine for his colds, his attitude towards them was far more fatalistic than towards his other ailments.[64] For one thing, despite the discomfort they caused him, Josselin's colds never appeared to him to be very serious illnesses, unlike other ailments such as severe agues or the chronic leg problem which tormented his final years. For another thing, Josselin's colds dragged on so long that to have allowed himself to take up a sick role during them would have been financially and professionally disastrous. In one case, a cold apparently lasted from 13 August 1646 until at least 3 January 1647! In addition, his colds even served as rather gratifying tests of faith and fortitude. For instance, he wrote in September 1647, 'This week I was somewhat troubled with a pose, but though rheumes and pose haunt me I praise god, they do not cast me down'.[65]

Josselin was prey to a host of minor symptoms which annoyed more than worried him. During his early years at Earls Colne he frequently mentioned rheumes in his eyes.[66] He also developed a sore tongue,

---

[59] Other marginal notes refer to such topics as the weather, Josselin's income, religious events, etc.

[60] E.g. *ibid.*, pp. 49, 103, 134, 200, 271.   [61] *Ibid.*, p. 63.

[62] *Ibid.*, p. 79.   [63] *Ibid.*, p. 603.

[64] He took hyssop syrup made by his wife for a cold: *Diary*, p. 218.

[65] *Ibid.*, p. 102.   [66] E.g. *ibid.*, pp. 29, 42, 56, 94.

pain in his chest which he concluded was wind, and occasional soreness in his bones.[67] At one point he developed swellings in both sides of his groin which mercifully abated within a week.[68] Some of the sensations he experienced were downright mysterious – for example, the 'coldness or moistness in the crown of' his head which he felt on 14 January 1649.[69] In addition to these problems, Josselin was a bad traveller. Frequently even short journeys left him feeling ill. Sometimes he experienced nausea and vomiting; sometimes he felt aguish and sore.[70] In one case, while returning from London he was overcome with wind and had to be treated in the home of an acquaintance.[71]

Like their contemporaries, Josselin and his family suffered from the dietary and sanitary conditions of their time. Indeed, it is remarkable that they were so infrequently 'ill in their stomachs'.[72] However, the humoral theory dominant in the period, which regarded evacuation as beneficial, helped them to bear their discomforts. For instance, when Ralph suffered from diarrhoea in April 1646, he 'conceived it a mercy'.[73] Again, in December 1648 he wrote 'After above 30 hours illness in my stomach I fell into a great looseness which I conceive did me much good'.[74] When 5-year-old Ann had an each-day ague in August 1659, the fact that she vomited and sweat gave her parents hope.[75]

Almost every member of the Josselin family had ague at one time or another. These attacks ranged from single fits to life-threatening illnesses such as the attack Ralph had in February 1648. During this illness he wrote that his friends were very worried about him – despite the fact that his wife gave birth to a son who died during Ralph's convalescence. At one point a week after his fits had begun, Josselin wrote a will.[76] His illness actually ended within fourteen days of its onset, but it frightened him considerably. Some attacks lasted a good deal longer than this. Jane senior developed a quartan ague in October 1668 which lasted until mid-March of the following year and was so serious that her adult daughter Jane was summoned home to look after her.[77]

In addition to the ailments mentioned above, Josselin suffered from two long-term illnesses worthy of mention. The first was an

---

[67] E.g. *ibid.*, pp. 72, 77, 103.
[68] *Ibid.*, p. 86.
[69] *Ibid.*, p. 152.
[70] E.g. *ibid.*, pp. 70, 81.
[71] *Ibid.*, p. 290.
[72] *Ibid.*, p. 27.
[73] *Ibid.*, p. 58.
[74] *Ibid.*, p. 149.
[75] *Ibid.*, p. 450.
[76] *Ibid.*, pp. 111–13.
[77] *Ibid.*, pp. 544–6.

inflammation of his navel which troubled him between early September 1648 and mid-April 1652.[78] This was a discouraging illness because his navel would appear to heal, then would become sore and moist all over again, despite the various treatments Ralph tried on it. Although never incapacitated by the discomfort his navel caused him, he was worried about it. In March 1649 he wrote that he had 'heard of one that after two years illness was killed with a rawness in his navel, but god shall heal me of this infirmity'.[79] However, as time passed he grew less concerned, writing in August 1651, 'my navel was a little but not much ill, it hath not been dressed near a year'.[80]

The second long-term illness Josselin suffered from was the swelling and ulceration of his left leg, variously diagnosed as scurvy and dropsy. This ailment incapacitated and probably eventually killed him. The first hint of a problem came in November 1672, when Ralph had a 'sciatica pain' in his hip.[81] This passed by the end of the following month, when he reported being able 'to take many steps without stick or stay'.[82] However, by 27 February 1673 'some red spots appeared on my lame thigh, which they conceived the scurvy'.[83] From that time on, the diary is a catalogue of pain, swelling, different treatments applied, fears and disappointed hopes. As the old sores healed, the swelling broke open in new places. By early 1683, after ten years of misery, Josselin was a very ill man indeed. His leg was swollen and painful. His belly also swelled. He was very short of breath. He developed a 'great and dangerous cough' and double vision.[84] Despite his infirmities, he continued to preach.[85] However, he must have feared that death was near, for he wrote on 1 June, 'I saw my countenance much changed...I did no[t think] I gathered strength nor lost any, but in the use of means continued in the same way. However I stay [myself] on my good god, that this sickness doth not issue in death, but in a trial to do me much good'.[86] This forlorn hope was never realised. Josselin died two months later, at the age of 67.

Josselin described in some detail his own last illness and those of his children who died in childhood. It is interesting that he does not give descriptions of the deaths of two adult children, Thomas and Ann, in the summer of 1673. Alan Macfarlane suggests that Thomas may have died of consumption.[87] However, Josselin himself wrote nothing to

78 *Ibid.*, pp. 141–277.
79 *Ibid.*, p. 159.
80 *Ibid.*, p. 253.
81 *Ibid.*, p. 566.
82 *Ibid.*
83 *Ibid.*
84 *Ibid.*, p. 642.
85 *Ibid.*, p. 643.
86 *Ibid.*, p. 644.
87 Macfarlane, *Family Life*, p. 119.

support this diagnosis, reporting only that 29-year-old Thomas had come home ill on 22 March 1673, and that he died on 15 June, having suffered very little.[88] We do not know when Ann returned to Earls Colne from London, but Josselin wrote that she was ill on 17 June.[89] By 20 July she was 'ill and deaf and thereby uncheerful'.[90] She died 31 July, aged 19.

As we have said, Ralph Josselin was concerned about the health of his family members, which included his servants. Since the smooth operations of his domestic life depended upon the labour of at least one maid-servant, the health of his servants was important to him.[91] Thus he reported the ill-health of servants in his diary, although he never went into much detail about their ailments.[92] For instance, when his maid Joan went home to her mother, 'very sick, urina nigra', he prayed 'God restore her to her health'.[93] The ill-health of a servant could certainly inconvenience the household. When Josselin's maid was very ill in March 1650, his wife was 'toild above measure'.[94] A servant's illness could also endanger the family, as in January 1649, when Ralph feared that his maid had smallpox.[95] In turn, the family's ailments could endanger the servant, as in August 1658, when the Josselins' maid caught the measles from 4-year-old Ann, and had to return home.[96]

Josselin was less forthcoming about the illnesses of neighbours and friends. Although it was his duty as a clergyman to visit the sick, he did not report doing so very often. Sometimes he was summoned to sick-beds, as in the case of 'a sick man one Guy Penhache who was much troubled in mind upon his life: he had strong temptations from Satan'.[97] In other cases, the sick person was his friend, as when in June 1646 he visited Mr Thomas Harlakenden who was suddenly ill.[98] Jane Josselin was more involved with sick friends and neighbours, often taking the role of nurse in their illnesses and confinements.[99]

Although Ralph Josselin was not as active in visiting the sick as his sociable contemporary, Samuel Pepys, he was interested in the ills

[88] *Ibid.*, p. 567.
[89] *Ibid.*   [90] *Ibid.*
[91] By the end of his life he was also employing a man-servant: *Diary*, p. 629.
[92] E.g. *ibid.*, pp. 39, 47, 118, 429, 539, 629.
[93] *Ibid.*, p. 39.   [94] *Ibid.*, p. 192.
[95] *Ibid.*, p. 154.   [96] *Ibid.*, p. 429.
[97] *Ibid.*, p. 18.   [98] *Ibid.*, p. 62.
[99] E.g. *ibid.*, pp. 91, 131, 215, 278.

which beset others. He was particularly fascinated by the deaths of other ministers. On 1 September 1644 he reported that 'Mr Pilgrim Minister of Wormingford fell down dead in his pulpit'.[100] He heard of the deaths of two ministers on 28 August 1646, and on 18 June 1657 he 'heard of Mr Whiting's death minister of Lexden, who putting his finger into a man's mouth whose throat was ill with a squinsey, and non compos mentis, he bit it vehemently on which it gangrened, and killed him about eight days after'.[101]

Perhaps similar to his interest in the calamities befalling other ministers was his preoccupation with the providence of God in afflicting those who broke heavenly rules. His satisfaction is apparent in his story of

One John Chrismas a miller in our town whose parents were godly and one in a way of doing well, but his heart leading him to tipple and game, and his wife being sharp to him, he got what he could together, and left her, his brother brought him home, but about a week after he was sick of the pox and died, a warning not to go out of god's way[102]

Josselin was even more smug in the following report:

I observe a providence. A man I was hiring one Peakes son, declined me to go to a Quaker I know not his motives, there he fell sick of the small pox, and his mother keep[ing] him came home and died, the lord watch over me and mine for good.[103]

In addition to their physical ills, Josselin and his circle were prey to a host of mental disorders. Some were essentially spiritual in nature. Josselin himself apparently suffered from a severe depression during the spring and summer of 1652, writing frequently of a deadness of heart which he felt powerless to combat.[104] However, in Josselin's world the distinction between mental and physical ills was cloudy at best. His friend Mr R. H. (probably Richard Harlakenden) had a spiritual crisis which Josselin felt should be treated with physical means. He wrote:

Mr R. H. in great agony of heart sent down for me, weeping, apprehending himself lost for ever. I feared his head most. Got a physician who let him blood, advised him to alter his course of diet [,] he promised it. I lay with him that night. God gave him rest, and I hope in time perfect health.[105]

---

[100] *Ibid.*, p. 18.
[102] *Ibid.*, pp. 393–4.
[104] E.g. *ibid.*, pp. 278, 280, 281, 282.

[101] *Ibid.*, p. 402.
[103] *Ibid.*, pp. 459–60.
[105] *Ibid.*, p. 476.

Another Harlakenden, William, died in 1675, after suffering from madness for a time. His insanity was actually cured by a physical complaint. Josselin wrote:

An illness in his feet from his running abroad brought the madness out of his head, but he recovered no great use of his reason spiritual or natural, only on discourse, he savoured of both.[106]

Then as now, unhealthy mental states brought on physical illness. When Josselin's daughter Jane had a relapse of ague, her mother felt the illness was due to 'fear and grief to see her mother so tormented as she was with a felon on her finger'.[107] And when Jane senior became faint and ill two months after the death of her daughter Mary, Ralph felt her disorder was caused by grief.[108]

Like their children, seventeenth century adults were victims of accidents. The Josselins were fortunate in this respect. Although Ralph reported quite a few 'near misses', only a few of the accidents he and Jane were involved in resulted in injury. Thus, on 27 October 1649, 'I was cutting wood my axe slipt and cut the leather at the toe of my shoe almost through without any hurt'.[109] Sometimes they did hurt themselves, as when Ralph hurt his eye 'very dangerously' and when Jane fell and bruised her eye.[110] However, their neighbours fared much worse. Josselin reported a case where

One Robert Davy of my town a butcher cutting out of meat, his son in law Kendall stood behind him, was strucken with the cleaver upon the forehead dangerously, beat out his eye etc...[111]

Despite this example, the overall impression given by the Josselin diary is that people had less to fear from accidents in seventeenth century rural England than they do in our gadget-ridden age, regardless of our supposed safety-consciousness. A far greater threat posed by the environment was disease – both infectious and non-infectious. The above discussion has concentrated on the ills people suffered from. The next section will describe what Josselin and his social circle did about their ailments.

Means and healers

Although Ralph Josselin's diary is replete with details about symptoms (particularly Ralph's own), it is much less informative about the

106 *Ibid.*, p. 583.   107 *Ibid.*, p. 297.
108 *Ibid.*, p. 212.   109 *Ibid.*, p. 183.
110 *Ibid.*, pp. 429, 579.   111 *Ibid.*, p. 33.

treatments used and healers consulted in times of illness. Indeed, considering the seventeenth century fondness for remedies (a predilection we share with the people of that time), the diary is tantalising in what it does not say. In all, Josselin reported approximately 762 cases of illness or injury happening to himself, his family members, friends, acquaintances and neighbours. In only seventy-nine cases did he mention the treatments applied. And in only twenty-one cases did he even suggest consultation of a healer. (By this term I mean someone whose part- or full-time occupation was to treat patients. The term includes physicians, surgeons, apothecaries, midwives and bonesetters. It does not include family members and friends.) What do these numbers mean? It is possible, but unlikely, that most symptoms went untreated. It is more likely that Josselin simply did not always mention the treatments applied. Concerning the consultation of healers, the diary is probably a bit more reliable. Such consultations, except when they involved the midwife or the local bonesetter, required either a journey or formal correspondence. In either case it would have been uncharacteristic of Josselin to fail to note an incident which cost him either effort or money or both.

Like many of his contemporaries, Josselin was fairly knowledgeable about medical matters. In 1649 he read two medical works: Leonard Lessius' *Hygiasticon, or the Right Course of Preserving Life and Health unto Extreme Old Age* (1634) and Daniel Sennertus' *Institutionum Medicinae* (many Latin and English editions).[112] He routinely examined his own urine during times of illness, interpreting its characteristics in order to determine the prognosis of the disease. For instance, when recovering from a severe ague attack, he wrote 'my water brake very ragged and a little red sediment [,] it argued as I conceive a remainder of ill humours in me and that nature was concocting and expelling them'.[113] His comment upon the maid Joan's 'urina nigra' mentioned above suggests that he may have examined the urine of other members of his household as well.[114] Josselin also commented upon other bodily excretions. As already indicated, he subscribed to the general humoral view of the body and its processes. Thus when he took two ounces of syrup of roses for ague, he wrote that it 'wrought very kindly with me, gave me 9 stools brought away much choler'.[115]

Together with his wife, Ralph Josselin diagnosed the ailments of his children. They decided that their baby daughter Jane had rickets, that

[112] *Ibid.*, pp. 154, 181.
[113] *Ibid.*, p. 117.
[114] *Ibid.*, p. 39.
[115] *Ibid.*, p. 112.

the second Ralph was livergrown, and that 6-year-old Jane had the 'spleen'.[116] When Jane and Thomas were shrieking in their sleep in October 1650, Ralph felt they probably had worms.[117] Having diagnosed a disease, Ralph and Jane either treated it themselves or sought out treatment they felt would be appropriate, feeling free to reject both new diagnoses and suggested treatments. Thus, when Jane took 7-month-old Ralph to Lady Honeywood's to consult with her about his problems, the diary reported the interview as follows:

my Lady fears he is in a consumption, but indeed he is troubled with the rickets, my Lady adviseth an issue to which my wife hath no mind god in mercy bless other means that are used.[118]

Indeed, the main authority on medical matters in the Josselin household was not Ralph but Jane. Ralph did not indicate whether or not she had read medical works, but he mentioned her role as nurse and medical consultant during many illnesses of family members, friends and neighbours. Jane made at least two of the medicines she used − a distillation of roses and hyssop syrup.[119] She dosed members of her family, acted as a surgeon when their burns, cuts and ulcers needed dressing, and helped out during her neighbours' and daughters' confinements.[120] She nursed her husband and children when they were ill, sometimes becoming ill herself in the process.[121] Indeed, nursing was so important a part of her expected role that Ralph was quite annoyed when she withheld this service, as was the case on 16 November 1676 when 'my wife on some discontent which I know not would not assist me in dressing my poor leg'.[122]

Jane was also summoned to the sick-beds of friends and neighbours. When her dear friend Mary Church hurt her leg in April 1647, Jane applied leeches to it.[123] When Lady Honeywood's child was ill in August 1648, Jane went to Markshall (the Honeywood's home) to help out.[124] Jane also treated herself, dosing herself with 'pills' for wind and tobacco for toothache on one occasion.[125]

The Josselins relied mainly on herbal remedies and 'simples', rather than the compound medicines favoured by apothecaries and physicians. Ralph used violet cake for an aguish feeling in March 1645, syrup of roses for ague in February 1648, and a mixture of plantain water and

[116] *Ibid.*, pp. 94, 200, 281.
[117] *Ibid.*, p. 219.
[118] *Ibid.*, p. 186.
[119] *Ibid.*, pp. 61, 218.
[120] E.g. *ibid.*, pp. 218, 412, 570, 584, 604.
[121] E.g. *ibid.*, pp. 189, 508.
[122] *Ibid.*, p. 595.
[123] *Ibid.*, p. 91.
[124] *Ibid.*, p. 131.
[125] *Ibid.*, p. 64.

loose sugar as a dressing for his sore navel in November 1648.[126] On one occasion he apparently employed a kind of sympathetic magic, applying honey to a bee-sting.[127]

Very occasionally, more complex remedies were tried. In April 1649 Ralph treated a cold both with mythridate, which he must have purchased, and with a 'Stybium vomit prepared at Cogshall' presumably by an apothecary.[128] During his final illness he took Daffy's Elixir, Talbor's Pills and a medicine prescribed by the London physician Dr Cox, with whom Josselin corresponded.[129] In an attempt to cure his leg, Josselin also made a trip to Tunbridge Wells, drinking the waters there between 13 July and 1 August 1675.[130] However, even during those last ten years of torment, Ralph relied mainly on simple herbal remedies, both as dressings and as internal medicines. He poulticed his leg with red rose leaves and milk, with bread, with burdock leaves, elote leaves and green tobacco leaves.[131] He ate nutmeg, took hartshorn drops and drank 'Mrs Spicer's ale'.[132]

A question which is often asked is 'Did these remedies work?' Certainly modern herbalists and homeopaths rely on substances which would have been familiar to the Josselins. However, the purpose of this study is not to determine by controlled experiments whether herbal or 'old-fashioned' remedies actually ameliorate symptoms like those the Josselins suffered from, but to explore the Josselins' experiences as related in Ralph's diary. The question of whether or not a medicine 'worked' was understood differently by Ralph Josselin than it would be by a modern patient. The modern patient wants to know whether a medicine will produce a cure, or at least make him or her feel better. Josselin and his contemporaries expected a medicine to show its strength by producing an immediate result – usually in the form of multiple stools or vomits. Thus a remedy could 'work' without curing the patient. This was the case when Mary Josselin, five days before her death, was given a clyster (enema) which 'wrought very well'.[133] Indeed, medicine was expected to make the patient feel sick. When two of Josselin's children, Thomas and Jane, were given physic in June 1650 (presumably in a state of health), they 'were sick even to death,

[126] *Ibid.*, pp. 36, 112, 147–8.
[127] *Ibid.*, p. 19.
[128] Stibium is black antimony, used as an emetic or poison: *Oxford English Dictionary*.
[129] *Ibid.*, pp. 584, 642, 643.
[130] *Ibid.*, p. 585.   [131] *Ibid.*, pp. 584, 591, 628, 629, 630.
[132] *Ibid.*, pp. 615, 644.   [133] *Ibid.*, p. 202.

so that our hearts trembled, fearing the issue, but the lord in mercy to us quickly blew it over, and they revived and are now well'.[134]

Of course, the Josselins hoped that medicine taken during times of illness would help to produce a cure. In May 1683, when Ralph was desperate for relief from his multiple ailments, he wrote to Dr Cox for prescriptions. He reported 'Cox sent me his old receipts: the Apothecary made [me] pay dear'.[135] Several days later he wrote 'I took my physick from Dr Cox...my wife apprehends it doth me no good, but I cannot be fully of that mind'.[136] Some remedies were more definite in their effects. Jane senior cured her wind and toothache with the pills and tobacco she took.[137] And when Ralph returned from travelling, aguish and sore, Jane's 'careful use of means', together with her tenderness and God's goodness, cured him.[138]

In most cases Ralph and Jane relied upon their own medical knowledge and skill to treat their own ailments and those of their children. However, they occasionally asked for the help of other people: friends, nurses, part-time healers and full-time medical 'professionals'. Lady Honeywood apparently acted as an informal general practitioner, advising the Josselins when their children were ill, and even looking after Ralph senior for over a month when his left leg first began to trouble him. During this time, Ralph wrote, she 'was my nurse and physician and I hope for much good'.[139] The Josselins also asked the Harlakendens at the priory for medical help, getting from them a medicine for worms during Mary's final illness.[140] In addition, neighbours other than the local gentry helped the Josselins during their illnesses. When Ralph suffered from a particularly severe ague fit on 13 February 1648, '2 hours before day...some neighbours came in'.[141] And when Jane became faint and ill with grief after Mary's death, she and Ralph 'sent for neighbours'.[142]

In addition to this informal help, the Josselins consulted two local women who acted as bonesetters. When John 'had a fall about the street threshold which made him limp', the 'shut-bone in his instep' was set by 'Spooner's wife'.[143] And when the second Mary's arm was dislocated by the maid, 'Mrs Withers came and set it'.[144]

When Jane Josselin gave birth she was routinely attended by the midwife and a number of neighbour women. In at least one case a

[134] *Ibid.*, p. 207.   [135] *Ibid.*, p. 643.   [136] *Ibid.*
[137] *Ibid.*, p. 64.   [138] *Ibid.*, p. 81.   [139] *Ibid.*, p. 566.
[140] *Ibid.*, p. 201.   [141] *Ibid.*, p. 111.   [142] *Ibid.*, p. 212.
[143] *Ibid.*, p. 314.   [144] *Ibid.*, p. 468.

nurse was present. In three recorded cases the Josselins hired a nurse to help out for the first few weeks after a baby was born, when Jane was still in bed. The nurse stayed for about a month after their third child was born, and stayed for five days after the death of the first Ralph.[145] She stayed only two weeks after the birth of their eighth child, but this was because she had promised her services to another woman.[146] The nurse was apparently summoned about a week before the child was expected. For instance, although in the last mentioned case the nurse left when the baby was two weeks old, Josselin indicated that she left on the twentieth day of her stay.[147]

The Josselins almost never consulted physicians and surgeons. Despite the fact that five Josselin children died between February 1648 and July 1673, only once was a physician called to a child's death-bed. Oddly enough, this one occasion was four days before the death of the first Ralph, then only six days old.[148] One wonders whether the physician also saw Ralph senior, then ill of ague.

Otherwise, the only member of the Josselin family to consult physicians, surgeons and apothecaries was, as far as we know, Ralph senior. This he did on only one recorded occasion in his early life, during a quotidian ague.[149] He did not see a physician thereafter until 1675, when he had already suffered with his swollen and ulcerated left leg for two years. During his long final illness, Josselin consulted the physicians Dr Talbor and Dr Cox. He apparently visited Dr Talbor, while he merely corresponded with Dr Cox. He also consulted two surgeons – the first unnamed, the second a Mrs Doughtie.[150] He used the services of an apothecary to make up Dr Cox's prescriptions.[151]

It would be incorrect to suggest that Josselin 'did not believe in' physicians. In a case already cited, the instance when Mr R. H. suffered an emotional crisis, Josselin sent for a physician himself.[152] Indeed, Josselin had at least one physician as a personal friend. Dr and Mrs Colier and their daughter arrived from London on 1 August and stayed with the Josselins until 19 August 1664. During their visit, John Josselin developed a violent fever. Josselin wrote 'it was a great mercy Dr Colier was with us'.[153] Nonetheless, it seems obvious that the Josselins only rarely felt that the services of a physician were necessary, even in the most extreme cases. Since Ralph never wrote about his feelings

[145] *Ibid.*, pp. 51, 116.   [146] *Ibid.*, p. 418.   [147] *Ibid.*
[148] *Ibid.*, p. 112.   [149] *Ibid.*, p. 14.
[150] *Ibid.*, pp. 594, 595, 614.   [151] *Ibid.*, p. 643.
[152] *Ibid.*, p. 476.   [153] *Ibid.*, pp. 510–11.

regarding physicians, one can only speculate about the reasons for his behaviour. The most likely explanation is that, for the Josselins, neither healers nor remedies were of ultimate importance in determining the outcome of an illness. Whatever happened was God's will.

Josselin rarely mentioned health or illness without mentioning God. In this he was a man of his time. The seventeenth century was rich in works of what might be called 'moral medicine' which explained all illness and disaster as God's punishment for sin or his way of testing the faithful. It might be tempting to argue that Josselin, the good vicar, was merely paying pious lip-service to convention. After all, he did resort to physical remedies as well as prayer. However, the diary leaves no doubt that Josselin's faith was real, and, from his point of view, rewarded. For instance, when Josselin had ague in 1643, his physician told him he would have one more harsh fit, 'but on Friday night seeking god for my health that if it pleased him I might go on in my calling, I was strangely persuaded I should have no more fits neither had I'.[154] As this example demonstrates, although Josselin occasionally consulted healers and used medicines, hoping that these would help, he placed far more confidence in the Divine Physician.

Josselin truly felt that the best remedy was prayer and the best preventive medicine was a sinless life. As Alan Macfarlane points out, Josselin held himself responsible for both his own ailments and those of his children.[155] This belief is taken to its logical extreme in Josselin's assumption that God had punished him for his fondness for playing chess by killing the infant Ralph.[156] Josselin's feelings of guilt and responsibility drove him to ever stronger devotion to God: after all, his family and friends were, in effect, hostages for his good behaviour.

Fortunately for Josselin, the divine pendulum swung both ways. His preoccupation with providence as it affected himself and his neighbours has been mentioned above. Believing that evil-doers were surely and swiftly punished, he was often relieved and grateful when potential disasters failed to harm him and his. For instance, on 31 March 1648, on a trip to Colchester, 'my horse threw me as I returned home, but through the good providence of god, I had no hurt at all'.[157] However, only good behaviour and prayer could predispose God in man's favour, and even those sometimes failed. Because of his limited capabilities, man could not always know how he had sinned in order to bring calamity upon himself. Thus, when both his wife and daughter were

[154] *Ibid.*, p. 14.   [155] Macfarlane, *Family Life*, pp. 174–6.
[156] *Diary*, p. 114.   [157] *Ibid.*, p. 121.

ill, Josselin wrote 'its hard to find out the particular cause of our troubles, but what good we omit, or ill we do that is hinted to us, its safe to reform, to thee oh...lord we come in Christ for thy healing in body and spirit'.[158] Therefore, Josselin and his family were perpetually at work to propitiate their stern heavenly father. They prayed as individuals, in family groups and with friends and neighbours to heal sickness, survive childbirth, avoid epidemics and, in one case, help a parishioner while he was being cut for the stone in London.[159]

Ralph Josselin's theological view of illness dovetailed nicely with his humoral orientation. Both approaches saw ill-health as a personal particular manifestation stemming from divine displeasure on one hand, or an imbalance of the individual's humoral make-up on the other. Each individual's ailment was different from those of others, requiring individual understanding for its cure. Thus a cold could be caused either by the sufferer's sin or by his having had wet feet. In either case, it could be dealt with by a combination of physical means and prayer. Without divine sanction, however, it could not be cured.

Sickness behaviour and attitudes

Despite the numerous references to ill-health contained in the diary, neither Ralph Josselin nor members of his family often took up a sick role. While they frequently complained and sometimes took medicines, their behaviour was analogous to that of modern people whose livelihoods would be threatened by too frequently taking sick leave. This is not surprising. When Ralph took to his bed, he had either to find a local clergyman willing to preach to his congregation or to leave his flock without spiritual comfort. As noted above, even when he became a near-invalid in his last years, he managed to preach on Sunday. Certainly, his living was by no means so secure that he could afford to neglect his duties. Particularly after the Restoration, Josselin remained at Earls Colne on sufferance.[160] A long illness might have helped to persuade the already suspicious authorities that the Non-conformist Josselin had to go.

Jane Josselin also could not afford to take to her bed when she felt unwell. Although she had a maid-servant to help with housework and childcare, her task was a heavy one. Her house was relatively large, her family at most times numbering seven or eight (including husband and servant as well as children). In addition to helping with the

[158] *Ibid.*, p. 374.
[159] E.g. *ibid.*, pp. 333, 407, 516.   [160] Macfarlane, *Family Life*, pp. 28–9.

cooking, cleaning and farm work, she nursed her husband, children and servant when they were ill, and also helped friends and neighbours, as indicated above. She was needed. Thus, although her pregnancies were uncomfortable and she frequently complained of aches and pains when she was not pregnant, she neither took up a sick role nor was regarded as sick by her husband unless her illness actually incapacitated her.

The diary does not always indicate when one of the Josselins was confined to bed. Jane senior spent about three weeks in bed after each childbirth. Ralph was confined to bed for about two weeks with his ague attack in February 1648. Thomas spent at least two weeks in bed with smallpox.[161] Mary spent between two and three weeks in bed with her attack of worms before she died.[162]

During acute bouts of illness, the Josselins were treated differently than during periods of minor discomfort. They were visited by friends and neighbours, remedies were actively sought and, in at least Ralph senior's case, the sufferer's urine was examined. Family members took care of one another. When Jane senior was seriously ill with a quartan ague in autumn 1668, her adult daughter Jane came home to tend her.[163] And when Elizabeth was reported to be fatally ill in London in March 1682, Jane senior hurried to be with her.[164]

The process of arising from a sick-bed was gradual and apparently conformed to certain expected conventions. Ralph reported when Thomas was able to sit up and when he first came downstairs during his recovery from the smallpox.[165] He mentioned when his wife arose from her bed and when she first left the house – usually to go to church – after giving birth.[166]

Conversely, Josselin sometimes commented when an illness did *not* confine the sufferer to bed or keep him or her from daily employments. In one of his many weekly reports of his family's health he wrote 'Mary and my wife, ill but not down sick'.[167] And when Ralph himself had a cold, pose and pain in the right side of his head in September 1646 he wrote 'yet praise be god I continued able to do my work'.[168]

Unfortunately, the diary does not mention special food or clothing used during times of sickness. It says virtually nothing about the expected sick behaviour and treatment of young children. Yet it

161 *Diary*, e.g. pp. 113, 447.
163 *Ibid.*, p. 545.
165 *Ibid.*, p. 447.
167 *Ibid.*, p. 198.
162 *Ibid.*, pp. 200–3.
164 *Ibid.*, pp. 636–7.
166 E.g. *ibid.*, pp. 168–9.
168 *Ibid.*, pp. 70–1.

certainly gives the impression that the Josselins had definite expectations of themselves and others during periods of acute illness. Sick people were expected to act sick – to stay in bed, be waited on and (usually) take medicine. People well enough to be out of bed were entitled to complain about discomfort, but were expected to carry on with their normal duties. The major exception to this rule, then and now, was chronic illness. Although Ralph was able to preach during the last ten years of his life, he behaved in other respects like a sick person, trying many remedies, consulting several healers, and expecting special services and consideration from family members.

As we have seen, the Josselins suffered from and died of a variety of illnesses. However, the ailments they had, with minor exceptions, were not the ones Ralph most feared. For instance, although his daughter Mary died of worms, he did not appear to be particularly concerned when he or others of his children suffered from that complaint. After her death, he even mentioned his relief that her disease had not been infectious.[169] Yet he was terrified of epidemic diseases, especially smallpox and plague. He mentioned his apprehension about smallpox no fewer than twenty-one times in the course of some thirty years. His fear remained even after several of his children had contracted the disease and recovered from it. Whenever smallpox was in Earls Colne Josselin mentioned the fact, and often gave details of those who died from it.[170] Always nervous about it, his fear reached a peak during a particularly virulent outbreak of the disease in 1651. When both Thomas and John developed rashes in early 1652, Josselin was certain they had smallpox.[171]

Although plague was a less frequent visitor to the vicinity, Josselin feared it terribly. During the great plague year 1665–6, he recorded figures from the London Bills of Mortality weekly. His comments on Earls Colne's virtual escape from infection ranged from the complacent 'god good in our preservation', to the frantic 'when will Coln lay it to heart', to the mystified 'and yet Colne, sinful Colne spared'.[172]

Josselin's fears were based on both medical and religious concerns. Plague and smallpox were deadly diseases. Although there were many remedies which promised to prevent or cure the plague, it was generally regarded as incurable. And while physicians argued the merits of 'hot' or 'cooling' regimens in the treatment of smallpox, the

[169] *Ibid.*, p. 204.
[170] E.g. *ibid.*, pp. 230, 238, 339.
[171] *Ibid.*, p. 273. [172] *Ibid.*, pp. 520–1.

disease mutilated those it did not kill and was, therefore, particularly horrific.[173]

More frightening than the failure of medicine to deal with epidemics was their sudden, mysterious onset and their collective nature. Convinced that epidemics were God's punishment for collective sin, Josselin was deprived of his usual weapons against disease: righteous behaviour and prayer. Even in his capacity as vicar he could not control his neighbours' thoughts and actions. Consider his reflections in August 1644 when the plague, 'that arrow of death', was at Colchester: 'What a mercy of God is it to respite our town Lord spare it, and let not our sins, our covetousness and pride of the poor in the plenty of their Dutch work cause thee to be angry with us'.[174] How fearful, to have to depend upon the relative virtue of all of one's fellow townspeople!

Josselin also may have seen epidemics as heralds of the end of the world. For instance, he described the late summer of 1647 as a time

of great sickness and illness, agues abounding more than in all my remembrance, last year and this also, fevers spotted rise in the country, whether it arise from a distempered and infected air I know not, but fruit rots on the trees as last year though more, and many cattle die of the murrain, this portends something…[175]

Whatever the reasons, epidemic diseases were for Ralph Josselin what cancer is for many modern Westerners. The mysterious terrors of their very names made the shivering and burning of ague fits seem desirable by comparison.

Conclusions

This paper has addressed the single question of what the Josselins felt and did when they became ill. Unambitious as this inquiry may seem, such a study should help to provide a foundation for a wider investigation of illness and medicine from the sufferer's point of view.

The Josselins' experience of ill-health can by no means be assumed to be typical for mid seventeenth century England. For instance, Ralph Josselin's near contemporary, Samuel Pepys, was both more secular in his attitude toward disease and more likely to consult a licensed physician or surgeon than was the vicar. The conclusions we can draw must therefore refer only to the Josselins themselves.

---

[173] See K. Dewhurst, *Dr Thomas Sydenham (1625–1689), His Life and Original Writings* (London, 1966), pp. 105–14.

[174] *Diary*, p. 15.   [175] *Ibid.*, p. 101.

Ralph Josselin was unwell, or at least uncomfortable, most of the time. It is no wonder that he at one time reflected that 'this life is a bundle of sorrows'.[176] The nearly continual colds which plagued him and his family, their unpleasant eye and skin disorders, and the endless discomforts of Jane's pregnancies surely encouraged the feeling that ill-health was a normal state of affairs. Indeed, Josselin commented on *good* health whenever he could, in his weekly reports, thus giving the impression that such a condition was at least worthy of remark.[177]

Although the Josselins occasionally consulted healers and more frequently used medicines, they did not expect to be cured by such measures. Rather they hoped for some help through them, but were not disappointed when remedies and healers failed. Their ultimate trust was in God, and they did not expect to feel completely well in any case.

For the Josselins, as for their contemporaries, death was familiar and expected. It could come at any time, as the result of any accident or illness. Thus it was natural to think of death for oneself or one's loved ones in almost any situation. For instance, nine days after giving birth, Jane was 'very ill, as if she would have even died, [and] she uttered as formerly these words thou and I must part'.[178] When 2-month-old John became ill, his father expected death and 'cried to my god with tears for him and he heard presently he sweetly revived'.[179]

However, for Ralph Josselin the expectation of death did not reduce the value of the loved one. If anything, it made his wife and children more precious to him because his fear of losing them was quite real. Certainly, Josselin did not fail to become emotionally attached to his children because of the likelihood that they would not survive. His grief for 8-year-old Mary produced the most moving passage in the diary, and his desolation is apparent in his reflections on the deaths of Thomas and Ann in the summer of 1673: 'god hath taken 5 of 10. lord let it be enough, and spare that we may recover strength'.[180]

And, in the same vein, despite Lawrence Stone's argument, naming a child after a deceased sibling did not, for the Josselin family, indicate 'a lack of sense that the child was a unique being, with its own name'.[181] There were probably two different reasons for the two examples of this practice in the Josselin family. In one case, two infants born within fifteen months of each other were named Ralph after their

---

[176] *Ibid.*, p. 538.
[177] E.g. *ibid.*, pp. 178, 238, 307.
[178] *Ibid.*, p. 51.
[179] *Ibid.*, p. 262.
[180] *Ibid.*, pp. 203–4, 568.
[181] Stone, *The Family, Sex and Marriage*, p. 70.

father. In this case the re-use of the name indicates not disregard of
the individuality of the first baby, but a special value placed upon the
name itself. In the second case the Josselins' eighth child was named
Mary nearly eight years after the death of her older sister of that name.
In this case it is fair to assume that the name was meant as a memorial
to the deceased older child rather than as a negation of her
individuality.

Despite their expectation of death, the Josselins were relatively
fortunate in surviving the hazards of their time. Ralph Josselin himself
lived to be 67. His wife, only ten months younger than he, survived
him. So did five of his children, the eldest of whom was nearly 38
and all of whom were over 19 at the time of his death. Considering
Lawrence Stone's findings, that in 1650 40 per cent of squires and their
social superiors left no son; that nearly 40 per cent of children born
in 1650 died before age 15; and that peers born in 1625 could expect
to live only until about age 31, Ralph Josselin and his family did very
well indeed.[182]

[182] *Ibid.*, pp. 67, 69, 71.

5

Participant or patient? Seventeenth century childbirth from the mother's point of view

ADRIAN WILSON

Introduction

The first act of the historian, the act which constitutes all the history (s)he subsequently writes, is to decide to write the history *of something*. That 'something' is naturally, normally, taken from the world around us, the world of which the historian is a part. And so it is that in roughly the last hundred years we have had histories of midwifery, of obstetrics, and of their professions – female midwives, male obstetricians.[1] The writing of the histories coincides with the existence of these present realities of which the histories have been written. Such history-writing forms a specimen both of 'tunnel history' and of 'present-centred history'.[2] Equally, and of special concern in the present volume, it is 'iatrocentric':[3] that is to say, histories of, say, obstetrics are inevitably written from the viewpoint of the obstetrician. The survival of evidence in handy packages (treatises of obstetrics/midwifery, written mainly by men) conspires with the attitude of the historian to perpetuate this state of affairs. There is an overwhelming tendency to see the story as a technical matter, to dignify the techniques therefore

[1] See, for instance, J. H. Aveling, *English Midwives: Their History and Prospects* (London, 1872); Herbert R. Spencer, *The History of British Midwifery from 1650 to 1800* (London, 1927); Walter Radcliffe, *Milestones in Midwifery* (Bristol, 1967).

[2] J. H. Hexter, *Reappraisals in History* (London, 1961), pp. 194–5, criticizes tunnel history; the concept of present-centred history was developed by Timothy Ashplant (personal communication, 1975), and is outlined in Adrian Wilson, 'The infancy of the history of childhood: an appraisal of Philippe Ariès', *History and Theory*, XIX (1980), 147–50.

[3] David Richards and John Woodward, 'Towards a social history of medicine', in Woodward and Richards (eds.), *Health Care and Popular Medicine in Nineteenth-Century England* (London, 1977), p. 16.

with a special status, and thus to end not only with a whiggish history of inevitable 'progress' (the present day being the age of perfected technique), but also with an account which excludes the viewpoint of the very people who must have been at the heart of the story: the women who actually gave birth to our ancestors.[4] We are entitled to suspect that the story will look very different, and will become palpably more human, if it can be written 'from below' — from 'the patient's view'.

It might be thought, by those of us belonging to the generation influenced by the new feminism, that this revolution of viewpoint has already happened. The old medical history which I have been criticizing was written by men, and mostly about men; we now have a new historiography, written increasingly by women and about women. Instead of the male practitioner — the obstetric surgeon, the 'man-midwife', the 'obstetrician' — being the central figure, and the female midwife being castigated out of hand as ignorant and superstitious, we now have accounts which take the midwife seriously, and which place her at the centre of the stage. It therefore appears that we have escaped from the male and professional point of view, and from this it seems to follow that we are beginning to get that history-from-below to which this volume is dedicated. Yet there are grounds for believing that the *patient's* viewpoint has still not been reached. The mother and midwife were formally distinct; even though they were both women, this does not imply that their viewpoints were identical; and the fact that we tend to assume a shared 'women's view' may be a product of our late twentieth century feminism. Moreover, there remains a tendency to see the midwife as a technical practitioner; and, what probably accounts for this, the entities being historicized remain medical, professional, and thus very possibly anachronistic.[5]

We may escape from these constraints, I suggest, if we set ourselves the task of writing the history of *childbirth*,[6] rather than histories of

---

4 For a recent example of this dignifying of techniques, see Edward Shorter, *A History of Women's Bodies* (London, 1983).

5 Jean Donnison, *Midwives and Medical Men* (London, 1977); Jane B. Donegan, *Women and Men Midwives* (Westport, Conn., 1978); Audrey Eccles, *Obstetrics and Gynaecology in Tudor and Stuart England* (London, 1982).

6 I have sought to do this in my thesis, 'Childbirth in seventeenth- and eighteenth-century England' (University of Sussex D.Phil. thesis, 1982), cited hereafter as Wilson, 'Childbirth'; to be published as *A Safe Deliverance: Changing Rites of Childbirth in Early-Modern England* (Cambridge, forthcoming). The subject has been treated for the case of France by Mireille Laget, 'Childbirth in seventeenth- and eighteenth-century France: obstetrical

midwifery, midwives, obstetricians, obstetrics-and-gynaecology, and so on. The word childbirth, and the concept of childbirth, span the centuries for which there is available evidence; and to take this as our object is to free ourselves from the pre-structuring of the story which I have been discussing, a pre-structuring which, as I pointed out initially, begins in the act of choosing a historical topic. A 'history of childbirth' would encompass *all* the different points of view: those of mother (patient), midwife and male practitioner.

In order to do this, some will say, we have to be supplied with convenient bundles of evidence written by these respective participants – mother's testimony, midwife's testimony and doctor's testimony, to be ranged alongside one another. If this were so, our task would be logistically very difficult as regards the mother, and virtually impossible in the case of the midwife. The testimony of mothers, such as it is, is confined to wealthy women and is scattered in family papers in dozens of different repositories, while the testimony of midwives barely exists before the eighteenth century. But in fact the historian does not work in this way; he does not, or at least should not, simply pillage 'the sources' for direct testimony; rather, the historian reconstructs human activities (beginning with those activities which produced the evidence in question), and this can and should include the reconstructing of the different 'points of view' which are involved. Thus the 'testimony' of a male author, though it is naturally written from one particular viewpoint, can serve as evidence for other viewpoints, provided we have grasped the nature of the author's *own* viewpoint. For example, to cite the main primary source on which I have drawn in this paper: the obstetric surgeon Percival Willughby, practising in and around Derby in the 1660s, wrote a book entitled *Observations in Midwifery* for the purpose of educating midwives; and he announced this aim repeatedly in the book. He illustrated the work with plentiful case-descriptions which show, more often than not, how he was called to the births in question, and this makes it possible for us to reconstruct the various different 'paths' (as I have termed them) by which he came into the delivery room at all.[7] Those paths make it clear that the

practices and collective attitudes', trans. Elborg Forster and Patricia M. Ranum, in Robert Forster and Orest Ranum (eds.), *Medicine and Society in France: Selections from the Annales Economies, Sociétés, Civilisations* (London, 1980), pp. 137–76.

7 Percival Willughby, *Observations in Midwifery* (Warwick, 1863; Wakefield, 1972), written in the 1660s; cited hereafter as Willughby, *Observations*. 'Paths' to childbirth are defined and outlined in Adrian Wilson, 'William Hunter

summoning of this particular male practitioner was a social act – that it was not the technical problems of childbirth but the expectations of women which led to his being called and which decreed what was expected of him once he had arrived. And thus, by considering this piece of male 'testimony' we are inexorably led back to a recognition, and thus to a reconstruction, of the way the birth was being managed *before* he was called.

In Britain in the 1980s the vast majority of births take place in a hospital; they are under medical control, with the (female) midwife acting largely as the agent of the (usually male) obstetrician; and they are seen as medical events, both in the sense that they are fraught with danger which is fended off with elaborate instrumentation, and in the sense that the mother is passive, almost a helpless spectator at her own delivery. The child's father may or may not be allowed to observe the birth (that depends on the medical authorities concerned) and even if he is allowed to observe, he will probably not be allowed to participate in any way. The other people in the room are professionals, usually total strangers, to whom this mother is the same as any other – a piece of routine to be managed, to be got through, in the course of a working day. All this is utterly different from the way childbirth was managed in this same country some three centuries ago. In the late seventeenth century childbirth was under predominantly female control; the mother herself chose who would be present; these were mostly non-professionals, although they participated in the management of the birth; and it took place at home, not in the separate, alien, sterile, impersonal territory of the institutional hospital. It looks, therefore, as though the seventeenth century mother was a *participant*, in contrast to the twentieth century mother who is a mere *patient*. Before deciding on this, however, we need to look rather more closely at the way seventeenth century births were managed.

  The task before us, then, is to reconstruct a set of human activities in the past: specifically, those activities which went into the management of childbirth in seventeenth century England. If we focus upon the technical means by which birth was managed, we find a picture of bewildering diversity (and I shall attend to this diversity in due course). But these technical measures were embedded within a social framework

and the varieties of man-midwifery', in W. F. Bynum and Roy Porter (eds.), *William Hunter and the Eighteenth-Century Medical World* (Cambridge, 1985), pp. 343–70.

which was much more consistent: a *ceremony of childbirth*, a pervasive popular ritual, which was maintained by (and had probably been created by) the women of England.[8] Just as we today have a medical and hospital ritual of childbirth, so our ancestors had their own lay and domestic ritual. It was this ritual which both required and gave meaning to the many specific activities and customs which I shall now describe.

The ceremony of childbirth

Before she fell into labour, a mother had already made her social arrangements for the birth; when labour pains arrived she set these arrangements in motion, summoning (with the help of her husband, a servant or both) the birth-attendants she had chosen in advance – her midwife, and a number of other women who were also designated to take part. Aristocratic mothers sometimes engaged the midwife to reside with them from late pregnancy onwards, to be near at hand as soon as labour pains came; most mothers, however, simply sent for the midwife at the onset of labour, and they could do this because most villages had their own midwife. In the larger settlements (those with 200 families or so) there were often two or more midwives; and it appears that different religious groups each had their own midwife, so that in a county town there might be a Presbyterian midwife, a Catholic one, and several others of the Anglican communion. Occasionally the labour proceeded so swiftly that the delivery was completed before the midwife arrived; usually, however, the midwife arrived in good time and promptly proceeded to take charge.[9]

The midwife, however, was only one of the several women invited to the birth. For this was an important social occasion, and it seems that perhaps six or more women typically attended. These other

---

8 The ritual of childbirth itself (as distinct from the rites of baptism and churching) seems to have escaped historians' notice, apart from one or two remarks in Alan Macfarlane, *The Family Life of Ralph Josselin, A Seventeenth-Century Clergyman* (Cambridge, 1970), pp. 84–5 (cited hereafter as Macfarlane, *Josselin*). On healing rituals in England, see Keith Thomas, *Religion and the Decline of Magic* (Harmondsworth, 1973), ch. 7; on domestic rituals in early-modern Europe, Shorter, *Bodies*, pp. 4–5; on rites of passage in England during the following century, Roy Porter, *English Society in the Eighteenth Century* (Harmondsworth, 1982), pp. 170–1.

9 Willughby, *Observations*, pp. 42, 239; Wilson, 'Childbirth', ch. 5 (numbers of midwives); David Harley, personal communication, 1983 (different religious groups); Macfarlane, *Josselin*, p. 85 (delivery without the midwife; the process of sending for the midwife and other women).

women comprised friends, relatives and neighbours, but they were no mere random selection. The mother had specifically invited each of them; to issue such an invitation was a compliment, to neglect it was a slight, and a mother might subsequently feel guilty that she had not invited some particular acquaintance. The popular term for these attending women itself reveals something of their identity. They were known as 'gossips'; the word was derived originally from 'god-sibling' and pertained to the function of witnessing the birth and the subsequent baptism of the child, but by the seventeenth century its usage had expanded so that it embraced, in effect, a woman's circle of close female friends.[10] Men, on the other hand, were conspicuously absent: childbirth was a woman's business and a female occasion. The husband sat downstairs and worried (as in *Tristram Shandy*), or whiled away the time with other men in a neighbour's house; even a small boy would be sent out of the room on the grounds that he was 'the only male' present. Every account of childbirth takes this exclusion of men for granted: those present were invariably described as 'the women', and it was never prescribed but simply accepted that the birth was a female affair.[11]

As the husband was taking his leave, the women were busy preparing for the birth, for all the gossips actively participated in the ritual which was now being constructed. At this stage they had two main tasks: preparing the room on the one hand, and the caudle on the other. The mother's bedroom (or whatever room she was lying in – perhaps in her own mother's house) was transformed from its everyday appearance into the *lying-in chamber*, by physically and symbolically enclosing it. Specifically, air and daylight were excluded, by shutting up all apertures, such as keyholes, and by darkening the room with curtains. Whatever the time of day, therefore, the room had to be lit with candles, and these were part of the standard requirements for a delivery. The *caudle* was a hot drink of wine or gruel

[10] Macfarlane, *Josselin*, p. 85, cites Ralph Josselin as recording that 'only five' women were present at a delivery of 1648; Willughby, *Observations*, p. 305, wrote in about 1672 that 'five or six women assisting will be sufficient', implying that the number was often greater than this. Mothers feeling guilty at not having invited someone: Michael Macdonald, *Mystical Bedlam* (Cambridge, 1981), p. 109. For the meaning of 'gossip', see the *Oxford English Dictionary* (hereafter *O.E.D.*) and, for instance, Nicholas Culpepper, *A Directory for Midwives* (London, 1675), p. 119.

[11] See Madeleine Riley, *Brought to Bed* (London, 1968), p. 106; Phillis Cunnington and Catherine Lucas, *Costume for Births, Marriages and Deaths* (London, 1972), pp. 22–3; Willughby, *Observations, passim*.

sweetened with sugar and flavoured with spices, which the mother drank throughout the delivery (and afterwards) to keep up her strength and spirits. With the midwife present, the last of the gossips arrived, the caudle brewed, the curtains up, the candles lit, everything was ready.[12]

Only now could the birth itself begin – now, that is, that this event of nature had been immersed in culture, in the ordered ritual which made the birth a social and human act. The steps we have been observing amounted to the setting-up of a *ceremony*, which had five defining features. First and foremost, it was a female ritual: men were excluded, and childbirth belonged to women. Second, it was a collective female ritual, an activity of a group, not of the mother alone nor of the mother and midwife, but of mother and midwife and gossips. Third, it took place in a special, consecrated space – it is almost appropriate to say a sacred space[13] – the lying-in chamber, demarcated from the outside world and ritually distinguished from its ordinary functions as a mere room. Fourth, there belonged to it the special drink called caudle – nourishment for the mother which also (as we shall subsequently see) served a ceremonial and social function. Finally, there was one woman (apart from the mother) who enjoyed a special status: the birth was managed by the group, to be sure, but one member of that group was distinguished as the *midwife*.

How did the midwife differ from the other women at the birth? First, it seems likely (though I have not verified this) that she alone was entrusted with the right to touch the genital parts of the mother. Second, she was paid a fee – perhaps a shilling or two if the mother was poor, something like six shillings for a typical delivery in a market town, and probably a handsome remuneration measured in guineas for an aristocratic delivery.[14] But the most important characteristic of the midwife was that she was in charge of the birth. It was she who told the mother when to bear down, and when to rest; whether to lie in bed or to kneel on the floor or to sit on a 'midwife's stool'; what to eat and what to drink in the course of the delivery. As we shall see, the midwife's power might sometimes be challenged, but the normal

[12] See Wilson, 'Childbirth', p. 131; *O.E.D.*, 'caudle'.
[13] Mircea Eliade, *The Sacred and the Profane*, trans. W. R. Trask (New York, 1959), pp. 20–65.
[14] Wilson, 'Childbirth', p. 38; Joan Lane, 'The administration of an eighteenth-century Warwickshire parish' (Dugdale Society Occasional Papers No. 21, Oxford, 1973), pp. 20–1; J. H. Aveling, *English Midwives: Their History and Prospects* (London, 1872), pp. 15–16, 31–4.

state of affairs was that she ran the show: this indeed was the substance of her office.

The authority of the midwife was, like the structure of the ritual as a whole, a constant feature of the ceremony of childbirth. But this very authority meant that in the technical management of the birth (the aspect which tends to interest our twentieth-century eyes), the constancy with which we have been dealing gave way to enormous variability. Different midwives managed the birth in very different ways: not only were there different postures, as we have just seen, but also some midwives used force and others left the birth to nature; some used magic and charms while others did not; and some, but probably not all, used herbal remedies to facilitate the birth. Correspondingly, midwives themselves were a very heterogeneous breed: although most were apparently married or widowed, at least one example of an unmarried midwife is known, and we find them described as young and old (aged even in their eighties), rich and poor, skilful and unskilful, compassionate and cruel, literate and illiterate.[15] Some were trained by serving as deputies under a practising midwife; most, apparently, set up in practice on the basis of having seen some deliveries in the capacity of gossips and probably buying a 'midwife's book' for elementary instruction. In theory, midwives were subject to licensing by the Church, and this licensing seems to have been introduced on a systematic scale (in the early seventeenth century) in an attempt to regulate their technical skills. In practice, however, Church licensing was not intensively enforced, it provided no effective test of skill, and it probably served merely to ratify local choices already made.[16] How a woman became a midwife, fascinating and important though that question is, we shall probably never know: the documentation of women's lives is just not good enough.

Once the child was delivered, the constancy of the ritual framework reappeared in the final act of the birth itself, namely the *swaddling* of the child. It was the responsibility of the midwife to ensure that swaddling was carried out, though any of the gossips might perform it; and it would seem that only when the baby was swaddled was it handed to the mother. Though we tend to see swaddling as part of

---

[15] Wilson, 'Childbirth', note 2 to ch. 6 and note 25 to ch. 1.

[16] Deputies: J. H. Aveling, *The Chamberlens and the Midwifery Forceps* (London, 1882), p. 37; Jean Donnison, *Midwives and Medical Men* (London, 1977), p. 8. Licensing: Adrian Wilson, 'The origins of Anglican licensing of midwives', *Journal of Ecclesiastical History* (forthcoming).

'child care' or 'infant management', in reality it was an integral part of birth. Consequently, it was discussed in midwifery treatises, always in such a way as to take it for granted that the child would be swathed up. Indeed, there was some tendency to perceive the swaddling-clothes as an integral part of the newborn child. It was these clothes which made the child human,[17] just as the wider ceremony of childbirth of which swaddling was a part made the delivery an act of culture, not merely of nature.

The childbirth ceremony usually *worked* magnificently, just as our very different ritual does so today, and for the same reason: most births, then as now, were normal and spontaneous. But a small minority of births – perhaps one in thirty – became obstructed. What was to happen now? Sometimes a second midwife was summoned, perhaps from the next village, perhaps from further afield; this second midwife might have mastered the technique of podalic version, in which case she could probably deliver the mother. On other occasions the second midwife was no more fortunate than the first, and thus we find instances of three and even four midwives present after protracted obstruction. Eventually, if none of the midwives could deliver the child, it would die; and the point now came when the mother's life, too, was in danger. In these desperate straits the only recourse was to send for a male practitioner – that is, for a surgeon, who could extract the dead child with suitable instruments. The task of the midwife was to deliver a *living* child, the task of the male practitioner to deliver a *dead* one; and it is not surprising to find that very few midwives used instruments, nor that male practitioners were regarded with fear and dread. To call the surgeon was to abandon the ceremony, to surrender hope for the life of the child, and to subject the mother to a terrifying and often painful operation. Consequently, women put off this step until the last possible minute; and there was sometimes conflict over whether, and when, to send for the man. It was in these circumstances, as we shall subsequently see, that the midwife's authority could be challenged.[18]

During the birth the mother was not only in an altered bodily state,

[17] Wilson, 'Childbirth', pp. 133–4; David Hunt, *Parents and Children in History* (New York, 1970), p. 130.

[18] This is a highly simplified account; for a more extended treatment of male 'paths to childbirth', see my paper cited in note 7 above, and on the attitudes of women to male practitioners in obstetric emergencies, see Wilson, 'Childbirth', *passim*, especially pp. 263–81.

but also in a special physical space (the lying-in chamber) and a special social milieu (the company of women); thus she was separated from mundane life in three dimensions. This complex structure had now to be dismantled: the mother had to recover from her bodily exhaustion, the lying-in room had to be returned to its normal functions and appearance, and the mother had to resume contact with the world of men. How was this done? What we find is that this process was a gradual one; that it proceeded in stages; and that each stage saw a change in all three of the dimensions just distinguished. The whole process was termed *lying-in*.[19] At first, for about a week, the mother kept to her bed and could be visited only by women; and these women drank the caudle left over from the delivery. Then she 'made her upsitting': the bedclothes were changed for the first time, and she could now move freely about the room, but for a further period of some days she could not leave the lying-in room. A third stage followed, when she could move about the house but was not permitted to go outdoors; according to the proper form, she could now receive male visitors provided that these men were her relatives. Together the three stages lasted for something like a month; the period was referred to as 'the month', or as 'her month', though as we shall shortly see it did not necessarily last for exactly thirty days. The mother could not attend the baptism of her child, which took place in church about a week after the delivery; instead, the midwife was prominent at this ceremony. And it seems that throughout 'the month' the newly delivered mother abstained from sexual intercourse with her husband.[20]

The lying-in period was terminated, for Anglican women, by a further ritual – the ecclesiastical rite of *churching*, which consummated and completed the process, and which is its best-documented moment because the churching ritual was ecclesiastical and official, bringing the world of women (to which birth and lying-in belonged) into contact with the literate world of men. Although churching had its official rationale (originally, purification; since the Reformation, the giving of thanks for a 'safe deliverance'), it seems that it also had a popular meaning, to do with the completion of lying-in. Thus it was probably

[19] *Ibid.*, pp. 134–8.
[20] *Ibid.*, pp. 138–9; Jane Sharp, *The Midwives Book* (London, 1671), p. 271; Lawrence Stone, *The Family, Sex and Marriage in England, 1500–1800* (London, 1977), p. 501; Randolph Trumbach, 'The aristocratic family in England, 1690–1780. Studies in childhood and kinship' (Johns Hopkins University Ph.D. thesis, 1972), pp. 21–3.

not from ecclesiastical diktat but rather from folk belief that a mother was thought (in parts of Wales) to be liable to kill the grass on which she trod if she ventured out of doors before her churching.[21] But how then was she to get to the church? It seems that she went surrounded by the company of women, led by the midwife, and wearing a white veil – that is, duly enclosed until the moment came, on the completion of the churching service, when she could throw back the veil and resume ordinary life.[22] Even Puritan mothers, though their preaching mentors objected to the 'popish superstition' of this ceremony (with its overtones of defilement-by-birth and ecclesiastical 'purification'), seem to have followed the lying-in ritual in its main outlines, though sometimes completing this without giving thanks in church. The ceremony of childbirth, from the original summoning of the gossips to the final giving of thanks, transcended doctrinal niceties and subordinated official ritual to popular custom.[23]

Without doubt the childbirth ritual in its more elaborate form was observed particularly amongst the upper classes. The humble cottager's wife did not have the physical space for a separate room, probably could not have recruited help about the house for a month's lying-in, and may indeed have had to go back to work out of doors at such times as the harvest. Yet there was much scope for flexibility: if a separate room could not be found in the house, the delivery might take place at the mother's mother's house, or perhaps at the house of a friend; or else the bed alone might be curtained off, creating so to speak a lying-in 'space' within a family room. What little indication we have of the observance of the ritual, limited and indirect as it is, does suggest well-nigh universal acceptance of some form or other of lying-in.[24] It appears that in two parishes of early seventeenth

---

[21] See Thomas, *Religion and the Decline of Magic*, p. 39 (and cf. p. 612).

[22] W. P. M. Kennedy, *Elizabethan Episcopal Administration* (3 vols., London, 1924), vol. 3, pp. 149–50; Wilson, 'Childbirth', pp. 136–7.

[23] *Ibid.*, pp. 137–8; Macfarlane, *Josselin*, pp. 86, 88. I know of no published research on the specific practices of non-Anglican women, nor for that matter on the observance of churching in the eighteenth century amongst Anglican mothers.

[24] John Landers, personal communication (1979), informed me of the practice of mothers being delivered in the houses of their own mothers: Willughby, *Observations*, p. 120, said that he delivered a woman who was staying in the house of a friend of his. The following evidence concerning the observance of churching in early seventeenth century London comes from Jeremy Boulton, 'The social and economic structure of Southwark in the early seventeenth century' (University of Cambridge Ph.D. thesis, 1983), pp. 336–9; to be published as *Patterns of Urban Life* (Cambridge, forthcoming).

century London for which parish clerks' day-books survive, over 90 per cent of mothers were churched after childbirth. The interval was *less* than thirty days (generally three to four weeks), suggesting that mothers did indeed improvise slightly within the form. What is striking is that this high observance was found in a context where it might least be expected: large, urban, Puritan parishes.

Until the eighteenth century male observers accepted without comment the female management of childbirth and the structure of its ritual; they treated it as natural, which is precisely what we should expect them to do. Percival Willughby believed that the chamber should be darkened; William Forster, writing in 1745, that a 'constant dew' – that is, sweating – was an 'absolute necessity' after labour. Midwifery treatises, though mostly written by men, were aimed at an audience of midwives, for it was still believed that the midwife was the appropriate childbed practitioner. And medical views of childbirth were structured by the categories of popular ritual: the timing and management of the 'upsitting', and the diseases of women 'within the month', were standard items for treatment in midwifery texts.[25]

But in the middle decades of the eighteenth century a new type of male practitioner came into being – the 'man-midwife', that is, a man who was expected to deliver a *living* child. These practitioners, not surprisingly, had a more independent viewpoint. As a result, they began to write treatises of 'midwifery' for *men*, and from about 1750 onwards they began to criticize various features of the female ceremony of childbirth. First swaddling was attacked (in terms which made it clear that this was a female practice, to be undermined by male 'reason'), then the lying-in room had to be ventilated, and eventually the point came when a male practitioner advocated removal of the gossips from the lying-in room.[26] Nor did this male onslaught, piecemeal though it was, go without effect. Caudle, it seems, became 'old-fashioned'; the social rules for admitting male guests were relaxed; and Mrs Delany coined the word 'confinement' to refer to

This relates to the parish of St Saviour's Southwark; for the other parish, St Botolph's Aldgate, I am indebted to Dr Boulton's personal communication (1983).

[25] Willughby, *Observations*, p. 65; William Forster, *A Treatise on the Causes of Most Diseases* (Leeds, 1745), p. 166; François Mauriceau, *The Diseases of Women with Child, and in Child-bed*, trans. Hugh Chamberlen, 6th edn. (London, 1718), pp. 308–9; William Smellie, *A Treatise on the Theory and Practice of Midwifery* (London, 1752), pp. 385–427.

[26] William Cadogan, *An Essay upon Nursing* (London, 1748); Wilson, 'Childbirth', pp. 140–1.

the lying-in process, as though acknowledging that this was now perceived as an unwanted restriction.[27] In the 1790s the radical artisan Francis Place exercised a new male prerogative of consumer choice: dissatisfied with the way the midwife handled his wife's first delivery, he saved a guinea for a male practitioner at the second birth, and recorded with satisfaction that this time there were no candles (the room was not darkened) and no 'stimulating messes' (the caudle was dispensed with).[28] Thus the traditional ceremony of childbirth was gradually transformed under the impact of the male practitioner – a point which underlines how distinctively female that ceremony had originally been.

Conclusion

In retrospect, we can see that the early-modern English ceremony of childbirth conforms closely to the classical description of 'rites of passage' developed by Arnold van Gennep.[29] Van Gennep suggested that *rites de passage* always involved three distinct stages – separation, transition and reincorporation – each characterized by human activities embodying these meanings but otherwise seemingly purposeless or unintelligible. Many of the component customs of the ceremony I have been describing do indeed fall within this framework: for instance, the demarcation of the lying-in room (separation), the isolation of 'the month' (transition) and the ritual of churching (reincorporation). Curiously, van Gennep himself was barely aware that his framework could be applied in this way. He did not mention the fact that childbirth management was undergoing historical change; he thought that in Western Europe the mother's churching was the sole ritual

---

[27] Trumbach, 'The aristocratic family' (note 20 above), p. 38; *O.E.D.*, 'confinement'.

[28] Mary Thale (ed.), *The Autobiography of Francis Place* (London, 1972), p. 184.

[29] Arnold van Gennep, *The Rites of Passage*, trans. M. B. Vizedom and G. L. Caffee (London, 1960; French original published 1906), pp. 10–11, 46. The ritual management of childbirth is considered in Clellan Stearns Ford, *A Comparative Study of Human Reproduction* (Yale University Publications in Anthropology No. 32; New Haven, 1945), and in Niles Newton and Michael Newton, 'Childbirth in crosscultural perspective', in John G. Howells (ed.), *Modern Perspectives in Psycho-Obstetrics* (Edinburgh, 1972), pp. 150–72. These studies are organized thematically, and thus do not attempt to reconstruct any specific ritual. More helpful, therefore, even though not dealing directly with childbirth, is John M. Janzen, *The Quest for Therapy in Lower Zaire* (Berkeley, 1978); Janzen's concept of a 'therapy-managing group' is directly comparable to the 'childbirth-managing group' which I have found for seventeenth century England. See Wilson, 'Childbirth', pp. 200–1.

component; and he suggested that the timing of this ceremony reflected physiological realities, seemingly believing that the customs of his own society (early twentieth century France) were rooted in an objective, scientific understanding of nature. Yet this is intelligible enough, for nothing is more difficult than to stand outside one's own culture. The anthropological stance is easy to take with a totally alien society, somewhat more difficult to adopt towards our own past (so that the ritual nature of seventeenth century childbirth has virtually escaped observation), and most difficult of all to take towards our own present.

At least one recent observer, however, has examined modern hospital childbirth from this stance. Peter Lomas, commenting critically and from a psychoanalytic perspective, finds that much of the paraphernalia of hospitalized childbirth serves as ritual rather than (as its practitioners believe) for instrumental purposes. The medical science on which are based such practices as shaving the mother's pubic hair can be used to show that these same practices do not have the efficacy which is claimed for them. The modern ritual, Lomas believes, exists for the sake of the attendants, not for the sake of the mother: ritual practices are immensely reassuring. (The mother, one gathers, is reassured in a different way, namely by *submitting to* the ritual, whatever it may be.)[30] The fact that the modern management of childbirth also takes a ritual form helps to substantiate an underlying theme of my argument: that early-modern childbirth was indeed managed by a consistent ritual, even though no contemporary described it in these terms.

To return to the original question, it is now apparent that the seventeenth century mother's viewpoint could conflict with that of the midwife, even though the mother had chosen her own midwife (probably from a large pool of alternatives, for there were many midwives in practice). Such conflict would arise particularly if the birth was difficult, and it is thus made visible for us by the testimony of the male practitioner.[31] Percival Willughby recounted a delivery of 1640

---

[30] Peter Lomas, 'An interpretation of modern obstetric practice', in Sheila Kitzinger and John Davis (eds.), *The Place of Birth* (Oxford, 1978), pp. 174–84.

[31] Willughby, *Observations*, pp. 226, 47, 146. It may of course be objected against testimony such as Willughby's that he was biased against midwives, and thus had an interest in recording cases such as these. See David Harley, 'Ignorant midwives – a persistent stereotype', *The Society for the Social History of Medicine Bulletin*, XXVIII (1981), 6–9; Adrian Wilson, 'Ignorant midwives – a rejoinder', *ibid.*, XXXII (1983), 46–9; Bernice Boss and Jeffrey Boss, 'Ignorant

at which he was standing by. After the child's head emerged, the aristocratic mother suffered great pain, and called out for Willughby's help, 'but the midwife would have had me put by, and said that my Lady must stay God's time and pleasure'. Willughby's physical presence in the house enabled him to exert *force majeure*: he came in and swiftly completed the delivery. In this instance the mother wanted the midwife to make haste, but she refused. Precisely the opposite conflict occurred in another delivery, some twenty-five years later, where the mother was of much lower social standing (a shepherd's wife). Here Willughby was called only in emergency – the child was dead – and the mother subsequently 'complained very sadly to me, how one of the midwives (that was a young woman) had afflicted her through much pulling and stretching her body'. The most spectacular instances in Willughby's treatise of such conflict between mother and midwife came in the deliveries of his special patient, Mrs Molyneux (later Wildbore), who after five deliveries by midwives lamented 'that they were all ignorant creatures', who in any difficult birth could only 'haul and pull the woman's body, and the child by the limbs'.

There could also be conflict between the mother and her gossips, since the decision to send for a male practitioner was sometimes taken collectively. Willughby recorded that one mother, after spending a day or more in great pain during a delivery, 'called all the women hard-hearted Jews, for that they did not send for me'. Her cry was heard, and the women relented, for within half an hour Willughby was at her side.[32] What is striking here is that 'the women' (whom Willughby clearly distinguished from the midwife), although they must have been chosen as gossips by the mother herself, nevertheless were contravening her wishes until she reached such a point of suffering that she called down a curse on them.

Such difficult births as these were of course not typical; most deliveries, then as now, proceeded smoothly and spontaneously, and the conflict which emerged in these cases was no doubt highly unusual. Yet what such conflict implies was in fact universal: mother, gossips and midwives had *different viewpoints*. For all that the childbirth ritual

midwives – a further rejoinder', *ibid.*, xxxiii (1983), 71; and possibly further rejoinders. On the reliability of Willughby's testimony, see Wilson, 'Childbirth', *passim*. The present argument by-passes this issue, since it is concerned not with midwives' skill but with conflict between mother and midwife; and because it does not depend on the frequency of such conflict, but rather on the simple possibility of its occurrence.

[32] Willughby, *Observations*, p. 38.

was a collective female event and a collective female product, it was a structured process comprising different roles. The midwife, after all, was a paid practitioner. That was what she shared with her later competitor, the 'man-midwife'. Correspondingly, the seventeenth century mother was perhaps less of a participant, and more of a patient, than we might wish to believe.

The historiographical framework of this paper has been developed jointly with Timothy Ashplant and Andrew Cunningham during many congenial discussions. I am most grateful to them for their help.

6

Piety and the patient: Medicine and religion in eighteenth century Bristol

In the concluding chapter of *Religion and the Decline of Magic* Keith Thomas describes the 'decline of magic' after 1660, replaced by a range of practical, scientific and medical methods to counter, or at least mitigate, the uncertainties of life, amongst which illness was the most persistent. Historians of medicine have generally endorsed Thomas' view that medical remedies grew in importance in the eighteenth century, at the expense of religious or magical means of healing. In and around the towns at least the qualified medical man replaced the minister as the chief healer, whilst patent medicines, endorsed by medical men, proliferated at the expense of home-made cures. In the key areas of witchcraft and mental illness moral and religious explanations of disease gave way, in official circles at least, to more secular, materialistic accounts. Thomas suggests that such developments resulted in a widening gap between popular and elite notions, as the rural poor clung to their traditional remedies and magical beliefs, now dismissed as vulgar superstitions by the educated.[1]

Thomas and other historians have been more confident in describing this process than in explaining it. Thomas rightly dismisses the notion that medicine or science had decisively demonstrated their superiority, concluding that 'in medicine as elsewhere, therefore, supernatural theories went out before effective techniques came in'. Thomas is forced to suggest, tentatively, a revolution of aspirations, linked to a new scientific worldview. Geoffrey Holmes, without facing up to the

[1] K. Thomas, *Religion and the Decline of Magic* (London, 1971), ch. 22. For magic and medicine see also M. MacDonald, 'Anthropological perspectives in the history of science and medicine', in P. Corsi and P. Weindling (eds.), *Information Sources in the History of Science and Medicine* (London, 1983), pp. 61–80; T. Ranger, 'Introduction', in W. J. Sheils (ed.), *The Church and Healing* (Oxford, 1982), pp. xi–xxiv.

question so directly, has assumed that growing material comfort and
affluence produced a society less tolerant of pain, and better able to
pay for medical care, but he fails to establish why this money should
be spent on orthodox medical men, whose ability to deliver results he
exaggerates. Nineteenth century medicine successfully built on the
reputation of science to ensure a professional monopoly for the
correctly qualified, but nobody has yet sought to uncover any move
of this kind in the eighteenth century.[2]

The most persuasive explanation yet offered takes up Thomas'
observation about the dissociation of popular and elite cultures, and
uses this to account for the willingness of the elite to rely on unproved
medical solutions, precisely because they were different from popular
remedies. The patient sought out the socially respectable practitioner
and was prepared to pay large sums for his products as a symbol of
his membership of the affluent classes. Moreover, such reliance on the
medical establishment avoided the use of spiritual and folk healing,
which had become associated in the previous century with religious
enthusiasm and civil strife. Therapeutic eclecticism was rejected by the
elite for social and religious motives.[3]

If social and religious motives were dominant, then different medical
approaches might characterize different social and religious groups.
Reliance on established medical therapy should be associated with the
established Church, whilst the dissenters should hold on more firmly
to eclectic healing methods, or adopt alternative medical systems.
Michael MacDonald has argued that such a process can be seen in the

2 Thomas, *Religion and the Decline of Magic*; G. A. Holmes, *Augustan England*
(London, 1982). For the importance of medical practitioners before 1700 see
M. Pelling and C. Webster, 'Medical practitioners', in C. Webster (ed.),
Health, Medicine and Mortality in the Sixteenth Century (Cambridge, 1979), pp.
165–235. For medicine and professionalism see M. Pelling, 'Medical practice
in the early modern period: trade or profession?', *The Society for the Social
History of Medicine Bulletin*, xxxII (1983), 27–30'; *idem*, 'Medicine since 1500',
in Corsi and Weindling (eds.), *Information Sources in the History of Science and
Medicine*, pp. 379–407; L. Jordanova, 'Social sciences and the history of science
and medicine', in *ibid.*, pp. 81–98; N. Jewson, 'Medical knowledge and the
patronage system in eighteenth-century England', *Sociology*, vIII (1974),
369–85; *idem*, 'The disappearance of the sick man from medical cosmology
1770–1870', *Sociology*, x (1976), 225–44.
3 R. Porter, 'Was there a medical enlightenment in eighteenth-century
England?', *British Journal for Eighteenth-Century Studies*, v (1982), 49–64;
idem, 'The "rage of party": a glorious revolution in English psychiatry?',
Medical History, xxvII (1983), 35–50'; *idem*, *English Society in the Eighteenth
Century* (Harmondsworth, 1982). Holmes, *Augustan England*, could easily be
fitted into such an approach.

case of mental illness before 1750, whilst John Pickstone has sketched out a thought-provoking map of doctor–patient relations in late eighteenth century England based on the different models of religious relationship found in the established Church, old Dissent and new Dissent. Such descriptions tend to portray a growing divergence between the secular approach of Anglicanism, and of old Dissent by the mid eighteenth century, and the populist evangelical approach of new Dissent, building on the continued strength of folk healing and popular thaumaturgy.[4]

This chapter examines the evidence on these topics offered by one town, Bristol, and in particular the material contained in the journal of a Bristol accountant, William Dyer, who kept a detailed diary from 1751 to 1801.[5] Although Dyer was as untypical as any diarist, I believe that an examination of the nature of illness and healing, and their religious significance, from the perspective of a patient, may help to illuminate the significance of medicine in eighteenth century England.

William Dyer

William Dyer was born in Bristol in 1730 and lived in that city for the rest of the century. After attending the school of two writing masters he was apprenticed at fourteen to an apothecary, but left after five months to become a junior clerk to a malt distiller. He left this post at twenty when he married an excise officer's daughter, and became clerk to a gunpowder works, as well as acting as a freelance accountant. He prospered steadily, moving into better houses as the years passed and always enjoying considerable leisure. In 1764 he noted that he was worth £50 'clear of the world', and later he became first partner and then sole owner of a colour-making works which never

---

[4] M. MacDonald, 'Religion, social change and psychological healing in England 1600–1800', in Sheils (ed.), *Church and Healing*, pp. 101–25; J. Pickstone, 'Establishment and dissent in nineteenth-century medicine', in *ibid.*, pp. 165–90; L. Barrow, 'Anti-establishment healing and spiritualism in England', in *ibid.*, pp. 225–48; P. Lineham, 'The Biblical Christians of Salford', in *ibid.*, pp. 207–24; H. D. Rack, 'Doctors, demons and early Methodist healing', in *ibid.*, pp. 137–52.

[5] Dyer's diaries are in Bristol Central Library (BCL) Bristol Collection 20095 and 20096. BCL 20095 is a two-volume digest of Dyer's original diaries 1751–1801 produced by him when he destroyed the originals, keeping only the diary for 1762 which is now BCL 20096. All references below by date only are from these diaries, and all the 1762 information is from BCL 20096 unless otherwise indicated. The abstracts in BCL 20095 are not always in exact chronological order, so the date given is sometimes approximate.

did particularly well, but was worth £450 when he finally sold it in 1792. In 1785 he refused an offer to share the rental of the Hotwell House with a leading attorney, and in 1789 he declined a partnership in a new Bristol bank with shares worth £4,000, in return for acting as cashier, because he did not wish to tie himself to a desk, even for only two or three hours a day, nor to reside at the bank. He served regularly on the Grand Jury, and in 1773 was suggested as a candidate to be City Chamberlain. Although not himself a man of importance he knew many of the leaders of Bristol civil life. Dyer seems to have taken his conservative political attitude from the aldermen, Ames and Elton, for whom he worked in his early years.[6]

Dyer also participated in the intellectual and social life of Bristol. Despite his utilitarian education, Dyer loved reading, helped to edit several publications, and advised friends on the contents of several other publications, as well as contributing to the local papers. Although he avoided both the polite world of assemblies and plays, and the city's taverns and clubs, he was a lifelong member of a friendly society and a subscriber to various humanitarian bodies. He organized the Bristol 'Society for the Rescue of Persons Apparently Drowned', and actively supported both the Dispensary and the anti-slave-trade movements. In Bristol Dyer attended book auctions and lectures, and on his frequent visits to London he inspected the British Museum, anatomical exhibitions and other curiosities, and attended a meeting of the new Medical Society of London in 1775, with an introduction from Lettsom. Dyer knew Joseph Priestley, James Ferguson and Edward Jenner.[7] A member of the modern, middle-class profession of accountancy, with humanitarian and intellectual interests, Dyer appears on the surface a typical, if serious, member of the later English Enlightenment.

[6] 10.11.1753 (school); 5.11.44 (apprentice); 1–3.4.45 (clerk); 23.12.50 (marriage); 28.4.52, 10.3.62 (leisure); 10.11.58, 1.9.64 (earnings); 9.72, 5.84, 11.2.92 (colour-works); 5.85 (Hotwells); 6.89 (Bank); 10.7.75 (Grand Jury); 20.5.73 (Chamberlain); 1.5.54, 28.1.55, 3.73, 8.10.74 (politics).

[7] For his editorial work see 7.12.74, 28.10.75, 5.7.90, 2.7.93, and BCL 20097, an edition of R. Tucker's diary he prepared for publication. Advising friends, e.g. 23.1.63, 25.9.65, 6.9.71, 11.2.75, 10.5.75 (letters to papers); 1.6.75 (Society for Rescue); 22.2.94 (Dispensary); 11.8.87, 30.1.88 (anti-slavery); 9–13.1.62, 14.12.62 (book auctions); 15–28.12.60, 8.12.69 (lectures); 6.3.64 (British Museum); 18.12.70 (anatomy); 6.6.75 (Medical Society); 6.11.64, 25.7.66 (Priestley); 28.2.60 (Ferguson); 26.8.86, 10.8.87 (Jenner).

The patient

Dyer conforms outwardly to our standard picture of the eighteenth century patient. The most important medical practitioner to Dyer and his relations was the apothecary, whose advice and visits preceded any other medical attention. A physician was only called in occasionally, on the apothecary's advice, and Dyer seems to have felt that the physician would merely corroborate the apothecary's prescription. Surgeons feature less frequently, to draw teeth and mend cut heads, although Dyer occasionally records with admiration a successful operation they had performed. He often regarded surgery as dangerous, and was particularly critical of surgery to remove breast cancer. In Dyer's view this was both dangerous and ineffectual, since the illness was in the blood and so needed an internal remedy. Although his brief training as an apothecary may have encouraged the tendency, Dyer's general preference for drugs seems consistent with the great commercial popularity of patent medicines, and the prosperity of apothecaries, in this period. The only sign of a new medical practice is the use of inoculation, first mentioned here as late as 1770, but common in the 1780s.[8]

Dyer's circle did not limit their custom to the regular medical practitioners in Bristol. Eye problems were a fertile field for quacks and specialists, and in 1778 a friend of Dyer's had a successful cataract operation in London, performed by 'Baron' Wesell; in 1770 Dyer's brother went to a 'Jew physician' in London for a cure for rheumatism in the arm. In 1757 his father-in-law consulted an unnamed Devizes doctor about Dyer's wife, and after viewing her urine the doctor prescribed a remedy and charged a shilling, his customary fee. Dyer bought the articles prescribed but does not record the result, although he notes that the doctor was reputed to have a hundred applicants a day. In 1781 Dyer described Mrs Thomas, a neighbour, who had died, as 'medical professor', reporting that she 'subsisted by administering some few nostrums'.[9]

Although Dyer did not himself resort to 'quacks', he never inveighed against them, and he had his own fund of remedies against

[8] 11.6.52, 4.6.53, 2.4.60, 22.12.74 (apothecary); 9.1.70, 10.7.77, 25.12.83 (physician); 12.10.52, 22.11.58, 25.5.65, 22.12.74 (surgeon); 26.1.75, 25.10.87, 12.89 (breast cancer); 10.2.70, 22.3.84, 3.86 (inoculation). Richer patients than Dyer probably used a physician as their family doctor, rather than an apothecary.

[9] 20.8.78 (Wesell); 13.8.70 (Jew); 5.9.57 (Devizes); 9.10.81 (Thomas).

illness. To prevent illness he and his wife took cold baths, and he was also interested in hot bathing. When in pain he resorted to chewing tobacco, and occasionally used opiates. He also purchased proprietary medicines, of which his favourite was Dr James's Fever Powder. Dyer assiduously recorded remedies suggested by acquaintances, particularly for chronic diseases such as rheumatism. In 1785 he noted down a remedy for cramp that used broiled house-snail, eggshells and other items which, when placed anywhere on the body, 'operated insensibly'. Use of orthodox medical preparations was not seen as incompatible with personal experimentation with other cures, and such an eclectic attitude was doubtless encouraged by the direct appeal to the purchasing public of the proprietary medicine advertisements. Jewson has portrayed the physician as the servant of his wealthy patron's medical notions, but the apothecary and medicine-seller were equally at the mercy of their less wealthy customers. Dyer's diary records several instances where apothecaries had evidently discussed remedies and shared prescriptions with laymen.[10]

Unfortunately Dyer's diary gives little sense of his own experience of illness, and how he came to terms with it, but his remarks about the illnesses of others suggests a series of assumptions about the meaning of disease. Illness might result from a bad life, for example a case of consumption caused by drunkenness, or a death from 'debauchery and irregularity'. Here of course lay common-sense was echoed by a school of medical writers on regimen. Some of his diagnoses reflect a simple lack of interest in causation, as when Dyer noted that a brother aged 8 had died of 'convulsions' caused by being 'too suddenly aroused from sleep'. But his most frequent observation was on the power of imagination over the body. He shared popular belief in the effect of the mother's mental state on the unborn child, noting in 1759 that a child was born with a mark on its lip because the mother had been frightened by seeing a cat with a rat in its mouth. Dyer valued the writings of the Paracelsian Van Helmont for their account of the power of imagination, but like the Paracelsians he did not see this psychosomatic view as invalidating drug-based treatment,

[10] 2.56, 18.5.57, (BCL 20095) 7.6.62, 16.6.62, 18.7.64 (cold baths); 15.7.56 (warm bath); 14.6.66, 1.10.70 (tobacco); 28.8.62, 1.12.62, 23.6.69 (opiates); 13.10.79 (James's Powder). Remedies noted include: asthma 6.87; rheumatism 16.8.93; cramp 10.85; 14.2.64 (apothecary). For Jewson see note 2 above. For comparison see N. C. Haltin, 'Medicine and magic in the eighteenth century: the diaries of James Woodforde', *Journal of the History of Medicine*, xxx (1975), 349–66.

but as indicating the need for a balanced study of both mental and material factors.[11]

Dyer's beliefs included notions from astrology and correspondence theory. In 1757 he thought that the regular abatement of his father's illness after sunset was clear proof of the influence of the planets, including the sun, on the body. In 1787 Dyer recorded the testimony of a friend that her child's afterbirth, kept in a box, had protected the child from fire, and that a caul taken from a child's face would preserve the owner from drowning while the child remained alive. Ships' captains apparently advertised for such cauls, offering five guineas. The mother also claimed that she could tell from the condition of the caul whether the child was well or not. Dyer commented 'these are mysterious connections between caul and child'.[12]

A supernatural element was also still present in some more conventional treatments. Spas were traditionally associated with saints, and the new spas discovered were frequently associated with dreams. Dyer noted that the Glastonbury waters in vogue in the 1750s, which he visited, had been revealed through a dream, and the literature on the well comments on this. Glastonbury had unusually strong religious ties, of course, but the use of the Bristol Hotwells for the cure of diabetes was also believed to have started as the result of a dream. Controversy still raged over whether the efficacy of spas lay solely in their material constituents, or whether God's blessing was partly or wholly responsible for cures. When Dyer took medicine, or decided what to prescribe for others, he sought God's guidance and blessing.[13]

[11] For an example of Dyer ill see 13–20.10.77; 4.87 (consumption); 4.85 (debauchery); early 1751 (convulsion); 30.8.59, 9.12.66 (mother's imagination); 16.2.62, 14.5.62, 28.10.87 (Helmont). For medical regimens see note 56 below.

[12] 31.5.57 (father), cf. 31.8.70 (collecting morning's dew in a phial); 24.7.87 (caul and afterbirth).

[13] 27.4.51 (Glastonbury). See also: *Wilt Thou Be Made Whole?* (London, 1756); *An Address to the Inhabitants of Glastonbury* (Bristol, 1751), p. 5; *A Complete and Authentic History...Glastonbury* (London, n.d.), p. 80 quoting the Bristol diabetes case. For the Hotwells see V. Waite, 'The Bristol Hotwell', in P. McGrath (ed.), *Bristol in the Eighteenth Century* (Newton Abbot, 1972), p. 115, quoting Dr G. Randolph. A spring near Bristol associated with 'Mother Pugsley', a reputed witch of the late seventeenth century, was widely supposed to cure eye diseases, see J. Leech, *Rural Rides of a Bristol Church-goer* (reprinted Gloucester, 1982), pp. 100–1; Bodleian MSS Gough Somerset 2 ff.127–8, 4.8.1701; *Arrowsmith's Dictionary of Bristol* (Bristol, 1884), pp. 211–12; G. Pryce, *Popular History of Bristol* (Bristol, 1861), p. 576. For wells generally see J. F. Champ, 'Bishop Milner, Holywell and the cure tradition',

The practitioner

Dyer was himself actively engaged in medical practice, although strictly as an unpaid amateur, receiving only the occasional present for his pains. His medical practice was of two kinds: electrical and prescriptive. The prescriptive work was essentially that of an apothecary, suggesting drugs and occasionally preparing them for friends, relatives and poor people brought to his notice. The scale of his work is hard to judge. The full diary for 1762 shows him frequently engaged in prescription and electrical healing, but the abstracted diary for others years suggests much less regular practice. This probably reflects a real decline in activity after the early 1760s, but no doubt his full diary for other years would reveal a lot of routine cases. Dyer's brief training as an apothecary presumably encouraged him to help others medically, but his diary shows that several of his friends, clerical and lay, were adopting similar roles.

Some of Dyer's work involved sharing prescriptions he had received from medical contacts in London. In 1763 he received the secret recipe for a cure of cancerous breasts, based on horses' corns. In 1764 and 1783 he provided a styptic against the flow of blood, and in 1775 a liquid to cure leg ulcers and wounds. His most frequent remedy, for himself and others, was Dr James's Fever Powder, but in 1762 he also recommended and prepared decoctions of bark, Balm of Gilead pills, quicksilver, a decoction of marshmallow and elderflower, and hemlock pills.[14] All these remedies were, of course, typical of standard medical practice, and Dyer's practice probably complemented professional medicine. When one patient was ill of a fatal fever the physician called in at a late stage merely endorsed Dyer's use of Dr James's Fever Powder. An itinerant practitioner called Captain Cheyne consulted Dyer on the use of this power, and in 1762 the two collaborated on several cases, once going out together to collect hemlock. Dyer planted hemlock in his garden and prepared pills from it, using a book on the subject by Dr Storck, which he also lent to a friend.[15]

Dyer did not use his remedies blindly; he noted, and worried about, failures, as well as recording successes. In the fever case one feels that he is justifying his own diagnosis to himself by quoting the physician,

in Sheils, *Church and Healing*, pp. 153–64. For God's blessing, see e.g. 8.9.62, 23.10.62, 20.10.77.

[14] 12.7.63 (cancer); 22.2.64, 5.83 (styptic); 26.1.75 (leg liquid); 1762 *passim*.
[15] 17.5.62 (fever); 2.7.61, 4.7.61, 16.10.61, 26.5.66 (Cheyne); 15.10.62, 8.9.62, 23.10.62 (hemlock).

and when a female patient died after taking his hemlock pills he discussed the case with the surgeon called to take off her water. As well as noting lay remedies, Dyer noted when they failed, for example when the use of a potato to cure an eye disease led to the loss of the eye. Like Wesley in his *Primitive Physic*, or the correspondents to the local papers who sent in tested remedies, Dyer was trying to establish a range of safe, effective cures in a field where actual success seemed the only sure test.[16] To *his* patients Dyer may have been only one of many practitioners employed, and he noted with disgust that the woman who died after taking his hemlock pills had consulted a cunning woman as well.

Dyer's most distinctive practice was in his use of electrical therapy, and here his fame extended beyond family and friends. He was consulted, for example, by the overseers of Chew Magna, about ten miles away, about a man with rheumatism, whom Dyer felt he cured. He had fewer hopes of success when a child from Haverfordwest, whom Bristol Infirmary had been unable to cure, was brought to him, since she was mute and deaf, and had 'all the symptoms of an idiot', but he tried his best. Most of his patients were poor, but he also treated the families of several local parsons, an apothecary and the wife of a Bristol M.P. In this last case the patient declined his treatment after a few days and turned to her apothecary who 'did as much good as electricity which was none'.[17] There was considerable medical interest in his electrical practice. In 1760 the surgeon Nichols came to see Dyer's machine when he had just purchased his own, and later sought his help in a case. Dyer noted that several surgeons bought machines and one was fitted at St Peter's Hospital, Bristol, but concluded that they 'never did much good therewith, probably from want of the will and labour to attend to the application'.[18] Electrical therapy in Bristol remained

[16] 17.5.62 (fever); 26–27.10.62 (hemlock pills); 21.11.89 (potato). The library of the Wellcome Institute, London, contains many eighteenth century remedy collections, e.g. MS 3576, probably of Bristol origin. Examples of cures in the newspapers are in *Bristol Gazette* 26.9.1771, 4.6.1772 etc. For Wesley's place in this tradition see Rack, 'Doctors, demons and early Methodist healing' (note 4 above); G. S. Rousseau, 'John Wesley and *Primitive Physic*', *Harvard Library Bulletin*, xviii (1968), 242–56; R. E. Schofield, 'John Wesley and science in eighteenth-century England', *Isis*, xliv (1953), 331–40.

[17] 27.3.61 ('numerous patients'); 19.3.61 (Chew Magna); 4.10.62 (Welsh); 22.11.60, 3.1.70 (parsons); 20.10.69, 22.1.70 (apothecary); 13.1.75 (M.P.'s wife).

[18] 17.9.60, 11.8.62 (Nichols); 17.6.60, (BCL 20095) 24.3.62 (Hospital). 19.6.64 the surgeon Abraham Ludlow did a post-mortem on an electrified patient.

most firmly associated with amateurs, including both Methodist and Anglican ministers.

Dyer's own use of electricity started in 1760, when he obtained his first machine from London. He had first seen an electrical experiment in 1758 at the house of another clerk, Thomas Adlam. But he tells us that in 1760 he 'proposed to try its effect on bodily disorders having read Lovett and also Wesley's treatises on the subject and this was the first medical machine made use of in Bristol'. He later reports the successful medical use of electricity by his close friend Richard Symes, rector of St Werburgh's, the doctor Captain Cheyne, Thomas Adlam and others. Several Bristolians had copies of Dyer's machine built, including another parson.[19]

Dyer was interested in the general phenomenon of electricity, helping to set up lightning conductors and joining in electrical experiments with friends. He revised the treatise on electricity, *Fire Analysed*, by Symes, both in its first draft in 1761 and again before publication in 1771. When in London he called on leading electricians, and he also visited Lovett in Worcester. Dyer claims to have persuaded Priestley to subscribe to a work of Lovett's in 1764, and in 1766 he went with Priestley to see Symes when the former came to Bristol to visit Adlam.[20] But for Dyer, as for Symes and Wesley, the medical implications took pride of place. Dyer used his machine chiefly in chronic cases such as those of rheumatism, gout, lumbago and lameness, but also for nervous complaints such as headache, weakness of the nerves, hypochondria and melancholy, and for injuries such as burns and eye complaints. He scrupulously noted the effects, which were often negligible, but he clearly felt that he was doing some good, and continued his electrical practice into later life, if at a reduced level of activity.

Dyer's view of matter and spirit

Why was Dyer so interested in electrical medicine? One explanation is clearly his pragmatic willingness to use any possible remedy, and the fashionableness of electricity as a new cure. But this pragmatism

[19] 17.6.60 (Dyer's machine); 21.9.58 (Adlam); 17.9.60, 27.9.66 (copies).
[20] 31.12.62 (experiments); 12.10.61, 31.1.71, 15.5.71 (Symes); 13.7.63, 6.3.64 (London); 5.8.60, 4.11.64 (Lovett); 6.11.64, 25.7.64, 25.7.66 (Priestley). J. B. Becket, a Bristol bookseller, quotes Ferguson on Adlam electrifying him in Bristol for a sore throat: J. B. Becket, *An Essay on Electricity* (Bristol, 1773), p. 99. Becket was an admirer of Priestley and Franklin, rather than Symes, Lovett, etc., although he quotes their works and discusses medical electricity.

had its social and intellectual implications. Dyer's practice suggests that he shared the view of medical populists, both laymen and anti-theoretical doctors, that medicine should not seek to explain the causes of medical effects, but concentrate on the collection of case-histories to show which remedies were effective, accepting the apparent facts without worrying about fitting them into an overall theory of medicine.[21] Such empiricism was the typical defence of proponents of new remedies, be they new springs, electricity or more exotic cures, against the claims of the established physicians that such cures were theoretically impossible, and hence either fraudulent or enthusiastically motivated.

In the case of Dyer, as in that of Wesley, we can see a further dimension to this empiricism, inextricably associated with religious empiricism. Dyer was a pietist,[22] that is to say one who stressed the regeneration of the individual and his spiritual or 'heart' experience (as Dyer put it), rather than the liturgical or doctrinal aspects of religion. Like his close friend Stephen Penny, another accountant whose writings Dyer revised, he bitterly regretted the doctrinal controversies among Christians, and sought to promote a pietistic ecumenism based on the practical effects of Christian grace in the regeneration, both moral and spiritual, of the inner man.[23] In this religious search Dyer and his friends ignored sectarian boundaries, reading the pre-Reformation devotional tradition of Kempis and St Theresa, the writings of such Catholic mystics as Madam Guion and Marsay, and the works of the Protestant mystics Behmen and Law. Dyer's efforts as an editor and publicist were devoted to the spread of such writings, in close collaboration with the evangelist bookseller Thomas Mills, who played a key role in the publication of the cheap 'Repository Tracts' at the end of the century.[24]

[21] For Wesley see references in note 16 above, and for an example his letter to the *Bristol Gazette* 7.9.1789 on hops and brewing, reprinted in *Wesleyan History Society Proceedings* (hereafter *WHS Proc.*), VIII (1911–12), 165–73. Such empiricism about remedies is distinct from the 'natural history of disease' tradition which led to much epidemiological work in the later eighteenth century.

[22] I have adopted the term 'pietist' in preference to 'evangelical' because the latter stresses not only the conversion experience but a public, conversion-oriented ministry, whereas Dyer's religion was more introverted. Many suggestive parallels with German pietism will be evident to those reading Johanna Geyer-Kordesch's essay in this volume.

[23] 20.6.52, 23.6.59, 25.5.60, 19.7.62, 9.10.91; S. Penny, *Letters on the Fall and Restoration of Mankind* (Bristol, 1765).

[24] 22.2.66, 24.6.68 (Kempis); 29.6.63 (St Theresa); 17.4.59 (Poiret); 1.10.90 (Marsay); 8–10.12.62, 22.3.65, 12.12.67 (Behmen); 13.6.59, 21.7.60, 9.4.61

The link between this religious attitude and medical empiricism was made clear by Stephen Penny in his *Letters on the Fall and Restoration of Mankind*, where he explicitly paralleled the material body's need of material medicine with the soul's need of restoration. Just as the only indication of a cure was the return of health, so it was with spiritual medicine, and the path to regeneration lay in prayer, faith and good works, not in doctrinal theory.[25]

Moreover electricity in itself was a particularly important discovery in the eyes of many pietists. Dyer shared with Symes a devotion to the ideas of Jacob Behmen, as interpreted by William Law. Electricity seemed to the English Behmenists to provide natural evidence for their claim that fire was the moving force of the universe – hence Symes's title, *Fire Analysed*. Electricity showed the presence of fire in all things, and revealed it as the animating principle of the whole creation. This provided the crucial link between the worlds of spirit and matter which such thinkers sought. Electrical healing revived the animal spirits and removed the obstructions to vital life, in a process which clearly paralleled the spiritual awakening of the individual by grace. Dyer's diary contains only hints of his belief in such notions, but there seems no reason to doubt that they underlay his medical practice.[26] In the 1780s Dyer became interested in the revival of alchemy and in animal magnetism, and he attended several cures performed with the aid of the latter in Bristol, although he does not seem to have practised with

(Law); 7.12.74 (Guion); 4.77 (Marsay's Life); 11.2.75 (newspaper insertion). For Mills see 5.3.75, 26.8.75, and C. A. Muses, *Illuminations on Jacob Boehme* (New York, 1951), pp. 56 *et seq.*; J. Smith, *Supplement to Catalogue of Friends' Books* (London, 1893), p. 250; C. Walton, *Notes and Materials Towards a Biography of William Law* (London, 1854), p. 595n; DNB under Lord Macaulay, who was Mills' grandson! Typical works published by Mills are Jacob Behmen, *The Way to Christ Discovered and Described* (Bristol, 1775), with a preface by Dyer's friend Edward Fisher of Compton Greenfield near Bath; *An Address to all Orders of Men...recommending the works of William Law with three letters addressed to the author T. Mills by the late William Law* (Bath, 1781).

25 For Penny see J. Smith, *Catalogue of Friends' Books* (2 vols., London, 1867), vol. 2, pp. 364–5.

26 For Symes see Walton, *Notes and Materials*, pp. 141n, 408 (and for Dyer p. 595n); G. S. Rousseau, 'Medicine and millenarianism: the immortal Dr Cheyne', in R. Popkin (ed.), *Millenarianism and Messianism in the Enlightenment* (Berkeley, 1984), n. 92; R. Symes, *Fire Analysed* (Bristol, 1771); *WHS Proc.*, ix (1913–14), 14. For Behmenism and Law generally see S. Hutin, *Les disciples anglais de Jacob Boehme aux XVIIe et XVIIIe siècles* (Paris, 1960); D. Hirst, *Hidden Riches* (London, 1964); J. F. C. Harrison, *The Second Coming* (London, 1979), pp. 13–31; S. Hobhouse (ed.), *Select Mystical Writings of W. Law*, 2nd edn. (New York, 1948); H. Taton (ed.), *Selections from Byrom's Journal and Papers* (London, 1950).

it himself. By this time Swedenborgianism had become an important ingredient in the religious background to such scientific and medical speculation.[27]

Although electricity was a particularly important example of the link between matter and spirit, it was not the only one. Dyer used the world of spirit as an explanatory device in the material world, and also used material evidence to prove the existence of the spirit world. His diary is full of comments on the reality of the invisible world. He was very interested in prophecy, frequently noting the predictions of his friend Rachel Tucker, whose spiritual diary he prepared for publication. He often recorded dreams, both his own and others', and found their ability to foretell the future, especially forthcoming deaths, 'undeniable proof of the invisible agency and an invisible world'. He speculated that this might be explained astrologically, although he also commented that the stars could raise false effects in the imagination, so that most dreams were probably misleading.[28]

Many of Dyer's friends and relations believed that they had seen apparitions, and he records several cases of conversations held with such spirits. After dining with the itinerant preacher Captain Webb, who claimed to have seen angels and talked with spirits, Dyer's wife heard footsteps entering her bedroom and felt a weight on her bed like a lamb, but when she sat up frightened there was nothing there, and the weight ceased. In 1786 Dyer himself heard two raps at his chamber door, when nobody was there, which he interpreted in retrospect as a warning of the death of his uncle. He mentions at least four other cases where rappings or touches from spirits portended the death of a near relative. Dyer believed in the possibility of second sight or divination. In 1760 Stephen Penny told him that he had conversed with a Mangotsfield man who had known the noted Thomas Perks. Perks' dealings with a spirit, 'Malchi', whom he had raised by conjuring, were reported in a letter from Arthur Bedford, vicar of Temple, Bristol, to the Bishop of Gloucester in 1703.[29]

[27] 8.9.81, 26.8.83, 1.12.84, 17.6.85, 22.2.87, 30.1.88, 20.3.89, 11.4.89, 23.5.89, 17.2.91; for another Bristolian interested in health and animal magnetism see G. Winter, *A Compendious System of Husbandry*, 2nd edn. (London, 1797), p. xi; *idem, Animal Magnetism* (Bristol, 1801). For background see G. Sutton, 'Electrical medicine and mesmerism', *Isis*, LXXII (1981), 375–92.

[28] 29.6.66, 26.10.70, 25.1.71, 30.1.71, 13.12.82 and BCL 20097 (prophecy); 1.8.70, 15.9.70, 23.1.88, 12.3.89 (dreams).

[29] 25.5.53, 23.9.59, 18.9.69, 26.6.84 (apparitions); 17.12.72 (Webb and wife); 17.1.86 (raps); 17.8.62, 26.11.80, 29.12.84, 6.1.93 (deaths); 9.3.74, 2.2.90 (divination); 20.12.60 (Perks). *A copy of a letter sent to the Bishop of Gloucester from a clergyman of the Church of England living in Bristol* (Bristol, 1704) was

Dyer also believed in the existence and power of the devil. In 1789 he recorded a case of diabolical disturbance in Hillgrove Street, Bristol, which had lasted several years until an apparition told one of the household to place a Bible open at the ninth chapter of Luke in the doorway. By this means, Dyer commented, 'strange as it seems the adversary had not power to enter the room'.[30] Dyer's friend Henry Durbin had a daughter who was several times considered possessed. In 1769 she had convulsions in her tongue, sang and crew like a cock, while otherwise in perfect health. Dr Drummond prescribed nervous medicines but they were ineffectual and Dyer noted that the case was suspected to be supernatural. In 1775 Durbin called a further illness a possession. Only in 1788 did Dyer commit himself to an opinion on the case, when Durbin visited his daughter, by now in a lunatic asylum, and decided to test whether she was possessed by silently adjuring the devil to come out of her. The girl recovered her sanity temporarily, although she later relapsed. Dyer comments 'query whether this was not due to a want of faith or at least a continuance of faith', and recalls Jesus' saying, 'this kind goeth not forth but by prayer and fasting'. A month later Dyer records that his friend Rebecca Scudamore had begun to pray for a madman she had visited in St Peter's Hospital, and that the man became calm and was released, although he died a few months after.[31]

These two incidents in 1788 probably owed much to the interest aroused earlier in the year by the exorcism of George Lukins, 'the Yatton demoniac', by Joseph Easterbrook, the vicar of Temple, and

often reprinted, or referred to: e.g. *HMC Joint Publication* 26 no. 1273 (a letter to Philip Doddridge 10.9.1743 with a copy certified as correct by Bedford 1.1.1740); BCL 396 (mistakenly dated 1763); BCL 10364; *Arminian Magazine*, v (1782), 425; E. Sibly, *A Complete Illustration* (London, 1788), p. 1121; H. Durbin, *Narrative of some Extraordinary Affairs* (Bristol, 1800).

[30] 23.5.89. The Hillgrove Street family were involved in an earlier case of the supernatural in 1781, for which see *The Glory of the Heavenly City and Blessedness of Departed Saints graciously comforted in a vision to a young lady of Bristol on 10th October 1781*, 2nd edn. (Bristol, 1782); Walton, *Notes and Materials*, p. 620n; C. Garrett, *Respectable Folly* (Baltimore, 1975), p. 149. The central figure here was the Behmenist Thomas Langcake (another accountant), whom Dyer knew well.

[31] 10.4.69, 22.1.75, 29.11.88 (Durbin); 29.12.88 (Scudamore). On 24.6.68 Dyer records that his servant maid had a fit after he read her a sermon on judgement on Sunday. Dyer's own brother was later in a lunatic asylum, and several other associates of mystical tendencies spent similar periods of confinement: e.g. Stephen Penny's sister (16.9.69). Two Bristolians who published very strange books, Edward Goldney (*Infallible Remedies*, London, 1770) and Henry Allen (*Letters*, n.p., n.d. [Bristol, 1774–5]), had been incarcerated earlier.

six Methodist ministers. In the ensuing controversy the chief critic was
the Yatton surgeon Samuel Norman, who claimed that Lukins was
a fraud, that insanity was physical, and that the supporters of the
exorcism were Behmenist and Methodist enthusiasts. When one of
Norman's brothers murdered another brother later in the year Dyer
commented 'and yet this Samuel Norman was the great adversary of
poor George Lukins, terming him an impostor and boldly affirming
there was no such thing as a possession. But what kind of spirit
activated Norman's unhappy brother when he committed the above-
mentioned awful deed?'[32] For Dyer, as for many others who saw the
personal hand of the devil in religious temptation and sin, possession
was a possible explanation of bodily suffering, particularly as it affected
man's rational faculties. But we should note that this did not exclude
the use of physical remedies as well as spiritual ones. Dyer electrified
Durbin's daughter to cure her convulsions of the tongue.[33] Both in
terms of remedy and of explanation the supernatural may have been
turned to only when the material failed, and even then material
remedies might still have a part to play.

Belief in the power of the devil and spirits extended, in the case of
Dyer and his circle, to belief in witchcraft. This need not necessarily
have been the case. For example the Somerset author John Beaumont,
whose writings Dyer studied, held such an extensive view of the powers
of the imagination and of spirits that he rejected the hypothesis that
human witches were needed as intermediate agents.[34] Dyer was
probably more influenced by biblical texts on witchcraft and by
popular beliefs about witches than the neo-Platonist Beaumont,

[32] 13.6.88, 30.9.88. For this case see G. Lukins, *A Narrative of the Extraordinary Case of George Lukins of Yatton* (Bristol, 1788); J. Easterbrook, *An Appeal to the Public Respecting George Lukins* (Bristol, 1788); S. Norman, *The Great Apostle Unmasked* (Bristol, 1788), esp. p. 28; S. Norman, *Authentic Anecdotes of George Lukins* (Bristol, 1788); T. Jackson (ed.), *Lives of the Early Methodist Preachers*, 3rd edn. (6 vols., London, 1866), vol. 6, pp. 127–8; J. Valton's MS Autobiography in John Ryland's Library, Manchester, vol. 9 (1787–93), part 2, pp. 24, 26–7, 31; *Arminian Magazine*, XII (1789), 155–9, 264, 324, 373; F. Grose, *A Provincial Glossary*, 2nd edn. (London, 1790), section on Popular Superstition, p. 4; *Gentleman's Magazine*, LIX (1789), 501.
[33] 10.4.69.
[34] J. Beaumont, *Considerations on a Book Entitled the Theory of the Earth* (London, 1693), p. 179; idem, *Gleanings of Antiquities* (London, 1724), pp. 189–92; idem, *An Historical, Physiological and Theological Treatise of Spirits* (London, 1705), pp. 296, 391–2. For the latest study of eighteenth century witchcraft see P. J. Guskin, 'The context of witchcraft', *Eighteenth-Century Studies*, XV (1981), 48–71.

although Dyer's position was never a simple matter of accepting popular superstition.

Dyer was a central figure in the Lamb Inn witchcraft case of 1762, and it was to preserve his account of this that he spared his original diary for that year. This was the most famous Bristol witchcraft case of the century, and drew national attention, coinciding as it did with the Cock Lane ghost affair in London.[35] The family of a Bristol innkeeper, Richard Giles, were plagued by poltergeist phenomena, both in the home and in the running of his waggoning business. His daughters suffered from fits, heard voices and saw visions, and had pins stuck into them. After their father was taken ill and died suddenly, the children's fits ceased, but then returned until their mother went to a local cunning woman who agreed to perform counter-magic. The family blamed the events on a witch from the nearby village of Mangotsfield supposedly hired for ten guineas a year by a rival waggoner. Critics of the affair claimed that it was a fraud arranged by Giles to lessen the value of the inn (of which he was a tenant) so that he could buy it cheaply, and they blamed his death on the prevailing influenza. Dyer and his friends formed the core of those who accepted the supernatural character of the afflictions, and eventually came to feel a witch was involved, although they were horrified at the use of counter-magic.

The subject attracted considerable attention in the Bristol newspapers, with the rival sides taking predictable stands. The critics cited Reginald Scot on past cases of fraud, and stressed the ability of conjurors to deceive the senses, while explaining away the biblical examples as natural cases of poisoning or insanity. Dyer's group clung to a literal biblical interpretation, and claimed that the sense evidence of so many unbiased witnesses could not be false, accusing their opponents of dogmatic and deistic rationalism. During the case Dyer read widely in such authors as Beaumont, Tertullian and Casaubon. The Bedford

---

[35] 13.7.63 shows Dyer reading a pamphlet on the Cock Lane affair. For the accounts of the Lamb Inn case in the Bristol papers see *Felix Farley's Bristol Journal (FFBJ)* 6.2.1762–13.3.1762 inclusive, 8–22.5.1762, 3.8.1765. John Wesley commented that the facts were 'too glaring to be denied' but as to whether they were natural or supernatural 'contend who list about this' (*Journal*, ed. N. Curnock (8 vols., London, 1909–16), vol. 4, p. 490). Two other Anglicans looking back at the affair were torn between belief and suspicion: see S. Seyer in BCL 4533 under 1762 and G. Catcott in BCL 22477 and BCL 12196 under 1761. For Durbin's view see BCL 7957 f. 272 and Durbin, *Narrative of Some Extraordinary Affairs*. BCL 20095 7.12.62 shows that Dyer, in retrospect, still felt the matter was one of witchcraft.

letter of 1703 was discussed, and the two cases explicitly linked by answers given by the spirit to questioning, in which it identified itself with the 'Malchi' that Perks had raised. When Henry Durbin's account of the 1762 affair was published, after his death, in 1800 the Bedford letter was appended.[36]

The protagonists in the case were Dyer, Durbin, Penny, a Quaker teacher George Eaton, and several clergymen, including Symes and Thomas Rouquet, his curate. All of the investigators stressed their openmindedness, and some do seem to have decided it was a fraud, but most were convinced. Traditional methods were used to test the children, such as planting special pins, holding the children down, and putting questions to them in a variety of languages, to be answered by raps. They did their best to avoid leading questions, although their critics were not convinced. The questioning inevitably shaded into asking the spirit about itself and the source of the witchcraft, a procedure which clearly worried the interrogators and was deplored by their opponents. In the case of Giles' death traditional criteria were employed to suggest bewitchment, such as unusual symptoms and the rapid course of the illness. Evidence of threats to Giles from the suspected witch, and the concurrent testimony of another Bristolian who claimed that spirits were talking to him about the Giles' case seemed sufficient proof.

In many respects the Lamb Inn case seems like a direct throw-back to the witchcraft cases of a century before, and the mother's response in turning to counter-magic was highly traditional. The position of Dyer and his friends was, however, slightly different. In the first place they were chiefly interested in the case as one of possession, not of witchcraft, but this of course reflected the preoccupation of the intelligentsia with the atypical religious aspects of witchcraft which was already clear by the early seventeenth century.[37] Secondly, none of the protagonists made any effort to act against the witch, nor to exorcise the spirit. After 1736 witchcraft was no longer an offence, and the Canons of 1604 forbade exorcism, which seems to have carried great weight with men like Symes. The only serious effort to pray over the girls was led by the Anglican clergyman closest to Methodism, namely Rouquet. Similarly in 1788, when Easterbrook, who had been raised

---

[36] See note 29 above for Bedford's letter.

[37] For possession see D. P. Walker, *Unclean Spirits* (London, 1981), and for the continued efforts of the intelligentsia to explain the causation of possession C. Webster, *From Paracelsus to Newton* (Cambridge, 1982), ch. 4.

as a Methodist, sought the assistance of the Bristol Anglican clergy sympathetic to the notion of possession in his exorcism, they all refused, including Symes, and Easterbrook had to look to Methodist ministers for help.[38] Finally, it is clear that many Bristolians were highly sceptical of the whole notion of witchcraft, although once the story got out many local tales of similar events came to the surface. Their opponents portrayed Dyer and friends as 'Puritans' from an earlier age strayed into more enlightened times, and Dyer felt that the 'serious' were surrounded by scoffers and disbelievers.[39]

How typical were Dyer's attitudes towards medicine and religion? His behaviour as a patient shows some of the standard features of eighteenth century practice, but his attitudes to illness and health, and his own medical practice, both seem to contradict the assumption that medicine was increasingly secularized and professional. I shall now consider how Dyer fits into the general Bristol pattern. How far was Dyer unusual in his medical and scientific outlook because of his religious attitudes, and how common was his religious position? How far does Bristol evidence for medical practice and ideas reflect the interests found in Dyer's case?

[38] For Rouquet see 22.11.76; A. B. Sackett, *James Rouquet and his Part in Early Methodism* (Wesley Society History Publications No. 8, Chester, 1972); C. Atmore, *Methodist Memorial* (Bristol, 1801), p. 445; *WHS Proc.*, IX (1913–14), 11–14, 123–5, XIX (1933–5), 88–9; J. Wesley, *Letters*, ed. J. Telford (8 vols., London, 1931), vol. 4, p. 142, vol. 6, pp. 187–91; J. Clark, *Hymns on Various Occasions* (Trowbridge, 1799), p. 171; *Memoirs of the Late Revd John Clark* (Bath, 1810); C. Evans, *Death of a Great and Good Man* (Bristol, 1776). For Easterbrook see note 32 above; *WHS Proc.*, II (1899–1900), 79, XIX (1933–5), 101–4; Wesley, *Letters*, vol. 5, pp. 82–3, vol. 8, p. 260; Atmore, *Methodist Memorial*, p. 110; and the funeral sermons by ministers of several denominations published after his death in 1791.

[39] *Farley's Bristol Newspaper* 29.1.1726, 5.2.1726, 14.5.1726, 12.11.1726, and *FFBJ* 25.11.1752 are generally noncommittal but comical about witchcraft cases, although J. Latimer, *Annals of Bristol in the Eighteenth Century* (Bristol, 1893), p. 249, quotes the *Gloucester Journal* of 8.11.1743 on a Bristol witchcraft case. The local deist writer 'Amicus Veritatis' attacked such beliefs in his essays on 'Credulity' in the *Bristol Weekly Intelligencer* 23.6.1750 and 14.7.1750, and J. F. Bryant, in his *Verses* (London, 1786), p. v, recalls the efforts of his tobacconist father to drive from the credulous boy all notions of supernatural existences. For Dyer's sense of isolation see 1.6.61, and cf. 15.5.71 on the scorn poured on Symes' book. On the other hand the locally printed chapbooks still dwelt heavily on the supernatural and divine judgement, e.g. *A Most Deplorable and Astonishing Relation from Reading* (Bristol, 1724).

Dyer and religious life in eighteenth century Bristol

As it has been widely assumed that the Methodist movement, and new Dissent generally, revived popular magical and animistic attitudes, the neatest way to fit Dyer into the current framework of medical historiography would be to label him a Methodist, a local example of the Wesley of *Primitive Physic*. Dyer shared Wesley's enthusiasms for electricity and cold bathing, although Wesley disliked Dr James's Fever Powder. Dyer knew both the Wesley brothers quite well, and many other Methodist preachers, and frequently attended Methodist meetings. Close friends such as Rebecca Scudamore and Henry Durbin were Wesleyan Methodists, while others like the bookseller Mills were members of Whitefield's Tabernacle.[40]

But Dyer would not have considered himself a Methodist, and his example, like that of many of his friends, illustrates the acute difficulty of distinguishing Methodism from a range of other pietist and evangelical movements within English Protestantism. Dyer was a loyal Anglican who attended parish services with devout regularity, notably those at St Werburgh where his friend Symes was rector, and also cathedral services. Dyer praised good Anglican preaching, particularly teaching which reflected the influence of William Law, whilst disliking rationalist preachers.[41] But Dyer also attended meetings of all the Dissenting groups in the city, including the Wednesday evening prayer

---

[40] 9.10.55, 20.3.88 (Wesley); 8.57 (Howell Harris); 5.12.51, 24.2.52, early 1754 (Methodist meetings). For Durbin see *Transactions of the Bristol and Gloucestershire Archaeological Society* (*TBGAS*) *Records*, xi (1976), 105–32, for a 1783 list of Bristol Methodists: J. Wesley, *Letters*, ed. D. Baker (2 vols. so far, Oxford, 1980–2), vol. 2, p. 642; *Arminian Magazine*, xx (1797), 200–2; *WHS Proc.*, ii (1899–1900), 40–2, 107, xix (1933–5), 83, 135, 167. For Scudamore see Smith, *Catalogue of Friends' Books*, vol. 2, p. 553; *Some Particulars Relative to the Life and Death of Rebecca Scudamore* (Bristol, 1790) (which Dyer revised for publication). For Mills see note 24 above.

[41] For Methodist links to other groups see J. Walsh, 'Origins of the evangelical revival', in G. V. Bennett and J. D. Walsh (eds.), *Essays in Modern English Church History* (London, 1966), pp. 132–62, and for Bristol, J. W. Raimo, 'Spiritual harvest' (University of Wisconsin Ph.D. thesis, 1974), pp. 187–93, 202n.3. Dyer describes his early religious development in a note at the end of 1757, and a good sense of his hectic and varied religious observations can be gained from the entries for early 1754. See also 24.2.52 (Symes); 10.2.58 (cathedral); 20.6.52 (Bishop Butler as his spiritual father because he confirmed him); 7.11.55, 14.8.74, 25.12.90 (pro-Law Anglican preaching); 11.8.82, 8.9.82, 3.10.82 (rational Anglicanism). For the complex links of Methodism to other Evangelicals in Bristol see Sackett, *James Rouquet* and L. E. Elliott-Binns, *Early Evangelicals* (London, 1953), pp. 332–7.

meetings run by William Morrish, a lay preacher. Dyer also had many Quaker friends, and his younger brother Samuel, whose education he sponsored, became a noted Quaker preacher.[42]

In other words Dyer practised that ecumenical pietism which he professed, valuing in all the groups that spiritual regeneration which to him was the essence of religion, and regretting the sectarian controversies which divided them. After a sympathetic account of Quaker principles Dyer finally concludes that their rejection of worldliness, which he supported, was paradoxically too much based on outward matters like dress, and too little on the inner workings of the spirit. Dyer's own metaphysical preference was for the doctrines of Law and Behmen, which he saw as the surest foundation for such a religious outlook, but he records disagreements with friends on the subject of Law's ideas, which Dyer did not perceive as destroying their fundamental unity of purpose.[43]

In Bristol at least there is some evidence that religious affiliations *were* broadly drawn along the lines Dyer perceived, with a pietistic alliance between dissenters of all kinds, Methodists and high church Anglicans on one side, and Presbyterians and low church Anglicans on the other. Dyer noted that Morrish had moved from the systematic

[42] 22.5.51 (Presbyterian ordination); 25.1.53 (opening of Tabernacle); 5.12.53 (new gallery in St James opened); 16.8.52 and early 1754 (Morrish). Symes also held evening meetings in his house for the like-minded (4.10.54). Dyer's brother Samuel has a biography in the Quakers' *Piety Promoted*.

[43] 21.9.80 (Quakers); 1.5.62 (disagreement on Law); 5.87, 1.10.90, 9.10.91 for ecumenical friends. Cf. his favourable comments on local non-Jurors 7.56 and in 1786. Many of Dyer's friends illustrate the complex religious affiliations of the time, particularly in relation to the Quakers. Stephen Penny was buried as a Quaker 'not in unity' (Smith, *Catalogue of Friends' Books*, vol. 2, pp. 364–5) but was also a Behmenist and Swedenborgian: see Walton, *Notes and Materials*, pp. 45–6, 597n; Hirst, *Hidden Riches*, pp. 200, 237, 247; *Memoirs of William Cookworthy* (London, 1854), p. 54 (Cookworthy was another Quaker Swedenborgian with strong Bristol links). The Quaker schoolmaster James Gough, of Bristol and Dublin, whom Dyer met (23.4.63), published lives of Lady Guion (Bristol, 1772), and Armelle Nicolas (Bristol, 1772) and *Select Lives of Foreigners Eminent in Piety* (Bristol, 1773), amongst other works (see Smith, *Catalogue of Friends' Books*, vol. 1, pp. 852–5). According to the 1982 edition of Wesley, *Letters*, vol. 2, p. 378 Wesley knew Gough and the Bristol edition of Gough's *Life of Guion* was abridged by Wesley. The Bristol Quakers retained a tie with the earlier mysticism of the French prophets, for whom see: H. Schwartz, *The French Prophets* (Berkeley, 1980), pp. 206, 289, 311; Raimo, 'Spiritual harvest', pp. 165–8; S. Hobhouse, *William Law and Eighteenth-Century Quakerism* (London, 1927). The chief Bristol figure was Thomas Whitehead, but May Drummond preached in Bristol and her *Internal Revelation the Source of Saving Knowledge* was reprinted in Bristol in 1736.

divinity of the old-style Puritans towards the ideas of Law, and the trend seems general. Many of the Anglican ministers like Symes were attracted by aspects of Methodism, which was still seen very much as a tendency not a party. Quakers, Baptists and Independents were similarly attracted to Methodism and to each other, and the Methodists in turn regularly lost members to these churches.[44] In such a fluid, pluralistic religious setting certain key themes seemed much more important than actual church affiliation, although the problems affiliation created could never be ignored.

One of the key dividing lines was the issue of the Trinity, on which Anglican Trinitarians of the high church could ally with Calvinist dissenters against the unitarian tendencies of Presbyterians and some other Anglicans. Dyer and his friends deplored such doctrinal quarrels, and Penny's *Letters on the Fall and Restoration of Mankind* first appeared in the Bristol papers as a plea for a non-sectarian pietism to end wranglings over the Trinity.[45] But behind this doctrinal dispute was a deeper issue (in which Dyer and his friends were broadly on the Trinitarian side) concerning the nature of revelation, the relations of matter and spirit, and the nature of religious conviction. Here Dyer represented the attitude of all those who feared the rise of deism and infidelity more than the risk of enthusiasm, and also, perhaps, those whose commitment to popular evangelism made them more sensitive to the persistent beliefs and fears of ordinary Bristolians. Suspicious as they might be of popular superstition, they could not afford to despise popular culture.[46]

It is possible to portray this mid-century alliance as a new development, representing a swing of the pendulum back from the widespread secularization of the early eighteenth century, and Wesley presumably saw his movement as such a revival. But in Bristol at least

[44] See notes 41–3 above, and for general comments on the influence of the mystics G. Rowell, 'Origins and nature of Universalist societies in Britain 1750–1850', *Journal of Ecclesiastical History*, XXII (1971), 35–56. Apart from Morrish and Symes, the main Behmenist influence on Dyer was the Rev. Fowler Comyns, who visited Bristol in December 1755.

[45] The Trinitarian dispute filled the Bristol papers in late 1765 and early 1766, with several pamphlets published by the main antagonists, Edward Harwood and Caleb Evans. For Penny's contribution see note 23 above. The significance of the dispute emerges clearly from the comments in C. H. Parry (ed.), *Memoirs of the Revd. Joshua Parry* (London, 1872), pp. 52–68.

[46] Although he stresses the Anglican fear of enthusiasm, MacDonald is well aware of this other facet of Anglican concern. See MacDonald, 'Religion, social change and psychological healing', pp. 121–2.

the evidence suggests a great deal of continuity of concern for these issues amongst those who wrote on scientific and religious matters, whilst presumably popular belief remained relatively unaffected by the mechanical philosophy. Wesley praised the ministerial devotion of Arthur Bedford, vicar of Temple until 1713, and of the Catcotts, father and son, the latter also vicar of Temple before 1779. Bedford's letter on spirits has already been mentioned, and he was a violent opponent of deism and Socinianism, and a critic of Newton's scientific and chronological work.[47] The Catcotts were the leading disciples in Bristol of the doctrines of John Hutchinson, another critic of Newtonianism. Hutchinsonianism attempted to link the worlds of matter and spirit, offering a direct physical cause for gravity in place of Newton's abstract mathematical one, and in doing so sought to show the primacy of biblical revelation, in particular of the doctrine of the Trinity and the reality of the Deluge.[48]

[47] On Methodism generally see Walsh, 'Origins of the evangelical revival'. For Bedford see note 29 above; Wesley, *Letters* (Oxford edn.), vol. 1, p. 254; Wesley, *Journal*, vol. 6, pp. 305–6; Bedford's letters in Temple Archives in Bristol Archives Office; *Animadversions on Sir Isaac Newton's Doctrine... Chronology* (London, 1728); *Scripture Chronology Demonstrated* (London, 1730); *DNB*. Bedford is also cited as one of the clergymen in a case of diabolic temptation in the chapbook *Heaven's Judgement on Gamesters, Drunkards and Seekers of Revenge* (reprinted Ellesmere, n.d.). Bedford's friend the Rev. Benjamin Bayly of Bristol, mentioned in the Perks case, was also interested in enthusiasm: see his *Essay on Inspiration* (London, 1707), discussed in H. Schwartz, *Knaves, Fools, Madmen and that Subtile Effluvium* (Gainesville, Florida, 1978), pp. 43–5.

[48] For the Catcotts see M. Neve and R. Porter, 'Glory and geology', *British Journal for the History of Science*, x (1977), 67–70, based on the Catcott papers in BCL 1154, 6495–6, 26063, and for Hutchinsonianism generally C. B. Wilde, 'Hutchinsonianism, natural philosophy and religious controversy in eighteenth-century Britain', *History of Science*, xviii (1980), 1–24; *idem*, 'Matter and spirit as natural symbols in eighteenth-century British natural philosophy', *British Journal for the History of Science*, xv (1982), 99–131; D. Greene, 'Augustinianism and empiricism', *Eighteenth-Century Studies*, i (1967–8), 33–68; G. N. Cantor, 'Revelation and the cyclical cosmos of John Hutchinson', in L. Jordanova and R. Porter (eds.), *Images of the Earth* (Chalfont St Giles, 1979), pp. 3–22. The Trinitarian theme is clearest in A. S. Catcott, *The Supreme and Inferior Elohim* (London, 1736). The Catcotts and their Hutchinsonian friends also saw electricity as a refutation of Newtonianism, whilst disliking the electrical doctrines of Franklin and Priestley: e.g. G. Stevens to A. Catcott 28.3.1752, 27.4.1752 in BCL 26063. The Catcotts were probably related to Symes, as A. Catcott was in correspondence with a relative Wroth Symes (BCL 26063 23.10.1773) and his brother was George Symes Catcott. Another relation, Anne Sherman, was interested in the mystics as well as Hutchinson (BCL 26063 late 1761 on). Dyer's friend the Rev. Arthur Hart wrote a long poem in praise of

These men did not necessarily agree with one another about metaphysics: for example Bedford attacked the elder Catcott's Hutchinsonian sermon delivered to the Bristol assizes in 1736, and also attacked early Methodism. The Catcotts were suspicious of both Methodism and mysticism.[49] But there were close intellectual parallels between the interests and methods of these men and the later pietists, and also biographical ties. Intellectually they all shared an aversion to the mechanist version of Newtonianism which won popular currency. They attacked this on empiricist grounds, as a form of dogmatic rationalism, and also on scriptural grounds as inconsistent with biblical revelation and thus destructive of religion. They sought to offer an account based on biblical evidence, as well as empirical proof, which would show the close ties of the worlds of spirit and nature, based on the analogies between the natural world and man's spiritual condition. The interest of such thinkers in the notion of analogy as a key to the natural world set them apart, and helps to explain their interest in animistic and correspondence theories.

A major figure in this intellectual tradition was the Bath doctor George Cheyne, and he also provided a personal link between various key figures. Cheyne came to the Bath area from a background in Scotland amongst the pietist school of Episcopalians centred on Aberdeen, who cultivated the French mystic traditions which so influenced Law and then Dyer.[50] Several of Cheyne's books were translated by the Wells physician John Robertson, a Hebraist and close friend of the Catcotts and other Hutchinsonians. Robertson was also

A. S. Catcott (BCL 26063 29.11.1737, 10.5.1738). Wellcome MS 3576, mentioned in note 16 above, includes notes from Dr Cheyne (see note 50 below) as well as the Catcotts, whilst in 1734 A. S. Catcott was on a milk diet, of the sort recommended by Cheyne (BCL 26063 20.7.1734).

[49] A. Bedford wrote *The Doctrine of Assurance* (London, 1738) against Wesley, but for Wesley's mild response see Wesley, *Letters* (Oxford edn.), vol. 1, p. 254. A. Bedford's *Observations on a Sermon* (London, 1736) produced replies from A. S. Catcott, Julius Bate, Daniel Gittins and John Hutchinson himself. For Hutchinsonian suspicions of Law see the *DNB* entry for George Horne, and Catcott's reservations about Dyer's edition of Guion (7.12.74).

[50] A full account of the intellectual traditions discussed below in relation to Wesley is given in J. Orcibal, 'The theological originality of John Wesley and Continental Spirituality' in R. Davies and G. Rupp (eds.), *A History of the Methodist Church in Great Britain*, vol. 1 (London, 1965), pp. 83–111. The best account of Cheyne is Rousseau, 'Medicine and millenarianism', but see also G. Bowles, 'Physical, human and divine attraction in the life and thought of George Cheyne', *Annals of Science*, xxxi (1974), 473–88. These provide a very different view of Cheyne from that of Porter, 'The "Rage of Party"'.

a correspondent of Wesley, who discussed Hutchinsonianism with him, concluding that such theories had demolished the foundations of vulgar Newtonianism even if he did not fully accept their alternatives.[51] Wesley was a great admirer of Cheyne. Down from Scotland with Cheyne came his brother-in-law, John Middleton, son of the Episcopalian writer Patrick Middleton. Middleton was the Wesleys' physician in Bristol, and Charles Wesley wrote a poem on his death, while the Wesleyan *Arminian Magazine* later reprinted a very long poem on Middleton's death as an awakened man.[52]

There is little room to doubt that these traditions affected Dyer and his friends. Cheyne was a key figure in the spread of Behmen and the mystics in England, and a major influence on William Law. The young Richard Symes was apparently a disciple of Cheyne. Dyer records in his diary the deaths of Cheyne, Middleton and the younger Catcott. His friend Stephen Penny, who lived in Portsmouth before he came to Bristol, was in correspondence with Law and interested in Hutchinsonianism. When the first Swedenborgian writings were published in England in 1749 Penny wrote enthusiastically to the publisher inquiring whether the anonymous pieces were by any chance

[51] John Robertson translated G. Cheyne, *De Natura Febrae* (London, 1725) and *Tractatus de Infirmarum Sanitate Tuendo* (London, 1726), edited J. Garden, *Comparative Theology* (Bristol, 1756) and wrote *The Ancient Manner of Reading Hebrew* (London, 1747), defending the Hutchinsonian approach of reading without points. There are many letters by him in BCL 26063 to the Catcotts. For his links with Wesley see Wesley, *Letters* (Oxford edn.), vol. 2, p. 342; *WHS Proc.*, v (1905–6), 15; *Arminian Magazine*, III (1779), 89–91, IV (1780), 352–8. Robertson was an Aberdeen M.D.

[52] Robertson refers frequently to Middleton in his letters (e.g. BCL 26063 17.4.1738). *Arminian Magazine*, VI (1783), 445, 502, 557 (the long poem on Middleton's death as an awakened man) notes that he died in the arms of his beloved friend Dr Robertson of Wells. On the Middletons of Aberdeen see G. Henderson, *Mystics of the North-East* (Aberdeen, 1934), p. 26 and *passim*; Patrick Middleton, *An Inquiry into the Inward Call to the Holy Ministry*, 1st edn. (Cambridge, 1741) and reprinted (Bristol, 1743), edited by his son 'J.M.'; *WHS Proc.*, III (1901–2), 14–17, XIX (1933–5), 36–7; Wesley, *Letters* (1931 edn.), vol. 1, pp. 358–60; C. Wesley, *Journal*, ed. T. Jackson (London, 1849), vol. 1, p. 248, vol. 2, pp. 61–3; Taton, *Selections...Byrom*, p. 211; C. F. Mullett (ed.), *Letters of G. Cheyne to S. Richardson* (Columbia, Missouri, 1943), p. 130; *idem* (ed.), *Letters of G. Cheyne to Countess of Huntingdon* (Huntington Library, 1940), pp. 21, 33; *Bristol Chronicle* and *FFBJ* for 20.12.1760. Middleton was also a friend of the Heylyn family. Law was the curate of Dr Heylyn in London, and Heylyn's library ended up in Bristol City Library (BCL 29739) after the suicide of his son John, who lived in Bristol, lodging for some time with Middleton (his diary is BCL 18871). Henderson, *Mystics of the North-East*, p. 189 records that Dr Heylyn was in Bristol in 1723.

by William Law, or else by a Hutchinsonian, as he discerned in all these groups a common concern to relate the Old as well as the New Testament to natural philosophy.[53] Wesley was strongly aware of the mystical tendencies in Bristol Methodism, whose introspective pietism did not entirely suit his evangelistic mission. Many who welcomed Methodism as a non-sectarian movement with its stress on spiritual awakening opposed its later development into an evangelistic church, and some of these people were attracted to the Swedenborgians or other congregations of like-minded pietists. Interestingly the roll-call of early Swedenborgians in London is full of accountants, instrument-makers, booksellers and others in the same intellectual and social milieu as Dyer.[54]

Medicine and religion in eighteenth century Bristol

For those who sought to relate matter and spirit, and stressed the analogies between the natural world and man's spiritual condition, medicine was of necessity a central issue. The drama of revelation and

[53] For Symes see note 26 above. Dyer's comments on Cheyne (30.3.52) are in marked contrast to the obituary of the 'dictator of physic' in the whig *Bristol Oracle and Country Intelligencer* 16.4.1743. 30.3.56, 30.12.60 (Middleton); 18.6.79 (Catcott). For Penny see 13.6.60; R. Hindmarsh, *Rise and Progress of the New Jerusalem Church* (London, 1861), pp. 4–5; note 43 above.

[54] Wesley was interested in the French prophets, and his publications included many from the Continental mystics, Quaker quietists and from Law, including *An Extract from Mr Law's Later Works* (2 vols., Bristol, 1768), but for his distrust of mysticism see *Letters* (1931 edn.), vol. 4, p. 341; *Arminian Magazine*, III (1780), 552–8. For the relations of mystics to Methodists in Bristol and elsewhere in 1775 see the account by Ralph Mather printed in Walton, *Notes and Materials*, pp. 595–6n. The Bristol Methodist Thomas Maxfield led a separatist movement away from Wesley, in part on the issue of illumination. Late eighteenth century Bristol Methodism was deeply divided on the issue of setting up a separate church, with Durbin one of the chief opponents (*WHS Proc.*, II (1899–1900), 42; XIX (1933–5), 135–42). John Whitehead, in his *Life of the Rev. John Wesley* (2 vols., London, 1793), vol. 1, pp. 353, 355–6, was strongly critical of separation, and he was another Bristol convert, whom one is tempted to link with the French prophet Thomas Whitehead mentioned in note 43 (see Smith, *Catalogue of Friends' Books*, vol. 2, pp. 915–16; *DNB*). Two leading early Swedenborgians in London were from Bristol: Manoah Sibly, brother of Ebenezer, and John Hindmarsh, who had taught at Wesley's Kingswood school near Bristol (Hindmarsh, *Rise and Progress*, p. 59). For the Swedenborgians and separatism see W. R. Ward, 'Swedenborgianism: heresy, schism or religious protest?', in D. Baker (ed.), *Studies in Church History*, IX (Cambridge, 1972), pp. 303–9. An interesting commentary on the vitality of such groups is provided by Robert Southey, himself a Bristolian, in *Letters from England* (3 vols., London, 1807), vol. 2, pp. 337 *et seq.*

redemption had to be played out in the health of the individual. The theme underlies the work of Dr George Randolph, whose account of the Bristol waters was the most thorough of the period, and highly respected. Randolph was a Hutchinsonian, and also an admirer of the young William Law, although he repudiated Law's later Behmenism. His accounts of spa waters start with attacks on the pretensions of mechanical theory to predict accurately the workings of the body, or the claims of the chemists to do any better. He proceeds rather by an examination of the proven cases of cure, and a historical account of the uses of the waters. His Bristol treatise ends with a discussion of the origins of spring waters which concludes that they show the presence of a great abyss, and hence the reality of the Deluge, which he explains by air pressure in true Hutchinsonian fashion.[55]

Although Bristol doctors held very varied political, religious and intellectual positions, a large proportion appear to have been high church Tories, like many of the minor clergy. C. B. Wilde has suggested that the Hutchinsonian solution to the matter–spirit debate reflected the social concern of Tory Anglicans at social developments in the country. An analysis of the regimens produced by medical populists, often Tory physicians, in the early eighteenth century has suggested that they were essentially vehicles to preach temperance and morality against luxury and corruption. Their stress on different regimens for different classes in society was intended to restore a threatened social stability. This response to the problem of 'luxury' has usually been related to the civic humanist tradition of political discourse, but I would suggest that the religious component is equally crucial.[56]

55 G. Randolph, *An Inquiry into the Medicinal Virtues of Bristol Waters* (Oxford, 1745) and 2nd edn. with additions (Bristol, 1750), esp. pp. 62, 164–74; *An Inquiry into the Medicinal Virtues of Bath Waters* (London, 1752); Sir J. B. Park, *Memoirs of the Late William Stevens* (London, 1859), p. 10; *Some Particulars...* R. Scudamore, p. 16; *Bristol Weekly Intelligencer*, 24.11.1750 'Lines written after reading Dr Randolph's Inquiry'; *FFBJ* 28.4.1764 (obituary). See the *DNB* for the Trinitarian activities of Randolph's relations, Thomas (1701–83) and Francis (1752–1831). BCL 26063 contains two letters of Randolph to the Catcotts, one undated, the other 4.3.1759, whilst Jones, Horne, Stevens etc. constantly refer to Randolph in their letters. Doctors Bave, Harington and Charlton of Bath appear to be part of the same tradition.

56 Wilde, 'Matter and spirit'. Cf. Hutchinsonian pleasure at the Tory victory in Bristol in 1756 (BCL 26063 29.3.1756). My information on regimen books is drawn from an unpublished paper by Cathy Crawford, for whose assistance on this point I am most grateful. On luxury see J. Sekora, *Luxury* (Baltimore, 1975) and J. G. A. Pocock, *The Machiavellian Moment* (Princeton, 1975).

Medical matters could have a much more direct political or religious significance. The ability of a Divine Right monarch to cure the King's Evil by touch raised in stark form the issues of material causation and political legitimacy. Two leading Tory doctors in Bristol, John Lane and Samuel Pye, gained notoriety in 1716 for their attestation that a local labourer had been cured by the Old Pretender. When Thomas Carte printed the story in his *History of England* there was a tremendous Whig outcry, both in Bristol and London, and strenuous efforts to disprove the story.[57] The interest in animal magnetism and astrological medicine of many quacks and laymen in the late eighteenth century did not leave local medical men unaffected. Ebenezer Sibly records that the much-respected Quaker doctor John Till-Adams was interested in astrological medicine, and Dyer refers to the same doctor reading Law's works to sick patients.[58] Till-Adams was a friend of the evangelicals gathered around Hannah More, who included Symes and Mills, as well as Sir James Stonhouse, physician turned clergyman, whose handbooks for the comfort of the sick were distributed cheaply by the evangelists.[59] There is some evidence to suggest that patients valued doctors of their

[57] T. Carte, *History of England* (London, 1747), vol. 1, p. 291; *DNB* under Carte; *Bristol Memorialist* (Bristol, 1823), pp. 65–70. For Pye as a Tory Anglican see BCL 11156–7 (Southwell papers); W. Barrett, *History and Antiquities of the City of Bristol* (Bristol, 1789), p. 471; *FFBJ*, 22.9.1759, 11.2.1760, and Feb.–Mar. 1765 for a quarrel over his medical methods. *Bristol Oracle* 23.1.1748 and *Bristol Weekly Intelligencer* 31.8.1751 (both Whig papers) both attack the King's Evil story, and the latter also the 'miraculous' claims for Glastonbury water.

[58] For Sibly and Till-Adams see *Ars Quatuor Coronatorum*, LXXI (1958), 48–53 and on Sibly, A. Debus, 'Scientific truth and occult tradition: the medical world of Ebenezer Sibly 1751–1799', *Medical History*, XXVI (1982), 259–78 and Muses, *Illuminations on Jacob Boehme*, p. 69 for his use of Law. For Till-Adams see 5.9.82; *Arminian Magazine*, v (1782), 325; BCL 9406; W. Matthews, *Miscellaneous Companions* (2 vols., Bath, 1786), vol. 1, p. 13; Bevan-Naish Collection, Woodbridge College, Selly Oak, MS 1227 (diary of S. Fox), ff. 95, 106, 120, 136, 191–2; P. J. Anderson, *Officers and Graduates of University and King's College Aberdeen* (Aberdeen, 1893), p. 103, where Dyer's friend Thomas Robins, cathedral precentor and admirer of Law, received a D.D. in 1783 on the recommendation of Easterbrook, Till-Adams and another minister. Ebenezer Sibly was an Aberdeen M.D., and in 1789 the Bristol Baptist minister in the 1760s Trinitarian dispute, Caleb Evans, received an Aberdeen D.D.

[59] For this circle see H. Roberts, *Memoirs of the Life...H. More*, 2nd edn. (London, 1834); Rev. J. Stedman (ed.), *Letters of the Rev. J. Orton and Sir J. Stonhouse*, 2nd edn. (2 vols., Shrewsbury, 1800), vol. 2, *passim* esp. p. 275; Sir J. Stonhouse, *Everyman's Assistant and the Sick Man's Friend*, 3rd edn. (Bath, 1794). Walton, *Notes and Materials*, p. 141 claims More, Mills and Symes met to discuss Law.

own religious persuasion, whose healing art might include religious support. All the denominations of the city had their medical adherents, including the Methodists, who attracted more medical men than might have been expected, given their failure to attract other professional or well-established groups.[60]

There is considerable evidence to suggest that patients still sought a spiritual interpretation of illness, as Stonhouse and others realised. In the early eighteenth century the state of public health, for example during the smallpox epidemic or under the threat of plague, was still seen in the sermons of both Anglicans and dissenters as related to God's judgement on national sins, requiring the reformation of manners and the revival of religion. Although other phenomena, such as earthquakes, were still interpreted providentially much later, this particular tradition seems to have ceased, but similar judgements were still passed on personal health.[61] Popular poems on health and illness portrayed the body as an economy, analogous to the world, so established as to punish sin with illness; and disease in general was seen as the outcome of original sin. Such notions could justify arguments for moderation in enjoyment of the pleasures of the world, but there was an equally strong tradition of distrust of this world, as the realm of Satan or at least a place of sorrow and temptation. Within the latter tradition illness was both a punishment and a salutary reminder of the need to look to the things of the spirit. Even death could be seen as a blessing, and a victory for the awakened, and this theme is repeated constantly in the many poems on the recently dead published in the local papers. Interest in illness and the death–bed scene remained intense, and sudden death without the chance of repentance was a dread occurrence.[62]

---

[60] For a bedside scene including a doctor of the denomination see *Piety Promoted* (4 vols., London, 1789), vol. 2, p. 325 on Dr Logan at Esther Champion's death in 1714. Apart from doctors the only other 'professional' or intellectual groups well represented among the Methodists in Bristol were printers and booksellers.

[61] M. Pope, *A Discourse on Afflictions* (London, 1703); S. Gough, *A Discourse Occasioned by the Small-pox and Plague now Raging in Europe* (London, 1711, for J. Penn in Bristol); W. Goldwin, *Sermon on Fast-Day for the Plague* (Bristol, n.d. [1722]). For Dyer's interest in earthquakes and other astronomical and terrestrial signs see 17.12.70, 12.5.71, 9.9.75.

[62] See note 5 above and 23.2.80, 2.86. An edition of E. Baynard, *Health: A Poem* was printed in Bristol *c.* 1750. Barrett, *History...of Bristol*, pp. 185, 611 refers to the effects on health of drinking and idleness. Barrett was a Tory surgeon. A classic example of the death-bed scene is that of William Fry (1723–76) in *Piety Promoted*, 9th part (London, 1789), pp. 79–83. For an example of illness correlated with spiritual changes see *The Life of Mary Dudley* (London, 1825), pp. 19–27.

If Jewson is right in seeing medical practice as patient-centred, needing to satisfy the patient's notion of illness, then doctors' theories and practices should have been sensitive to such interpretations of illness.[63] The stress on regimen, in particular control of the intake and output of food, together with bleeding, purging and emetics, would appear remedies suitable for patients needing to expiate guilt for the sins which had made them ill. The doctor could act simultaneously as judge and comforter. The expression of this relationship in a medical vocabulary, rather than a directly religious exhortation to morality or godliness, and the replacement of the minister by the doctor as the main figure clearly represent a major change, but I would not see this as simply a matter of secularization, nor even as the retreat by religion from areas where enthusiasm might blossom. The most important factor was probably religious pluralism. Whatever the strength of their personal religious convictions, and their effect on their medical outlook, the doctors of eighteenth century Bristol could not afford to express their ideas in overtly religious vocabulary, as this could only alienate potential customers.

Similarly trends can be seen outside the field of doctor–patient relationships, in the development of Bristol's medical institutions. Bristol's first hospital, St Peter's, was established as a workhouse as part of the campaign to reform manners in 1697, and soon developed an important surgical side, in which the cure of venereal disease served as a constant reminder of the links between poverty, morality and disease. The Infirmary, started in 1737, was publicized from its earliest days by the Anglican clergy as a centre for the moral and religious reform of the poor, as well as their physical recovery, and religious tracts were placed in the wards and given to those who recovered. The Infirmary was a consciously ecumenical effort, attracting many Quakers, Anglicans and Presbyterians as supporters, and its management was held up as an example of what Christian ecumenism could achieve. Even here there may be an undercurrent of opposition between the Infirmary supporters and St Peter's Hospital, managed by the Corporation of the Poor which was dominated by Anglican Tories hostile to the Whig City Corporation.[64]

[63] For Jewson see note 2.
[64] For St Peter's Hospital see J. Johnson, *Transactions of the Corporation of the Poor* (Bristol, 1826). For the Infirmary see G. Munro Smith, *History of Bristol Royal Infirmary* (Bristol, 1917), and the many sermons preached on behalf of the Infirmary: e.g. J. Castleman, *Sermon...Infirmary* (London, 1744), pp. 23 *et seq.*; W. Davies, *Sermons on Religious and Moral Subjects* (Bristol, 1754), p. 263 (Davies became chaplain to the Infirmary).

The fashionable Hotwells spa, despite its hedonistic lifestyle, was still the subject of religious interpretations, as we have seen, while a Wesleyan preacher, John Dolman, ran the rival New Hotwells as a godly alternative. The Methodists were the chief force behind the two Dispensaries established in the city. In 1747 Wesley set up a Bristol Dispensary shortly after his London one, and published *Primitive Physic* to help the good work. The Dispensary seems to have soon closed, but Wesley's book was often reprinted in Bristol. In 1775 the Whitefield Methodists at the Tabernacle established a Dispensary, whose committee met at the bookshop of Dyer's friend Mills. Dyer himself started the local branch of the 'Society for the Rescue of Persons Apparently Drowned' in the same year. Although there are few discussions of the religious purposes of the society, which was of obvious utility in a port, there are indications that support for teaching resuscitation was based at least in part on horror at the spiritual consequences of sudden death, or even worse of suicide.[65]

Bristol's role in improving the care of the mentally ill also owed much to religious motivations. The chief pioneer was the Baptist layman Joseph Mason, who treated his patients both physically and spiritually, combining humane care with daily prayer meetings, often administered by Baptist ministers from Bristol.[66] Perhaps because they were themselves accused of madness so often, the Bristol Methodists seem to have become champions of those accused of insanity.[67] The

[65] J. Dolman, *Contemplations amongst Vincent's Rocks* (Bristol, 1755), 2nd edn. (Bristol, 1772) and see note 12. For Wesley's Dispensary see A. Wesley Hill, *John Wesley Among the Physicians* (London, 1958), pp. 11–13, 46–8; Wesley, *Letters* (Oxford edn.), vol. 2, p. 225; *Letters* (1931 edn.), vol. 7, p. 17; references note 16. For the Tabernacle Dispensary see R. Smith, 'Biographical Memoirs' of Bristol Infirmary in Bristol Archives Office (BAO) in 14 vols.: vol. 1, f. 72; vol. 2, 682–90, 876; vol. 3, 7–9, 13 *et seq.*, 55; vol. 14, 226: *Bonner and Middleton's Bristol Journal*, 18.11.75, 30.12.75; *Plan of the Friend in Need* (Bristol, 1791). The doctors who helped with the Dispensary in its early days were mostly Nonconformists and Methodists, including Till-Adams. In the 1790s the millenarian William Bryan nearly became the Dispensary druggist: see 22.2.94 and J. F. C. Harrison, *The Second Coming* (London, 1979), pp. 71–2. For Society for the Rescue of Persons Apparently Drowned see 2–6.6.75, 26.6.75, 18.7.75; *Bristol Journal* 1.7.75, 29.7.75, 12.8.75, 26.8.75; BAO 04217 f. 35; J. J. Abraham, *Lettsom* (London, 1933).
[66] H. T. Phillips, 'Old private lunatic asylum at Fishponds', *Bristol Medico-Chirurgical Journal*, LXXXV (1970), 41–4; MS Mason's diary for 1763 in Bristol University Medical School Library; C. Evans, *The Hope of the Righteous in Death* (Bristol, 1780), preached at the chapel Mason had erected at his own expense at Stapleton.
[67] The Durbin family are recorded as helping people accused of madness in *The Genuine Trial of Grant Cottle* (Bristol, 1771) and E. Keate, *The Unfortunate Wife* (London, 1779), pp. 21–4.

former Methodist preacher Richard Henderson turned his school at Hanham near Bristol into a lunatic asylum, and his methods were applauded by Wesley, More, Stonhouse and Till-Adams.[68]

Henderson is famous chiefly because of his son John, whose brilliant promise and early death (unfulfilled) fascinated late eighteenth century intellectuals. John Henderson's intellectual quest led him deep into the occult sciences, including Behmenism, astrology and witchcraft, while his humanitarian concerns were expressed by his unofficial medical practice amongst the poor.[69] Although Henderson, through his friendship with Dean Tucker, Hannah More and Samuel Johnson, has attracted much more attention, it may well be that William Dyer, the obscure provincial, is a more significant representative of a strand of thought far too long neglected.

We shall not be able to establish with confidence the relationship between religion and medicine in eighteenth century England until we understand much more about the religious history of the period, and can penetrate the surface divisions of Anglican and dissenter. Nor can we appreciate the nature of eighteenth century medicine until we dismiss simple ideas of establishment medicine and quackery/magic. In both cases greater attention to the attitudes of the layman, and the reasons for his religious and medical choices, seems the most promising way forward. Those historians who have sought to explain the religious and medical changes under the broader headings of popular and elite culture have offered intriguing signposts towards such a goal, but the crude dichotomy of popular and elite is quite incapable of encompassing the ambiguities of position of middle class, provincial town-dwellers such as Dyer. Any account which ignores that crucial class cannot offer a satisfactory picture of eighteenth century society.

I have been greatly assisted in writing this paper by comments from those who heard an earlier version at seminar series in the Wellcome Institute, London, and the Wellcome Unit, Oxford, and by the advice of Michael MacDonald, Irvine Loudon and Harriet Barry.

68 'Bristol in the evolution of mental health', exhibition catalogue (Royal West of England Academy, 1961), p. 33; *Arminian Magazine*, v (1782), 322–5; Roberts, *Memoirs...More*, p. 217; *WHS Proc.*, III (1901–2), 158; Atmore, *Methodist Memorial*, pp. 183–4; J. Cottle, *Early Recollections* (2 vols., Bristol, 1837), vol. 2, p. 325; *Gentleman's Magazine*, LVI (1786), 738.

69 See note 68 above and *Gentleman's Magazine*, LVI (1786), 555, 677–80, 735, 739, LIX (1789), 210, 295–7, 789, 1031, 1122; *Notes and Queries* 1st ser., X (1854), p. 26; *Arminian Magazine*, II (1778), 662–3, XVI (1793), 140–4; Rev. J. Agutter, *Sermon...Death J. Henderson* (Bristol, 1788), esp. p. 5; J. Boswell, *Life of Dr Johnson* (2 vols., Everyman edn., London, 1906), vol. 2, pp. 518–25.

7

Cultural habits of illness: The Enlightened and the Pious in eighteenth century Germany

JOHANNA GEYER-KORDESCH

Doing justice to the patient's view is a precarious undertaking because it is a journey to uncharted regions. To help find our bearings, maps for analysis may be borrowed: those histories which have interpreted for us the work of physicians, their knowledge of diseases, or the medical profession's turning towards the hospital as a place wherein patients and their diseases are most efficiently scrutinized. But even if a patient is liable to accept with one part of his mind the medical version of what ails him, many another aspect of illness will turn to haunt the mind and the emotions, and precipitate an interpretation inconsistent with the more or less neat, and therefore also reassuring, pattern of medical analysis, with its diagnostic and prognostic functions.

In attempting a foray into such a land of variations, the only guideline will be the subjective view, the actions and thoughts of individuals as they are faced with suffering and bodily weakness. Subjective reactions are certainly conditioned by society and by personal values which temper what is done or left undone. The quirks of human nature are often most apparent in the face of unknown or dangerous situations. Whether one is stoic, frightened, resigned, disparaging or resolute can be conditioned, or it can be a response which breaks the mould. All it ultimately tells us about is how life was dealt with, but this, in itself, is an aid to interpretation.

The society examined here is that of northern, Protestant Germany, in the epoch termed the Enlightenment. As with any period, it was differentiated in its composition. The language of science and learning was Latin, the common parlance German. The religion was Protestant, but open to sectarian diversity, ranging from those smaller enclaves of religious belief which accommodated the classes not in power to the antagonism between Calvinism and Lutheranism. Nationhood in the nineteenth century sense was non-existent. Doctors were few and far between, at least those with a formal degree.[1] Enlightenment was a new ideal, envisioned and propagated by those with sufficient learning and the desire to have their habits set off from more traditional behaviour. Beliefs were still strongly held, but some already tagged with the term 'superstition', and spiritual and physical misery, as in all time, was tangible. Given this very diversity, it is justifiable to proceed according to phenomenological reality: to explain specific cases and to try and illustrate as many of the non-medical factors involved as possible.

Let us begin with the 'enlightened' men of the century and their attitudes to illness. Well-known personalities have provided comments on illness, mingled in with discussion of their more overt goals and purposes in life.[2] From the Lutheran clergy to the learned in other fields they are nervously aware that bodily affliction can ruin lives dedicated to matters seemingly more impersonal. The 'house of the soul', as the body is sometimes described,[3] must be kept in proper order for the realization of social and religious aims. Thus Philipp Jacob Spener (1635–1705), one of the great figures of Lutheran Pietism and a man of great abstemiousness, drank his glass of Hungarian Tokay every day for reasons of health. Johann Georg Sulzer (1720–79), a man of letters and a publicist on aesthetic theory, knew enough about the common rules of health to realize that when one is hot and sweaty, one does

---

[1] The relatively low figures of student enrolment for the medical faculties in the eighteenth century should caution us about claims regarding the extensive influence of learned medicine. For the enrolment of medical students, see E. Th. Nauck, 'Die Zahl der Medizinstudenten der deutschen Hochschulen im 14.–18. Jahrhundert', *Sudhoffs Archiv*, xxxviii (1954), 175–86.

[2] Obviously no systematic examination of lay attitudes to illness in the eighteenth century exists. I have approached the problem by reading into the extensive autobiographical and biographical literature of the period. Bibliographies are provided in: Ralf-Rainer Wuthenow, *Das Erinnerte Ich: Europäische Autobiographie und Selbstdarstellung im 18. Jahrhundert* (Munich, 1974); Günter Niggl, *Geschichte der deutschen Autobiographie im 18. Jahrhundert: Theoretische Grundlegung und literarische Entfaltung* (Stuttgart, 1977); Marianne Beyer-Fröhlich, *Deutsche Selbstzeugnisse*, vol. 7, *Pietismus und Rationalismus* (Leipzig, 1933); Werner Mahrholz, *Deutsche Selbstbekenntnisse: Ein Beitrag zur Geschichte der Selbstbiographie von der Mystik bis zum Pietismus* (Berlin, 1919).

[3] Mainly traceable to Pietist and sectarian works. For example Christian Friedrich Richter, *Die Höchst-nöthige Erkenntniss des Menschen...* (Leipzig, 1719). (This book went through eighteen editions in the eighteenth century.)

not stay for any length of time in a draught.[4] And yet, at a dinner invitation at the house of an '*empfindsame*' (a woman of sentimental perceptions) aristocratic lady, having dressed too warmly and becoming aware of his perspiring discomfiture, he sets himself at risk. She is inclined to open the windows of the dining hall to cultivate a romantic enjoyment of the glowering approach of a thunderstorm. Sulzer is perfectly miserable, but pays his stoic due to the manners of the times and to aesthetic appreciation. The fever originating in this episode contributes to his death seven years later.

There are cultural and individualistic traits to illness and ill-health which crack the ardently nurtured concepts of strict science. In the following I will explore two modes of 'patients' views' of particular import to the eighteenth century. They have already been indicated through the persons mentioned above: Spener and Sulzer. Biography provides the material, but my concern is not with individual lives. The approach to illness is not random and I wish to discover patterns, how these are expressed and what they mean. A cultural habit is like a gesture or a turn of phrase: it illuminates an attitude which extends beyond the individual. What seems eminently personal is not really so very atypical. Even an eccentric is only looked upon with favour in certain circles. I am therefore not concerned exclusively with the usual analysis of what constitutes the behaviour of a particular group, a 'subculture'. I am looking for a typology, an articulated approach to suffering which is recognizable and can be shared. In the *Commedia dell'arte*, for example, an individual actor articulates a stock set of characteristics. The typical expression of the role allows for easy identification by the audience: the lover, the fool, the doctor, the patient. On the other hand the individual interpretation of a character in a role presents a challenge. Perception and imagination can alter fixed roles. So, too, the sufferer transcends the particular circumstances of his or her illness as soon as he or she puts pen to paper, describes and lingers over feelings and thoughts. I do not wish to escape this fine interplay of role-casting and reflection, of narrator and audience.

[4] This and the following information from Johann Georg Sulzer, *Lebensbeschreibung von ihm selbst aufgesetzt: Aus der Handschrift abgedruckt... von Johann Bernhard Merian und Friedrich Nicolai* (Berlin, 1809), p. 54ff (cited as *Lebensbeschreibung*).

Patterns of being ill among the Enlightened

Enlightenment has a universal claim and yet the personalities and concepts which defined its image did not derive either from a mass culture or from popular ideas. The men (and in rare cases women) who invented the Enlightenment were trying to undermine prevalent modes of authority, those which cited tradition as the legitimate source of power and social stratification. The Enlightened propagated talent and belonged to that ambiguous region of writers, academics and some civil servants, later even clergymen, whose economic underpinnings were often precarious while their pen never wavered. Common-sense, the ideology of reason, and above all the legitimacy that a logical argument bestows upon 'self-evident' truths, swept away old irrational beliefs. The occult, the demonic, even man's subsidiary position before God and nature began to give way. The becoming humility or fearful dependence evident in the image of man as microcosm related to the powerful macrocosm of the forces of good and evil diminished as alchemy, astrology and magic waned. Pestilence, hunger and war had been fearfully present throughout the seventeenth century. They were no less malignant in the eighteenth. Art historians use the term 'baroque' (*Barock*) when they refer to this age, and it reminds us, as 'Enlightenment' does not, of splendid representational forms, courtly decadence, and an intruding, but prevalent, contemplation of death (*vanitas*). The Enlightenment's mental concerns did not share this pessimism, upholding instead the intrepid possibilities of virtue and reason.

The shift in ideology which initiated belief in autonomous reason and its optimistic correlates came from the well-educated middle classes and their centres of power: the educational establishments and the professions. In the reign of Frederick the Great these included philosophy and especially aesthetics, as the Academy in Berlin gained prominence.[5] The term which most efficiently expresses and summarizes the self-consciousness of the Enlightened was one which became fashionable at this time. The learned exponent of the new values was called and called himself a '*Weltweiser*';[6] this amalgamation of

[5] For the history of the Academy under Frederick II, see Adolf Harnack, *Geschichte der Königlich Preussischen Akademie der Wissenschaften zu Berlin*, vol. I.1, *Geschichte der Academie Royale des Sciences et Belles Lettres Friedrichs des Grossen (1740–1786)* (Berlin, 1900).

[6] This term is consistently applied throughout the eighteenth century. The epithet is used, for example, for 'Sulzer den Weltweisen'. The term means

'worldly' and 'knowledge' suggested someone in the know, competent, someone attuned to the world, not so much as a savant, but as a 'politick man'.

Johann Georg Sulzer had an established reputation in the Prussian capital, Berlin, among those who discussed literature, philosophy and the sciences.[7] He had been given financial gifts and land by the King and (since 1750) was a member of the Academy. Then a serious illness befell him. In the autobiographical manuscript later published by Friedrich Nicolai and Johann Bernhard Merian he relates the course of his suffering. The dramatic onset of Sulzer's illness in 1772 at a dinner party has already been described. It was the beginning of an ailment (probably tuberculosis) of which he could not rid himself until his death seven years later in 1779. The last part of his autobiographical account reveals how preoccupied he was with his health, always weighing the duties and projects upon which he was engaged against his remaining strength. He seeks relief not through medication or consultation but rather through a strategy of careful living. As he succumbed to fever in 1772 he trusted his own diagnosis, thinking he had 'a proper three-day fever'.[8] His condition worsened and he 'lets himself be transported into the city'[9] to seek medical advice. The physician told him to remain in bed, and there he is overcome by his symptoms – a high fever, and the expulsion of putrid matter so abhorrent in its smell 'that almost no one could come near me'.[10] His physician was able to reduce the fever, but his violent coughing continued. A persistent fever ('raised temperatures') weakens him for another eighteen months and he still coughs up phlegm 'in the sixth year after this fatal disease'.[11] He tries 'untold numbers of highly recommended medicines' all in vain.[12] In 1775, on the advice of Albrecht von Haller, he is told to spend the winter in Naples, but goes to Nizza instead because he had just finished reading 'the Englishman Smollett's journey through France and Italy'.[13] Needless to say, Sulzer uses his visit to produce a travel book (which appears a year after his death). Upon his return, from 1776 to 1778, he becomes increasingly ill and comments upon this state of affairs with the following words:

'someone learned in the ways of the world, in express contrast to those suffused with godly wisdom...'. See J. and W. Grimm, *Deutsches Wörterbuch*, vol. 14 (Leipzig, 1955), pp. 1724–7.

[7] *Hirzel an Gleim über Sulzer den Weltweisen* (2 vols., Zurich, 1779); J. H. Formey, *Eloge de Mr Sulzer* (Berlin, 1779); Sulzer, *Lebensbeschreibung*.

[8] Sulzer, *Lebesbeschreibung*, p. 56.   [9] *Ibid.*

[10] *Ibid.*   [11] *Ibid.*   [12] *Ibid.*   [13] *Ibid.*, p. 58.

I not only had to endure frequent and varied afflictions, but these assailed me in such a manner that I awaited my death from one month to the next. The constant idea [*Vorstellung*] that I am near death brought me to a nearly invariable state of indifference toward life, so much so that I now think I may envision death approaching without anger or resistance on my part.[14]

This remark is very revealing. It reflects an attitude applauded and reiterated by J. H. Samuel Formey (a member of the Berlin Academy and the eulogist of many of its distinguished members) in his *Eloge de Mr Sulzer*. He writes that shortly before Sulzer's death, on the occasion of his last visit, he was touched by the demeanour of this 'decorated athlete', crowned in the contest between pain and dignity.[15] 'His eye was serene' and in his conversation he would return to the vivacity indicative of health. Formey admired the detachment attained by the philosopher, who, he adds, did not spoil it by claiming the pride of the Stoic. Formey then writes a few words on the promises offered by way of religion, but the point is obviously one of manners, showing the imperturbable philosopher who is subjected to suffering but can endure and remain aloof. This is the point that Sulzer himself made by dwelling in such a detached manner upon a most agonizing seven years.

The mundane, the urbane, the *Weltweiser*, not only adopts but is appreciated ('prize-crowned') for this, his triumphant moderation in the face of his own physical decomposition, the evident signs of his own mortality. Is there justification for maintaining that this social manner of dealing with illness was particular to the Enlightened? Sulzer and Formey are in agreement precisely when their views are the objects of public attention, in the published representation of how life is to be lived, in their model support of philosophical detachment. Whatever ideology of reason the Enlightenment brings, here is its style of manners; and the most reasonable short-cut to health, the praise of the efficacy of 'modern' medical sciences, does not enter its hall of fame.

There is a history to this, and it begins with the epoch of the new 'bourgeois' predominance.[16] If the Baroque of the seventeenth century

---

14   *Ibid.*, p. 60.
15   This and the following quotes from Formey, *Eloge de Mr Sulzer*, pp. 43–4.
16   The Marxist-oriented theory of the 'rise of the bourgeoisie' is still influential for the interpretation of the German Enlightenment: Franz Borkenau, *Der Übergang vom feudalen zum bürgerlichen Weltbild* (Paris, 1934); Leo Kofler, *Zur Geschichte der bürgerlichen Gesellschaft* (Berlin, 1948); Hans Medick, *Naturzustand und Naturgeschichte der bürgerlichen Gesellschaft: Die Ursprünge der bürgerlichen Sozialtheorie als Geschichtsphilosophie und Sozialwissenschaft bei S. Pufendorf, John Locke und Adam Smith* (Göttingen, 1973).

expressed itself in its ornateness, the careful rhetoric of speeches and poems, the festivals at court, the correctly elaborate clothes of its men and women,[17] then the waning of the seventeenth century, its turn towards the Enlightenment, brought with it a different pose in worldliness.

The outward signs of the new interest, the new dictates of behavioural fashion, are most easily discernible on the book market. In the last decades of the seventeenth and the first of the eighteenth century fashionable book titles appear whose claim to attention is the phrase '*politische Klugheit*'.[18] The political world, that of government, is not directly addressed. The phrase is meant to lure those who are aware of a significant change: that success now depends increasingly upon combining talent with the proper smoothness of manner. Behaviour has become a key to careers and advancement. As the traditional hold of the aristocracy on court and bureaucratic positions loosens, the middle ground of worldly posts turns into a battlefield of talent and patronage, a terrain fought over by the so-called lower aristocracy and the sons of the *dritte Stand* (middle classes) who have access to education. '*Klugheit*' was equivalent to worldly prudence, and educators like Christian Weise (1642–1708) in his teaching career at Zittau and Weisenfels emphasized behavioural modes of prudent accommodation.[19] Even men not born to it were to practise the

---

[17] Richard Alewyn (ed.), *Deutsche Barockforschung* (Cologne, 1965); H. Wölfflin, *Renaissance und Barock*, 2nd edn. (Munich, 1907); F. Strich, 'Der Europäische Barock', in F. Strich, *Der Dichter und die Zeit* (Bern, 1947), G. R. Hocke, *Manierismus* (2 vols., Reinbek, 1957–9); W. Flemming, 'Deutsche Kultur im Zeitalter des Barock', in *Handbuch der Kulturgeschichte*, vol. 1 (Konstanz, 1960); Wilfried Barner (ed.), *Der literarische Barockbegriff* (Darmstadt, 1975).

[18] For example: Christian Thomasius, *Kurtzer Entwurff der politischen Klugheit sich selbst und anderen in allen menschlichen Gesellschaften wohl zurathen und zu einer bescheidenen Conduite zu gelangen* (Frankfurt, 1707); Julius Bernhardt von Rohr, *Einleitung zu der Klugheit zu leben: Oder Anweisung, Wie ein Mensch zur Förderung seiner zeitlichen Glückseligkeit seine Actiones vernünftig anstellen soll* (Leipzig, 1715); Christoph August Heumann, *Der Politische Philosophus, Das ist Vernunftsmässige Anweisung zur Klugheit im Gemeinen Leben* (Leipzig, 1724). For discussion of the concept and literature, see: Barbara Zaehle, *Knigges Umgang mit Menschen und seine Vorläufer: Ein Beitrag zur Geschichte der Gesellschaftsethik* (Heidelberg, 1933); Arnold Hirsch, *Bürgertum und Barock im deutschen Roman: Eine Untersuchung über die Entstehung des modernen Weltbildes* (Frankfurt, 1934), p. 72ff; Wilfried Barner, *Barockrhetorik: Untersuchungen zu ihren geschichtlichen Grundlagen* (Tübingen, 1970), p. 138ff; G. Frühsorge, *Der politische Körper, Zum Begriff des Politischen im 17. Jahrhundert und in den Romanen Christian Weises* (Stuttgart, 1974).

[19] Hans Arno Horn, *Christian Weise als Erneuerer des deutschen Gymnasiums im Zeitalter des Barock: Der 'Politicus' als Bildungsideal* (Weinheim, 1966).

language of manners, and in dress and demeanour show their capacities for equality in politeness. This was essential in the double-dealing world of court and bureaucracy where dissimulation was a stage requisite.[20] Christian Weise's publications grew out of his practical experience with the young men whom he taught. His books sold very well as manuals, such as that for correct and polite letters (*Politische Nachricht von Sorgfältigen Brieffen*, 1693) and in the forms of entertaining pedagogy, such as novels and plays.[21]

The world of books here fitted a projected need, a decisive shift in the distribution of jobs and wealth. Illness seems separate from this, but it was not. In 1727 the book entitled *Der Galante Patiente* appeared.[22] The author, Johann Daniel Longolius,[23] was himself typical of the readership to whom he appealed. The son of a Protestant minister in a small Saxon village, he was well educated (classical and oriental languages). He went to the university of Leipzig where he 'became Baccalaureus philosophiae and bethought himself to qualify as a useful and politick schoolmaster'.[24] Characteristically he had also attended the finishing classes in dancing and fencing, formerly useful only to noblemen. His father's illness cut his plans short and he was forced to earn his keep as *Hofmeister* (teacher of languages and manners) to the children of a minor aristocrat. Later he studied medicine in Halle, but never really made it his profession. His book the *Galante Patiente*, bears the subtitle a 'philosophical manual of how a sick person should behave charmingly and decorously'. The first two chapters depart nicely from pedantic advice, amusing the reader with a train of thought about those ill with illusory complaints. Those who play sick 'eat well, drink well, sleep well, and field their arguments very well... only their work will not be done quite as well'.[25] In some situations, Longolius

20 Karl-Heinz Mulagk, *Phänomene des politischen Menschen im 17. Jahrhundert: Propädeutische Studien zum Werk Lohensteins unter besonderer Berücksichtigung Diego Saavedra Fajardos und Balthasar Gracians* (Berlin, 1973), esp. p. 138ff.
21 Dieter Kimpel, *Der Roman der Aufklärung 1670–1774*, 2nd edn (Stuttgart, 1977): 'Verwandlungen des barocken Pikaro-Romans im frühaufklärerischen Politischen Roman' (p. 25ff). Contains bibliography.
22 Johann Daniel Longolius, *Galanter Patiente oder philosophischer Unterricht wie sich ein Kranker so wohl gegen sich selbst, als gegen andere nett und galant aufführen soll*...(Budissin [Bautzen], 1727).
23 An autobiographical sketch is given in Longolius' introduction to Cornelius Bontekoe, *Abhandlung von des Menschen Leben, Gesundheit, Kranckheit und Tode*...(Budissin [Bautzen] and Leipzig, 1719).
24 *Ibid.* (no pagination for introduction).
25 Longolius, *Galante Patiente*, p. 14.

counsels, 'a good posting will alleviate the difficult symptoms and the
malum hypochondriacum of a scholar living in obscure circumstances
more definitely than all possible medicine'.[26]

The theme of the failed intellectual, of the hypochondriac, of those
who use sickness to bow out from demands, is the price of worldly
optimism and worldly pressure to make good. If Longolius touched
lightly on the subject, it was because its dimensions had not yet assumed
their later proportions. The famous popular book on the subject by
Johann Ulrich Bilgauer was to be published in 1767.[27] Its title page
makes two things clear: that it will explain the causes and effects of
hypochondria for a nonspecialist readership and, secondly, that Bilgauer
proposes to demonstrate that this illness '*heutigen Tages*' (today) is so
endemic that it can be counted as a cause of depopulation. Hypochondria,
and its bed-fellow melancholia, were painfully present in the eighteenth
century, as in other times, and this has been noted by historians.[28] But
they view melancholia in the light of a continuous tradition, and link
it almost exclusively with the religious enthusiast. The book *Melancholie
und Aufklärung* (1977) sees psychological illness as the dark side of the
Enlightenment. It ascribes to religion what Longolius in his witty way
attributed to the up-and-coming Enlightenment figure, the man who
needs charm and adroitness to make his mark upon his worldly
contemporaries. Longolius' *Galante Patiente* alerts us to the link
between the behavioural expectations of the Enlightened and their
ways of escape into hypochondria, even as Formey pointed out that
Sulzer '*der Weltweise*' showed himself to be a philosophe and
gentleman because he *denied* pain. This is also Longolius' train of
thought when he asks rhetorically (in his introduction) why it is of
importance to propose '*Galanterie*' for the ill 'who must die and

---

[26] *Ibid.*, p. 13.

[27] Johann Ulrich Bilgauer, *Nachrichten an das Publikum in Absicht der Hypochondrie,
oder Sammlung verschiedener und nicht so wohl für die Ärzte, als vielmehr für das
ganze Publikum gehörige, die Hypochondrie, ihre Ursachen und Folgen betreffende
medicinische Schriftstellen, und daraus gezogener Beweis, dass die Hypochondrie
heutigen Tages eine fast allgemeine Krankheit ist, und das sie eine Ursache der
Entvölkerung abgeben kann* (Copenhagen, 1767).

[28] Extensive bibliographies are to be found in Gerhard Sauder, *Empfindsamkeit*,
vol. 1 (vol. 2 has not appeared) (Stuttgart, 1974) and Hans-Jürgen Schings,
*Melancholie und Aufklärung: Melancholiker und ihre Kritiker in Erfahrungs-
seelenkunde und Literatur des 18. Jahrhunderts* (Stuttgart, 1977). Sauder,
pp. 147–54, surveys the main tendencies, stressing the 'aesthetic' poses of
melancholia, and its 'imaginary' or hypochondriac aspect. Schings
concentrates on melancholia amongst the religious.

become old, suffused with signs and bitter complaints, with their thousandfold unclean excretions'.[29] Melancholia, hypochondria and pain are existentially apparent for the Enlightened as well as the Pious. The mark of the enlightened man, however, is their denial.

In other words, death and illness for the Enlightened were not negligible quantities. The 'Baroque' period point of view saw death and illness as an integral part of man's inconsequential and shadowy existence. But for the Enlightened these were existential components which could be vanquished. Manners and reason could concur in a strict discipline to conquer the psychological and social intrusion of disease. This type of discipline is the fruit of an internalized mode of behaviour. It does not negate experiential reality, but imposes upon it a different authority. Going one step further one could claim that the demands of the *Weltweise* or philosophe to suppress the dictates of an ailing body align him with the most dominant element of society of that time. The aristocratic dictum of placing oneself above the rest was not only a claim by birthright. It demanded behavioural patterns, the epitome of which was the nobleman in his honoured role as military officer. None but the titled held office. In military Prussia – and elsewhere – the aristocratic officer still led from the front line as an inspiration to his men, and he stayed there until mutilation or death took its course.[30] Pain, or, in a different context, other spontaneous reactions, were to be subordinated to class behaviour. In trying to live up to this dictate the man of bourgeois origin put himself on the same level as his social rival. Christian Weise's initiation of the bourgeois into the world of power, the 'politic' world, had brought its price. It is very close to Stoicism and very far from religion, and earns the Enlightened a worldly triumph at the price of the responses of the body.

A most remarkable episode illustrates the conjunction of these behavioural patterns. In 1777 Sulzer's health was at a new low.[31] He was having difficulty in standing for long periods, but this was precisely what was required in the presence of the King of Prussia. Frederick the Great, renowned as one of the most accomplished of enlightened

---

[29] Longolius, *Galante Patiente*, introduction.

[30] '*Tapferkeit*' (heroism) was not an abstract term in the combat of earlier centuries. See *Memoiren des Freiherrn D. G. von Natzmer*, ed. Eufemia Gräfin Ballestrem (Berlin, 1881) (original manuscript: 1722–30). This type of warfare and its heroic 'privilege' is well described in Jean Henri Dunant, *Erinnerungen an Solferino*, 1st edn (Geneva, 1862), the book which led to the founding of the Red Cross.

[31] Sulzer, *Lebensbeschreibung*, p. 61ff.

monarchs, adept at music and a philosophical author in his own right, commanded Sulzer to attend him. Sulzer asked permission to lean on someone or against something. It was the only concession made, and for some hours a discussion ensued in topics of religion, on the clergy and on sovereignty. It was held in French. Only when the interest of the King waned, did he remark 'je vois que vous êtes fatigués, je vous ferai appeler un autre fois'.[32]

As clearly evident, behaviour in illness is dependent on forms of social interaction. Longolius' book, *Der Galante Patiente*, provides another insight into the world of this 'enlightened' patient, both male and female. He deals with the material arrangements attendant on the sick-bed and prescribes ideal behavioural patterns. Because the book belongs to the genre of 'politic' advice books it shows us the behavioural aspirations of the enlightened middle class. The sick-bed as described in the book is not just a functional place, such as that in a clinic, devoted to recuperation, but at the centre of many types of behavioural expectations. First of all, the patient should command a room of his own which is furnished specifically to accommodate his needs. The advice is detailed:[33] the right heating, not too cold, not too hot; the bed away from the door and not too near the stove; small tables for medicine, to be kept very clean; no pictures on the walls (too much of a luxury); no stylish clothes; no brooms to whip up dust; no snuff; a chair for visitors; not too many visitors; cutlery and plates; and – as for the healthy – a comb, toothpick, knife and an implement to clean the ears. Longolius then takes up dietary prescriptions which prohibit any inclinations to compensate the ill for their suffering through exorbitant food:[34] no meat; plenty to drink; some fresh air; no tobacco; plenty of sleep induced through silence and a peaceful atmosphere. The patient should avoid '*Nachsinnen und Raisonnieren*' (speculative thinking and reasoning at length).

The fifth chapter reviews the behaviour of the patient towards his physician(s).[35] Right at the outset Longolius comments that patients are not to view their doctors either as 'half in the nature of a prophet' nor as 'merely the purveyor of samples of urine'.[36] Then he advises truthfulness and exactness when asked about symptoms. The same painstaking care is to be taken with all the recommendations of the

---

[32] *Ibid.*, p. 66.
[33] Longolius, *Galante Patiente*, ch. 3, p. 25ff., for the following recommendations.
[34] *Ibid.*, p. 31ff.   [35] *Ibid.*, p. 38ff.   [36] *Ibid.*, pp. 47–9.

doctor since some patients have wonderful manners with the physician but neglect their pills entirely.[37] The matter of money is not ignored, and Longolius reminds the patient that it is not good enough to reward the physician with what it would cost to buy a new pair of heels for old boots.[38] Rather the surest guide for the honorarium would be to follow the official tables published by the respective sovereign territories for remedies and for physician's costs.[39] When changing physicians, a problem which Longolius treats as common, he reminds the patient that a great deal of tact is useful. Besides the good manners necessary for managing a physician, a problem grave enough to merit a complete chapter, the hired or voluntary help required for the sick also deserved the reader's attention.[40] Longolius forbids his patient vehement oaths or even irony when either the hired help or friends do not care for him 'subtly enough' or try to console him too much. On the other hand the nurse is provided with a few rules of conduct as well: he or she should not command the house like a lord or demand the best in food and drink. Nor should the nurse depart when the case reveals itself to be a contagious disease.

In the last chapter Longolius treats the last things.[41] A will should be made before illness debilitates the patient too much. And when visitors come to see the ill or the dying no one should forget that contemplation and reflection before God does more than save the soul: it may also restore the body to health because of the soul's intimate union with it. If the soul gathers strength it becomes 'less fearful and steadier in its ability to minister to the body and can expunge more happily the evil lodged therein'.[42] With these words Longolius bowed respectfully before Georg Ernst Stahl and the Pietists in Halle.

If, in the foregoing summary of Longolius' advice the tone has been laconic, touching sometimes satirically on the foibles of human existence, then this is the tone of the original. But advice to the '*galante Patiente*' was also specific: it was possible to put it into effect. In the case of a person suffering from the long and wearisome diseases of the eighteenth century, putting it into effect would mean that he or she shared a 'modern' outlook: willingness to abandon agencies of advice incorporated in the traditional, oral, and direct transfer of skills, and instead to acquire knowledge set out in a book. This book belonged to the kind of literature which advertised itself – the very laconic tone

---

[37] *Ibid.*, p. 51.   [38] *Ibid.*, p. 60.
[39] *Ibid.*
[40] *Ibid.*, p. 62ff, for this and following information.
[41] *Ibid.*, p. 69.   [42] *Ibid.*

of the work underlines this – as a vehicle of enlightened modernity. To respond to such a book or to use its interpretation of the locale of disease was to align oneself with the new. How far the majority did so is quite beside the point. Longolius states a claim, which was that of the ambience and fashion of the Enlightenment. The style of writing in this book, its mixture of the concrete and specific along with its ironic references (the urine analysis of doctors; the asides on foibles of philosophy; and the strident, undisciplined dealings by the patient) imprint not only a social norm, but also the fashion by which it is acquired.

Longolius' book was trend-setting. It suggests cultural changes in patterns of being ill which are not strictly identifiable with medical progress. Even if the items enumerated for use in the sickroom and the behaviour of the bedridden were in accordance with 'modern' techniques (Longolius studied medicine at the University of Halle), the cultural meaning of the book rests in its worldly pattern. The patient's sphere here exhibits all the attributes of showiness, and the book's recommendations are certainly 'ostentatious' for the time. The sick room comes close to being fashionably dressed, just enough of a shade beyond the useful or the scientific in such a way as to speak the language of those arrived among the Enlightened.

Illness, then, whatever the disease, gave rise to social patterns beyond those we associate with medical consultation or such professional items as nursing. In the context of the German Enlightenment, in the Protestant north, secular patterns have shown certain contours. Among the thin crust of the educated, those to whom the term 'Enlightened' must primarily be applied, the weakening of the body and its ailments called for a philosophic stoicism (Sulzer, Formey's assessment of Sulzer, Frederick the Great) which merged with new habits of worldliness. Men of the world, fashionable men, kept quiet as to their disabilities. Dissimulation, even where the ailment was outrageously apparent (Sulzer's audience with the King), belonged to the code of manners of those in the urbane court cities (Berlin, for example) whose philosophy sought to distance them from the bitter messages of illness and death. Only hypochondria and melancholia were 'interesting' diseases, linked, however, as much by tradition as by any medical insight, to the image of the philosopher. For those wishing to be Enlightened, illness could be disparaged, or tolerated in a sick-room usefully arranged, self-contained in its secular and even 'puritanical' arrangement. Not so the other side of enlightened society: the sectarian religious enthusiasts and the Lutheran Pietists of the eighteenth century.

Religious enthusiasts and illness

The term 'Enlightenment' is selective. Historians have separated the religious enthusiast from his enlightened, usually Deist, counterpart as strictly as the Victorians separated the sexes. The ideological disparities and the problem of secularization inherent in the period remain undisputed. But the manner in which these tensions expressed themselves was not always in accordance with our assumptions about the patterns. Enlightened medicine, for example, is evaluated in terms of the learned doctor's 'modern' vocabulary of science: that is, the ability to investigate physical nature from a scientifically sanctioned method, 'ratio et experientia', leading to an appreciation of 'systems' (Friedrich Hoffmann and Georg Ernst Stahl), of inductive science in medicine (Hermann Boerhaave, Albrecht von Haller), anatomical and iatrochemical advances (the University of Leiden and Franciscus de la Boë Sylvius). And yet, in respect of these concerns, illness remains a subordinate item, a molecule in the grand logic of scientific revolutions.

Not so for other dimensions of thought and belief. Enlightened lay circles in Berlin had invented something else, had woven illness into the mentality they were creating – a worldly one, whose terms of behaviour were 'philosophical', an overtly social expression of subjugating the body to the mind. The Pious, on the other hand, could not enter upon such a solution. Under the aegis of enthusiastic religion the process of reasoning, the search for systematic explanation, had never been credited as spiritually helpful.[43] In fact systematic theology was considered to be a great enemy of religion.[44] Reason is a faculty mindful of proper order and proper categories, while crisis, emotion,

---

[43] This is most apparent when considering the strong influence of the 'mystic' tradition, often mentioned in Church histories of Lutheran Pietism. Oddly enough Church history traces the *ideas* of mysticism and its sectarian adherents but fails to acknowledge its distinct *emotional* appeal. For the influence of mysticism on Pietism, see: Heinrich Bornkamm, *Mystik, Spiritualismus und die Anfänge des Pietismus im Luthertum* (Giessen, 1926); Erich Seeberg, *Gottfried Arnold: Die Wissenschaft und die Mystik seiner Zeit. Studien zur Historiographie und zur Mystik* (Meerane, 1923; reprinted Darmstadt, 1964); Horst Weigelt, *Spiritualistische Tradition im Protestantismus: Die Geschichte des Schwenckfeldertums in Schlesien* (Berlin, 1973); Martin Schmidt, 'Speners "Pia Desideria"', in *Zur Neueren Pietismusforschung* (Darmstadt, 1977), p. 158ff.

[44] See the polemical writings of Johann Conrad Dippel (1673–1734) and the emphasis on 'Erfahrung' and 'Bekehrung' in the life and writings of August Hermann Francke (1663–1727).

conversion, breakdown, are immediate and tend toward irregularities. Religious conversion necessarily presupposes change, as the emphasis on ' re-birth' unequivocally shows. Enthusiasts have ever embraced this unsettling strain.

It needed, for it was dangerous, the anchor of written words. The most voluminous, and consistent, contribution to psychological writing of the eighteenth century stemmed from the re-born.[45] The ability to describe states of mind and of the emotions and the willingness to link them, or rather to infuse them, with symptomatic expressions of the body was thus a product of religious culture. Historically, its written record reached maturity and versatility, like a voice aware of its range, among the Pietists, the Separatists ('*radikal Pietisten*') and the communities gathered around Nikolaus Ludwig Count Zinzendorf (1700–60) in Herrenhut and in other territories controlled by a tolerant and pious aristocracy.[46] If the first tentative notes sound in the 1670s, the melody never breaks until it is changed into something very different under the hand of Goethe's classical orderliness, or that of his enemies, the Romantics.

In the eighteenth century enthusiastic religion was in tenor anticlerical and undogmatic.[47] These components made for instability: orthodox ritual and church authority could not be mustered easily against those

[45] Werner Mahrholz, *Deutsche Selbstbekenntnisse* (Berlin, 1919) and his *Der Deutsche Pietismus: Eine Auswahl von Zeugnissen, Urkunden und Bekenntnissen aus dem 17., 18. und 19. Jahrhundert* (Berlin, 1921); Heinz Kindermann, *Durchbruch der Seele: Literaturhistorische Studie über die Anfänge der deutschen Bewegung vom Pietismus bis zur Romantik* (Danzig, 1928); Erich Jenisch, *Die Entfaltung des Subjektivismus: Von der Aufklärung bis zur Romantik* (Königsberg, 1929). This phenomenon has been studied under separate academic disciplines. The literature on the subject is therefore to be found under various headings: autobiography; the contribution of Pietism to the development of the German language; and psychology – although this is usually approached from a 'modern' point of view, only the older 'philosophical' studies approaching 'Seele' from an eighteenth century perspective.

[46] In the eighteenth century the domains of the Counts of Sayn-Wittgenstein-Berleburg and of the Counts of Isenburg-Büdingen were particularly important. See also: Christa Habrich, 'Mediziner und Medizinisches am Hofe des Grafen Casimir zu Sayn-Wittgenstein (1687–1741)', *Deutsche Apotheker Zeitung*, XVIII.XIX (1983), 138–44; Werner Wied, 'Berleburg und Herrenhut: Der Besuch des Grafen Zinzendorf in Berleburg im Spiegel des Tagebuches des Grafen Casimir v. Berleburg', *Wittgenstein*, vol. 45, No. 3 (1981), pp. 95–116.

[47] This interesting observation is documented and discussed in Wilhelm Bender, *Johann Konrad Dippel, Der Freigeist aus dem Pietismus: Ein Beitrag zur Entstehungsgeschichte der Aufklärung* (Bonn, 1882).

searching their souls for religious affirmation. The signs of 'true religion' could not be those of Sunday church-going.[48] The religious search of the Enthusiast meant that he or she was seeking an inner-psychic assurance. The Enthusiast turned inward for emotive conviction: he or she *felt* religion. Subjectivity, under these circumstances, was at the very source of religious truth. Tangible evidence, that of the feelings, was needed as proof of God's presence. Deism, the favoured solution of the Enlightenment, which put the Creator at a respectable distance to Creation, bowing before Him as First Source and Regulator of the Universe, was not an option for Pietists or Enthusiasts. The religious struggle to confirm God in the soul evoked feeling: sorrow, joy, despondency, despair, release, dissatisfaction, love. Subjectivity and tangibility (senses and emotion) did not centre on the mind so much as on the body. Historically the case can rest with the word most often used in the context of conversion and re-birth: *Erfahrung*.[49] *Erfahrung* means experience, but not the kind which results in common-sense learning, in which one 'learns' to explain, but rather in the different sense of renewed exposure to sensibility. The very range of one's feelings bears witness to one's attachment to a Presence not tangible in any other way. Nothing objectifiable can really emerge here, but descriptive proof and identification of similar yearnings and experience become possible, uniting those aware of the problem.

One has to appreciate this fact deeply, if the contribution to cultural forms of perception proceeding from these circles is to be understood. Enthusiastic religious groups did, as medical science did not, provide the substantive basis for the psychology of the period. It would be reductionistic to claim that this contribution related purely to the soul, or that it was yet a science ('psychology'), because of the necessarily holistic, or 'psychosomatic' approach of their experience. The body was the medium of that *Erfahrung* without which it was useless to proceed. Illness was a part of this context, not an extraneous element. It was not something which befell one, but rather another condition, another passage in the personal contemplation of the 'pilgrim's progress'.

A good illustration of an *experiential* diagnosis of illness can be found

---

[48] August Gottlieb Spangenberg, for example, theologian and religious radical, refused to receive the sacraments in company with 'nominal' Christians: Gerhard Reichel, *August Gottlieb Spangenberg, Bischof der Brüderkirche* (Tübingen, 1906), p. 75.

[49] This is a subjective category, not one of 'observational' proof. It is in evidence in all conversion experiences.

in the autobiography of August Gottlieb Spangenberg (1704–92).[50] Spangenberg's life was intimately related to the religious revivals of the period. He studied theology in Jena, becoming *Adjunctus* to the professor of theology Johann Franz Buddeus (1667–1729), a man highly sympathetic to Lutheran Pietism, but not a radical, who had been at the University of Halle until 1705. In Jena Spangenberg had already drawn close to men less established, more readily persecuted, branded with the fires of an unorthodox enthusiasm, such as the 'Gichtelianer', followers of the Separatist Johann Georg Gichtel (1638–1710). Spangenberg went to Halle, called to a position in the theological faculty, but was soon expelled because of his unwillingness to disengage himself from Separatists.[51] He eventually joined Zinzendorf's 'Herrenhut' community and spent the main part of his life of over ninety years in their service, travelling to England and to the communities of Moravian Brethren in America. He had a typical *Bekehrungserlebniss*, the emotive experience of inner conversion central to the Pious, in 1722.[52] This is how he describes one of his early states of illness:

Because of concentrated and extended reflection I developed the habit of thinking consequentially now on this subject, then on another, soon on a third, and this did not cease even while sleeping. My dreams became an orderly succession of thoughts because one reflection proceeded from the previous one, and this blunted not only my bodily strength, but also endangered the powers of the soul to such an extent that I had cause to fear that it would impair grace growing within me. As I became increasingly distressed over this, an experienced friend advised me not to lose heart [den Muth nicht sinken zu lassen]; even though this condition would not disappear rapidly, in the course of time it would alleviate itself, if I would intimately attach myself to my Saviour in all the subjects upon which I had to think, and if my meditation would remain 'within Him' [immer in ihm geschähe]. I followed his good advice and found it held true ever after.[53]

These were not words lightly spoken. At that time Spangenberg was under extreme duress, having committed himself to a rigorous spiritual discipline of uninterrupted prayer and no unnecessary conversation.[54]

[50] Reichel, *Spangenberg*; Marianne Beyer-Fröhlich, *Pietismus und Rationalismus* (Leipzig, 1933): 'Aus: Lebenslauf unseres seligen Bruders August Gottlieb Spangenbergs, genannt Joseph, von ihm selbst aufgesetzt', pp. 52–67.
[51] Reichel, *Spangenberg*, p. 72ff.
[52] *Ibid.*, p. 24ff.
[53] 'Lebenslauf unseres…Spangenbergs', reprinted in: M. Beyer-Fröhlich, *Pietismus und Rationalismus*, p. 58.   [54] *Ibid.*, p. 55.

He was also just then divided between his loyalty to moderate Pietism (his attachment to Buddeus and his academic position) and his wish to serve the 'least of his brethren', the outcast members of radical enthusiast religion.[55] He describes very accurately what might be called a nervous breakdown. It has all the symptoms of a critical illness. The manner of his description illustrates how his analysis differs in approach from that of the Enlightened. First of all, it is precise in recording physical and mental symptoms. He records the autonomous mechanism of an overstrained mind, sleeplessness with disturbed dreams, loss of bodily strength, fear that the very object of his desires, his growth in grace, would crash to nought in this condition. He shows us that body and soul are not for him separate entities (both lose strength when he overtaxes their capacities). He is perfectly aware of what is happening. His solution is also typical: to go for advice to an 'experienced friend'. Here there is a marked difference to what Sulzer and Formey saw as ideal behaviour while afflicted: to endure, cognisant, lonely, but somehow triumphant. The method of alleviation for Spangenberg – and he knows his health is impaired – was to seek community and to 'throw his burdens upon the Lord'.

The major difference by contrast to the Enlightened, however, still rests with the principle of *Erfahrung*. Spangenberg meets his disabilities head on. The sign of his 'losing strength' becomes a measure for his 'losing grace' – his main fear. The physical tells him about the spiritual. For Sulzer illness was limitation. For the Pious, it is 'experience' translatable into another vocabulary. The significance of their illness may not be readily apparent to the Pious, but nonetheless the natural or physical can be interpreted. Illness, therefore, acquires a different explanatory mode. It is to be examined not for its physical symptoms alone – although scarcely anyone had a better pen for their description – but rather for its symptomatic indications of a person's spiritual progress. Count Zinzendorf, Spangenberg's close associate, the protector and leader of the Moravian Brethren in their German communities, gives us another instance of this.

Zinzendorf had a Pietist background almost from the cradle.[56] His father died when he was very young and he was brought up by his

[55] Reichel, *Spangenberg*, especially the years after 1722 when Spangenberg was in Jena and Halle.
[56] August Gottlieb Spangenberg, *Leben des Herrn Nicolaus Ludwig Grafen und Herrn von Zinzendorf und Pottendorf* (8 vols., n.p., n.d.; the introduction is signed Barby, 26 July 1775).

grandmother, Frau von Gersdorff, a staunch supporter of August Hermann Francke. His godfather was Philipp Jacob Spener. When his mother remarried, it was to the General D. G. von Natzmer, a leading Pietist at the court in Berlin. He was sent to Halle, to Francke's *Pädagogium*, with instructions 'to break his pride', having evidenced a precocious intelligence and having all the advantages (temptations for arrogance) of a high-born aristocrat.[57] His educational supervisor, sent with him as *Hofmeister*, was severe, and keenly determined to curb his evident Pious enthusiasm. The family did not want a religious maverick. The opposition thus loaded on his youthful shoulders was hard to bear. Zinzendorf later describes what happened to him as a boy in a letter of 1728:

all my secret burdens showed themselves in a severe bodily illness, in which I could not hold still any of my extremities and could not control my writing pen, until I was brought home for a time to Hennersdorf.[58]

Zinzendorf was aware of the psychological origins of his afflictions, but he had difficulty coming to terms with illness. Spangenberg writes about Zinzendorf's illness of 1733:

What particularly pained our Count during this time were the impediments to the work so dear to him, the work in the community. To these impediments I attribute his illnesses, in particular those affecting his eyes, to which he was much subject. In this respect it was very difficult for him to adopt the right balance; to know when to preserve his strength or when to risk working. When he rested and tried to let the illness take its course, he would soon think of one thing or another in which evil must be averted or useful actions instituted. He could then not remain quiescent, but got up, and disregarded his illness. But this often had bad consequences in that his pain increased to the extent that he became for a time totally incapable of doing any work whatsoever. This, however, caused him emotional disturbance [darüber wurde dann sein Gemüth krank] and he censured himself with so many reproaches that he was hardly to be comforted over all the things he thought he had left undone. In order to compensate, he then tore himself once more from the sick-bed and went to work, but achieved only another reversal of his health.[59]

[57] Spangenberg treats this obviously difficult episode in a very fair manner (both he and Zinzendorf had reason to complain about Halle): *Leben...Zinzendorfs*, p. 36ff; Zinzendorf's own version in a letter to Mag. Johann Liborius Zimmermann of 29 May 1728, which is also an autobiographical document, is reproduced in Beyer-Fröhlich, *Pietismus und Rationalismus*, pp. 34–9.
[58] Beyer-Fröhlich, *Pietismus und Rationalismus*, p. 37.
[59] Spangenberg, *Leben...Zinzendorfs*, vol. 4 (1773), pp. 776–7.

This description of Zinzendorf by one of his close associates clearly indicates the ambivalence he felt over the physical impairment of his spiritual drive. Patience in sickness, tolerance of frailty and adversity, the creed of obedience in suffering – all of which were staples of a religious orientation – are acknowledged, but subverted by an active impatience to transcend physical limits. What was true of Spangenberg is true of Zinzendorf: enthusiastic religion burns up the whole man. The minutiae of self-observance were clearly articulated: pain, emotional disturbance, patience and restlessness, a sense of spiritual duty, severe demands on discipline and energy. Illness is not separate, an invasion, but part and parcel of the interaction of demand, the soul's on the body and the body's dependence on emotional and mental capacities. The vocabulary of *abwarten*, *Vorwürfe*, *trösten*, *sich herausreissen* (to wait, to reproach oneself, to comfort, to tear oneself away) tells a tale quite the opposite to that of Stoicism, speaks of an immersion in immediate, articulated experience (*Erfahrung*) as the pious man unlocks the innermost chambers of the heart and mind for his own scrutiny and before the only relevant Person.

Zinzendorf was not ignorant about medicine,[60] nor were these Enthusiasts and Separatists the type of fundamentalist who rejects scientific progress. Several prominent figures of these circles were learned physicians with doctorates from Leiden or Halle, such as Christian Friedrich Richter (1676–1711), Johann Conrad Dippel (1673–1734) and Johann Samuel Carl (1675–1757). But their medical knowledge did not go in the direction of establishing a medical science apart from a more comprehensive interpretation of nature.[61] They all adhered to a belief in nature as a foil for the prime, invisible, but materially effective movement of the spirit, both the Divine Spirit and the individual spirit for whom the body was a vessel, or *Leibeshütte* (literally: 'hut of the soul'). It was a complex system of beliefs, different from orthodox interpretation, but it suggests the congruence between the explanations used by the Pietists and a broader interpretative

---

[60] 'Mit einem gewissen Gelehrten, der in die Physiologie und andere Theile der Medizin sehr gute Einsicht hatte, unterhielt er sich oft; denn er liebte diese Wissenschaft, und das war bei ihm, so lange er lebte, wahrzunehmen.' Thus Spangenberg on Zinzendorf's 'life-long love of medicine', in Spangenberg, *Leben...Zinzendorfs*, vol. 1, p. 100.

[61] Characteristically all these 'learned physicians' wrote religious tracts; Dippel and C. F. Richter polemically defended a non-materialist position in medicine against Cartesian and other 'physical' explanations.

plane. The experience of illness they are able to detail so well shows how their perception of physical 'signs' (symptoms) was linked to the interpretation of spiritual state.[62] It is perfectly inconsistent to apply the cliché that these Protestants disregarded their body or sought mortification of the flesh. Their bodies and their emotions, what the Cartesian followers chose to call material things, were anything but that. Illness and the body's state were sign languages, motifs in the spiritual tapestry out of which salvation was woven.

August Hermann Francke gives us another, a third, instance of the religious approach to illness. In his last illness, which had already afflicted him for some years (he died in 1727), Francke shows us one remedy for the conflict Zinzendorf experienced and with which Francke was well acquainted: that of spiritual drive and its chastisement through loss of bodily strength. He terms his illness the *malum*, the evil which befell him, and he describes his obedient search for alleviation through medical advice.[63] But he does not let things rest there. In a manner similar to Zinzendorf his activism or duty in religious works challenges his frailty. He tries for balance but then enters his plea in long pages of written prayer and scriptural meditation. His pain – and he records its details – is surmounted in an effusion of prayer and an offering of faith beyond any reach of the rationales of medicine. Here again, in 1727, illness is lifted from the usual confines of objective analysis and its reality is psychologically transposed. Francke records how his intense struggle leaves him, for a time, the conqueror of pain.

Lutheran Pietists and the more radical Brethren and Separatists left a mark upon the eighteenth century equal to the Enlightenment's bid for the 'natural', philosophical, and secular (medical) conceptualization of illness. Spangenberg, Zinzendorf and Francke have served to show how other motives and other beliefs gave the encounter with illness a different history. Their articulateness, the confessional purpose of their writings, provided the eighteenth century with a new pattern. These religious leaders were not isolated quietists, nor was their psychological acuteness confined to clerical elitism. It was the Enlightenment which argued downward to the (as yet) 'uncivilised' or

---

[62] Contrary to our own 'modern' position, it was much more 'natural' or evident to these persons to perceive the body and soul as 'one'. Alchemia and the teaching of '*Sympathie*', as well as magic, all have non-materialist roots and were believed effective. These were not yet 'superstitions'.

[63] Archiv der Francke'schen Stiftungen (Handschriftenabteilung), Halle, German Democratic Republic, A 116, manuscript pagination: 748–65.

'uneducated'. That premise appears between the lines of its educational treatises.[64] The religious movements, and in particular their radical offshoots, permitted a less rigid approach. To explore one's own soul encourages descriptive talents (however restricted) and upon these lay case studies rested a truly popular nosography of illness. Thus these religious outpourings, tracts, letters, exemplifications, biographies and other forms of communication – it was all intensely discursive – gave birth to the psychological novel of the eighteenth century with its frequent description of introspective states. So too, that special German genre, the *Bildungsroman*, borrowed and elaborated the biographical and psychological intensity of the Enthusiasts. Three seminal and justly famous literary works, all of them still in print,[65] rest upon the foundations of pietist and sectarian experience. In this context it is most important to note that the literary expression of illness and psychological insight was the work of men *not* to be counted among Berlin's urbane Enlightened. All those we mention below had close encounters with enthusiastic religion and were born into relative poverty and uncertainty.

Adam Bernd (1676–1748),[66] author of *Eigene Lebens-Beschreibung* (Leipzig, 1738), declines to give us the name of his father. We know only that he cultivated and sold cabbages. Johann Heinrich Jung-Stilling (1740–1817),[67] author of *Heinrich Stillings Jugend: Eine wahrhafte Geschichte* (1777) and its sequels, *Jünglings-Jahre* (1778), *Wanderschaft* (1778), *Häusliches Leben* (1789), *Lehrjahre* (1804) and *H. Stillings Alter* (1817), was the son of Johann Helman Jung, a tailor, surveyor and teacher from the village of Grund in the Duchy of Nassau-Siegen. Karl Philipp Moritz (1756–1793),[68] the author of *Anton Reiser: Ein*

64 The didactic tone and the proscribed virtue of the Enlightenment is best caught in the moral weeklies. See Wolfgang Mertens, *Die Botschaft der Tugend: Die Aufklärung im Spiegel der deutschen Moralischen Wochenschriften* (Stuttgart, 1971).
65 Adam Bernd, *Eigene Lebens-Beschreibung* (ed. with notes by Volker Hoffmann) (Munich, 1973). Johann Heinrich Jung-Stilling, *Lebensgeschichte: Vollständige Ausgabe*, ed. G. A. Benrath (Darmstadt, 1976); Karl Philipp Moritz, *Anton Reiser: Ein Psychologischer Roman*, 2nd edn. (Insel Taschenbuch 433, Frankfurt am Main, 1980).
66 Bibliography, H.-J. Schings, *Melancholie und Aufklärung*, p. 340.
67 *Allgemeine Deutsche Biographie*, 'Johann Heinrich Jung-Stilling'; Bibliography: G. A. Benrath (ed.), J. H. Jung-Stilling, *Lebensgeschichte* (Darmstadt, 1976), p. 763.
68 *Allgemeine Deutsche Biographie*, 'Karl Philipp Moritz'; Hans Joachim Schrimpf, *Karl Philipp Moritz* (Stuttgart, 1980): review of life and current work on K. P. Moritz; includes extensive bibliography.

Psychologischer Roman (published in four parts (1785–1790), beginning with the *Jugendjahre*), grew up in poverty, his father playing the oboe in a regimental band. Common to the lives and writings of these men was their early immersion in enthusiastic religion, so strong that their creative powers were spent putting its influences onto the page. Bernd and Jung-Stilling (the last part of whose name derives from the designation 'die Stillen im Lande' (the Quietists, a descriptive term for Pietists) exemplify the lay imagination and influence possible within enthusiastic religion. Their homes became centres for religious – and medical – advice.

Their autobiographical works are a new phenomenon, a surprise among the literature of the Enlightenment. These books subvert or countermand the main themes of Enlightenment literature.[69] Wherever one looks in the German Enlightenment, to plays or to novels, the trials and woes of main characters turn on the issue of virtue, of the triumphant search for a moral code this side of heaven. Man- and womankind reach the extremes of endurance in the name of a humanity which holds fast to the concept that it is self-made.[70] Providence pushes things along, but goodness is its own reward, and the evil-doers get their just deserts. Not so the works of the Pious. They revel in pain – Bernd is hugely apologetic in his introduction for *not* being an optimist.[71] Year by year (the structure of his *Lebens-Beschreibung*) he focusses on anguish and a display of depression. Moritz too relishes his failures. Instead of a literature akin to

---

[69] Themes of endurance and virtue triumphant: Ch. F. Gellert, *Das Leben der Schwedischen Gräfin von G.* (Leipzig, 1747/8); Sophie von la Roche, *Geschichte des Fräuleins von Sternheim* (Leipzig, 1771); Karl Friedrich Tröltsch, *Liebes- und Lebensgeschichte der schönen und tugendhaften Henrietta* (Leipzig, 1752). These themes became a literary genre: see Dieter Kimpel, *Der Roman der Aufklärung (1670–1774)*, 2nd edn (Stuttgart, 1977). The same is true of the Enlightenment genre, the '*bürgerliches Trauerspiel*', in which tragedy occurs because virtue is compromised (G. E. Lessing, *Miss Sara Sampson* (1752)); or in which the heroine dies in order that her virtue be preserved (G. E. Lessing, *Emilia Galotti* (1772)).

[70] This theme is turned around in G. E. Lessing's *Minna von Barnhelm* (1767) when Minna finally persuades Major von Tellheim that *his* virtue is not compromised, and that he is therefore worthy of her hand in marriage.

[71] Adam Bernd, *Eigene Lebens-Beschreibung samt einer aufrichtigen Entdeckung, und deutlichen Beschreibung einer der grössten, obwohl grossen Theils noch unbekannten Leibes- und Gemüths-Plage, welche Gott zuweilen über die Welt-Kinder, und auch wohl über seine eigene Kinder verhänget; Den Unwissenden zum Unterricht, Den Gelehrten zu weiterm Nachdenken, Den Sündern zum Schrecken, und den Betrübten, und Angefochtenen zum Troste* (Leipzig, 1738), introduction (no pagination).

mathematics, doing the sums of virtue triumphant, these Pious men are seeking to record their inner tensions. This was autobiography with a vengeance. In point of fact it subverted this genre. Up to that date biography and autobiography were very sober and reticent affairs.[72] For the educated they listed, by and large, teachers, schools, posts and other information. Only religious confessional writing (specifically recounting the conversion experience) went into feelings, reversals, escape from worldliness.[73] Not accepting these boundaries, Bernd, Jung-Stilling and Moritz (the best and most influential examples) wrote up their lives as readable novels. They combined the sense of veracity expected from autobiography with the pleasure of embellishment possible in the novel. By this strategy they could effectively introduce psychological description. Inner feelings and experience were thus assured of notice and a large readership. The introspection that Spangenberg, Zinzendorf and Francke (along with innumerable others) had written about and claimed as legitimate areas of investigation was now becoming increasingly a literary interest. Karl Philipp Moritz was well aware in whose footsteps he was treading: he gives his autobiographical figure a fictional name, 'Anton Reiser' even though no one was likely to be fooled, and subtitles the book, with an expert's touch, '*ein psychologischer Roman*', a psychological *novel*. He thus unites a threefold appeal to the popular imagination: a thinly disguised autobiography, a minute examination of inner experience, and the suspense of plot, character and development. It was a small step from there to his founding of the *Magazin zur Erfahrungsseelenkunde* (1753–93), a journal, literally, for the knowledge (*Kunde*) of the experience (*Erfahrung*) of the soul (*Seele*). The journal was the first of its kind: a periodical mainly devoted to illnesses of an emotional and mental nature. The contributions solicited were from laymen. The journal was of a piece with the non-medical readership, at the same time claiming medical relevance. Via the religious enthusiast's inclination to scrutinize the soul, increasingly popular as a subject, it collected symptomatic descriptions of illness from anyone who was willing.[74]

Illness had been a central theme of the *Eigene Lebens-Beschreibung* of

---

[72] Günter Niggl, *Geschichte der deutschen Autobiographie im 18. Jahrhundert* (Stuttgart, 1977), p. 14ff.

[73] *Ibid.*, p. 6ff.

[74] *Magazin zur Erfahrungsseelenkunde als ein Lesebuch für Gelehrte und Ungelehrte*, ed. Karl Philipp Moritz (10 vols., Berlin, 1783–93) (Neuherausgegeben und mit einem Nachwort versehen von Anke Bennholt-Thomsen und Alfredo Guzzoni; Antiqua Verlag reprint, Lindau, 1978).

Adam Bernd. In the introduction he states that he will portray in detail his own suffering, his *Leibes- und Gemüthsplagen* (bodily and emotional affliction), in order to help 'the common people', who, when afflicted 'do not know themselves, and cannot describe in words to those from whom they seek help, their condition and their illness'.[75] Bernd was also writing *against* a specific tendency, clearly evident to him as destructive of his own experience and insight. He mentions it more than once in the introduction, as the 'current philosophical, naturalistic, and irreligious world' which, for all its concentration on 'constipating spleen and feverish black bile' cannot recognize either the devil's or divine intervention in the life of the soul (*Anfechtung*).[76] He challenges the bland naturalism of materialist explanation in its denial of the turmoil and depths of the soul's suffering, the experience of depression and melancholia into which his pages plunge the reader. He dips his pen in irony against the dangers of the Enlightenment and its francophile materialism:

In its despair Naturalism, like cancer, has eaten so far around itself that even the treatises of the learned have become infected; those [i.e. the learned] for whom everything must appear natural, ungarnished, and wrapped in a French negligé, similar to the garment in which Bouffleur is said to have found his mistress, if it is to appeal to them at all.[77]

Illness, the soul's illness, the continuum of emotion and restlessness, of breakdown, and the varied symptoms and descriptions evident in the confessions of the Pious made them disbelievers of the Enlightenment's optimism. It is well to note that the unwillingness to believe does not originate from atheists, or from aristocratic decadence, but from a religious popular culture, from those usually deprived of learned articulateness. The 'common people' such as Bernd, Jung-Stilling and Moritz did not readily have access to education, yet they learned an effective language through the habit of self-observation. They could effectively use the legacy of the Enthusiasts, Separatists and Pietists. If Bernd, Jung-Stilling and Moritz are unusual, their habits were not, as the many extant records of religious enthusiasts' descriptions of illness show.[78] Christa Habrich has pointed out that lay observations from

---

[75] Bernd, *Eigene Lebens-Beschreibung*, introduction (no pagination).
[76] *Ibid.*   [77] *Ibid.*
[78] See the excellent references in Christa Habrich, 'Pathographische und ätiologische Versuche medizinischer Laien', in Wolfgang Eckart and Johanna Geyer-Kordesch (eds.), *Heilberufe und Kranke im 17. und 18. Jahrhundert: Die Quellen- und Forschungssituation* (Münster, 1982).

these circles are knowledgeable enough to be classed among the pathogenic and aetiological descriptions of illness in learned medicine.[79]

But one more issue should be raised. The close congruence of illness and psychological *Erfahrung* which led the Pious to invent a new vocabulary, charting the intricate possibilities of feelings and emotion, also prepared the way for a departure in a different direction. An artist of Olympian dimensions, such as Johann Wolfgang von Goethe, was able to turn the Pietist tradition, extant over three-quarters of a century, away from its religious roots. In his sixth book of *Wilhelm Meisters Lehrjahre* he inserts the *Bekenntnisse einer Schönen Seele* (1795), the 'testament of a rare soul'. In his book *Die Deutsche Autobiographie im 18. Jahrhundert*, Günter Niggl explains the subtle shift which Goethe effected.[80] All the structural elements of Pietist conversion literature are incorporated, including the typical phrasing for emotional experience. Even contemporaries of Goethe suspected he had simply incorporated into his fiction the writings of Susanna Katherina von Klettenberg (1723–74), a pious aristocratic friend of the family's in Frankfurt am Main. The *Bekenntnisse* begin with illness and its effect on the tender soul of a girl of eight: 'in dem Augenblick war meine Seele ganz Emfindung und Gedächtniss' (with this moment my whole soul was suffused with feeling and memory).[81] The delicate tale of a psychological pathography is then fully expanded, but, as Niggl points out, beneath the masterly use of the Pietist tradition there lurks a refined narcissism.[82] The '*schöne Seele*' is able to live out a luxurious separation from worldly demands. The descriptive capacities unfolded in the drama of the religious enthusiast seeking a tangible reference point within for the God he or she craves to know, are here used to effect to describe refinement. The term 'beautiful' soul (*schöne Seele*) in a sense gives the game away. Illness and sensitivity are instrumental – at the end of the eighteenth century – in creating the signs and mannerisms of a truly disassociated elite. Significantly, via Goethe's sleight of hand, we also perceive how the articulation of illness and sensitivity are wedded to a different realm: to the domain of the unworldly, unmarried, independently wealthy and specifically *female*

---

[79] I have differed from Christa Habrich's analysis in seeking to depict a non-medical context. The lay descriptions of illness and their medical affinities certainly deserve more attention in medical history.

[80] Niggl, *Die deutsche Autobiographie im 18. Jahrhundert*, p. 126ff.

[81] *Ibid.*   [82] *Ibid.*, p. 127.

sphere. Goethe's literary re-invention of psychological sensibility utilized the tradition of religious struggle, but it was devastating, almost diabolical, because the religious centre became vacuous. The art of worldly psychologizing achieved its first intricate triumph. Troubled Adam Bernd's 'truth' that pain had meaning, faded back into the enclaves of enthusiastic religion, no longer culturally incisive enough to raise the religious sceptic's voice against established perceptions.

Summary

In seeking to describe cultural habits of illness no tightly knit scheme of interpretation has been applied. No specific illness, pathogenic or aetiological pattern was analysed or even searched out. No medical nosography or medical system was taken into consideration. Instead, I have sought an open-ended identification of what might have been underlying considerations for behaviour among distinct sets of individuals in the eighteenth century. The first examples are of the Enlightened, culturally at home in the urbane city of Berlin under Frederick the Great. They belong to a small group of the learned poised to establish the dominant culture of the German *Bildungsbürgertum* (the educationally adroit among the middle classes). Their manners and habits of dealing with illness illustrate, on the whole, how effectively they sought to escape the nuisance of frailty and disease. The ethic was one of Stoicism, the means a philosophical frame of mind. Only in the attributes of the sick-room does the mentality of decorous functionality, a sober usefulness attributable to a 'modern' Enlightenment, show itself. Among the Pious, on the other hand, illness is subsumed to a different pattern. An intimate, and often overstrained, search to establish a religious identity outside the orthodox legitimization of ritual and the authority of dogma, leads to an affirmation of personal experience. The inward-turning scrutiny of the soul and the acknowledgement of frailty and illness combine with a third element, that of a desire to write it all down, to create a truly remarkable corpus of psychological introspection. The fact that recruits to enthusiast religion were almost by definition outside the normal social hierarchies (even if they were aristocrats) lets us glimpse the emergence of an extensive popular culture, whose contribution to the eighteenth century was decisive. The Pious produced the varied instrumentarium through which a vocabulary for feelings and states of mind became established. It was not a matter of a learned or erudite system, filtering down as it were, but a self-taught articulation of mental and emotional struggle. This found literary expression towards the middle of the century in the curious blend of autobiography and 'novel' that men from an enthusiast background wrote. Description of illness was central to these experiential soundings. None of it was directly derived from the eighteenth century medical canon, as scientific medicine moved in the direction of a different nosography and definition of illness and disease. The cultural meaning of illness has a different tone to it than the hospitals or medical faculties would care to give it. I have argued along the lines of possible interpretations, not in order to diminish the contribution of medical science, but to show where another kind of logic would lead.

8

'The doctor scolds me': The diaries and
correspondence of patients in eighteenth century
England

JOAN LANE

I have gone through much Medical discipline, as Venaesection, scalding
fomentations, Cathartics & a[t] length a large Vesicatory on my Stomach,
which gave me some check to the fury of my Distemper...
Reverend Joseph Greene to his brother, 13 June 1782.[1]

The value of diaries and correspondence as source materials for many
aspects of research has long been appreciated by historians to reveal
contemporary information about daily life, fashion, architecture,
politics, travel, spiritual reflections, agriculture, industry, weather and
even folk-lore. In the past historians with an interest in these categories
have used letters and journals as indispensable accounts of attitudes and
thoughts, facts, events and personalities not recorded elsewhere, and
to support or contradict alternative information. However, these same
accounts also contain a substantial amount of material about patients,
medical practitioners and contemporary responses to illness and health
in a particularly immediate and first-hand way. Recovering the medical
information from such sources is a slow rather than a difficult
procedure, but provides facts and opinions about the patient's illness
and health not to be found anywhere else in eighteenth century
material. Recent work to reconstruct community life in the past has
already shown the value of this new approach in research. The purpose
of this essay is to illustrate how fragments from diaries and letters may
be considered alongside each other and in relation to other sources to
provide a picture of eighteenth century medicine from the recipients'
view.

Diaries and correspondence differ from each other in four important
respects: purpose, content, psychology and survival rate. The purpose

[1] *The Correspondence of the Reverend Joseph Greene*, ed. Levi Fox (Dugdale Soc.,
XXIII, 1964), p. 134.

of an English eighteenth century diary could be little more than a factual record of a farm, estate, business, military campaign or parish, with almost no medical and personal details. Diaries of this kind were far more important in the eighteenth century, with its low level of bureaucracy requiring the individual to keep his own account of such things as when servants began employment, their wages and dependability, when a particular crop was sown in which field, when animals gave birth and what journeys were undertaken for business, for which later centuries were to devise a variety of more formal records. Diaries were also used, especially in the early part of the eighteenth century and before the advent of most local newspapers, as an objective as well as a subjective record, to note events of importance, and they seem to have been most commonly used for this purpose by country diarists; thus royal births and deaths, civil or other disorders (the Forty Five Rebellion, the Priestley Riots or the Nore Mutiny), were all likely to be chronicled, sometimes with comment, in the eighteenth century diary. Most diaries contain a random mixture of information, but are of only limited use to the historian if the writer were obsessed with a single theme or personal injustice, driving out other topics. Religious musings and lawsuits particularly unbalance the journal if they preoccupied the diarist. Although religious discipline was a strong motive in the seventeenth century diarist, it is noticeable that spiritual diaries in the eighteenth century were a minority, even amongst those kept by Anglican clerics, who recorded the daily problems of running their parish, their search for patronage and their financial worries of tithes and stipends rather than their religious doubts and certainties. Journals such as those kept by Ralph Josselin were essentially of the seventeenth century, although the Nonconformist desire to practise moral stock-taking and self-analysis, with abject repentance, continued, especially among female Quakers, throughout the eighteenth century, but almost as a separate genre from the diary. Although turbulent, the eighteenth century was confident, expansionist, outward-looking and materialistic, and the letters and diaries of the period reflect these qualities.

Some diaries were in fact commonplace or memorandum books rather than journals, kept not daily but erratically, noting great events, local climatic disasters or plants thriving out of season. Commonplace books also contained useful household and beauty hints, cures, recipes and a miscellany of material of current interest or future use to the writer. In this respect, like diaries, they noted a successful medical treatment and its outcome that could be used again in a future illness. Rather than cures for human beings (although remedies for the bite of a rabid dog were common) many of these memorandum books contained a range of veterinary cures, especially for the horse, reflecting its indispensable role in transport, commerce, industry and social life at this period, as well as a scarcity of competent farriers and veterinarians that necessitated home treatment for the sick animal. These commonplace books provide sporadic but useful medical information, rather than comment, so that, for example, in 1704 John Coggs noted the name of his aged uncle's medical attendant – 'his docter his name is Wellstide; he live in the Old Change London'[2] – a useful scrap of information, at least. Interesting though such notebooks are, they are not diaries, which imply a daily commitment by the writer, ill or well, busy or under-occupied; even when nothing at all happens in a day the true diarist comments on the lack of events, although uniform length of entries and punctuality is rare. The most dedicated diarist, however, sometimes failed to write his or her journal when a family death occurred; thus Joseph Farington, one of the most prolific diarists, wrote only a word or two each day in March 1800 when grieving after his wife's death. Some commonplace books have survived better than diaries or correspondence because they usually contain no personal details that later, more sensitive readers might find embarrassing and so be censored or destroyed by the writer's descendants. Commonplace books were also often inherited and cover many decades, although sporadically written, in contrast to the diary full of much detail across a shorter time-span. The occasional commonplace book is a mine of facts about local medical personalities; John Downing of Coventry kept such a book (1755–1800) in which, because of his own family medical connections, he noted as interesting the marriages of nine practitioners and three of their daughters as well as the deaths of two practitioners and two men's wives. This information is more than usually valuable since the parish registers for the city before 1800 were destroyed in the Coventry blitz of 1940.[3]

The purpose of the eighteenth century diary could be either self-revelation or self-justification, putting on paper thoughts that were unsuitable to the writer's worldly status: for example, criticism of an employer, spouse or parent by the junior in the relationship, and political opinions that were unacceptable if not treasonable, as well as

[2] Bodleian Library, Oxford, MS Eng. misc. f. 78.
[3] Coventry City Record Office, A 128/17.

secret faults the writer regretted. The diary could be the writer's confidant and, read by later generations, his champion. Throughout the eighteenth century many diarists (but for obvious reasons, fewer correspondents) were heavily critical of the Hanoverians, many despising their rule but equally fearing a Jacobite revival; others confided to their journals their sympathy for the American colonists or the French revolution. Some diarists used their journals to give vent to sharp, even savage criticism of contemporary figures; so Bonnie Prince Charlie was described by one who watched his march as a 'Nursling from Rome'.[4] Accounts of George III's periodic bouts of madness were widely noted in diaries, with pithily expressed concern for the nation as well as sympathy for the patient; for example, 'The King's determined illness, its probable event, and all its consequences, must, in one way or another, interest every mortal, and…cast a degree of uncertainty over everybody's plans.'[5]

A diary was above all else a repository of the writer's secret hopes and fears, ambitions and disappointments, and in this category diarists included their medical problems, cures, unsuccessful or satisfactory treatments, opinions of medical practitioners and their advice, as well as, in some instances, how they felt towards the whole experience of death, of being ill themselves or of tending an indisposed member of their family, often during a period of many weeks. An important aspect of such comments is their unselfconsciousness, for the writer did not know how the patient would progress in the future.

The purpose of letters, of course, was to inform one person distant from another about events, the form being stylised in 1740 in Richardson's *Pamela*, a whole novel composed of letters. Status differences did not preclude correspondence and members of different social classes corresponded fairly often in the eighteenth century. For example, the agent of a country estate wrote to his master in London, reporting not only about tenants, crops and livestock, but family health as well:

8 May 1727: yesterday about 3 o'clock the poor nurse fell down in the stone court, it being wet and slippery, and broke both the bones of her arm about 3 inches above her right hand. I sent immediately for Mr Fryer, who came

4   *The Diary of Richard Kay (1716–51) of Baldingstone, near Bury*, ed. W. Brockbank and F. Kenworthy (Chetham Soc., 3rd ser., 16, 1968), p. 103.
5   *Extracts from the Journals and Correspondence of Miss Berry, 1783–1852*, ed. Lady Theresa Lewis (3 vols., London, 1865), vol. 2, p. 438.

and set it before eight. We do not suffer Master Robert to suck for these five or six days, for these things are always attended with a feaver...

11 May 1727: the nurse is intirely free from pain, and has not been at all feavourish as we could perceive, so that in a day or two the child may suck without any manner of danger. Her breasts have been very regularly drawn all this time, and Master Robert has born the loss of the pap with a great deal of patience.[6]

A provincial schoolmaster with an aristocratic pupil could also be responsible for reporting his charge's ill-health to the child's parents in London in 1750 when a visit to the capital was proposed:

This day in ye morning as soon as Master West was up, we had a sad complaint from his of ye Tooth-ach, which we found accompani'd with a gentle cough, but without any inflammatory or feverish symptoms: This Evening, by keeping him constantly under our inspection, & a little kitchen physick, we found all our grievances dispers'd, except y^t his Eye-lids (according to his own account) smart a little; but this complaint we apprehend will be of very little continuance, and not in ye least hinder his Journey.[7]

Senior and junior members of the same family, such as parents and children, often corresponded, but the most interesting letters as a source of medical history are those between equals — sisters, brothers or cousins, or in marriages with an exceptional degree of equality. Most letters tend to survive in the papers of the recipient, but some families, such as the Milbankes and the Noels (the Lovelace papers) carried on a voluminous correspondence with each other, keeping copies of controversial items and copying out extracts to forward to each other from the letters of yet other relatives, rather like a family news-sheet. Placing these family letters in location and time can be difficult: addresses were frequently abbreviated (Holland House becomes H. Ho.) and personal names were reduced to a formula, so that Dr James Vaughan becomes 'the great Dr V'. Nick-names were widely used, almost a code within the letters, so that Harriet Stewart, the illegitimate daughter of Lady Bessborough and Lord Granville Leveson Gower, was called 'Arundel' in her parents' correspondence. Dates were often confused in letters, whereas a printed diary was more likely to record

---

[6] *The Letters of Daniel Eaton to the third Earl of Cardigan, 1725–32*, ed. Joan Wake and Deborah C. Webster (Northants. Rec. Soc., xxiv, 1971), p. 117.

[7] *Greene*, p. 70.

an accurately dated event. Correspondents recognised the problem of writing the date correctly, so that, in one of his many letters to John Bentley, Josiah Wedgwood in 1778 wrote at the top of his page '2nd of May I think, but Sunday morning certain'.[8] The correspondence of families scattered across the English colonies in the eighteenth century was often of a very high calibre and, when relations were separated for many years, their letters provide a remarkable, continuous insight into the writers' personalities and style of life, as they try to convey to their readers an impression of living in India or America or the events at home. Interestingly, letters often survive in spite of the writer's instruction to the recipient to destroy the missive; certain diarists, such as Trollope, destroyed their own journals in later life. Some personal papers have been bundled and labelled by later members of the family (the Verney and the Granville correspondence, for example), and occasionally endorsed with a comment on the contents, not always flattering. A packet of letters to the Duchess of Sutherland was labelled 'Unreadable. Insufferable piety' in a later hand.

Only between the closest correspondents were the most personal medical confidences exchanged; while many letters told of a third person's illness in great and exaggerated detail, only the most intimate writers described their own ill-health, their concern about the true nature of their illness or fears of death. When sisters or other female relations corresponded there is an encouraging prospect for the historian that they will be found to discuss medical matters. The papers of the Noel-Milbanke and Leveson Gower families are excellent examples of this, the women of the families exchanging medical details with great frequency: their fears about pregnancy, smallpox and inoculation and also interesting snippets of quasi-medical gossip about contemporaries, much of it highly defamatory. Thus in 1774 Judith Noel received a letter from her sister reporting:

I have been told as an *absolute* fact that Miss Proby is *with Child* by Mr Storer, & that she is coming down here [Bath] and it is reported that Lady Sarah Bunbury has been *equally* intimate with her Nephew Charles Fox. He is certainly capable of any *action*...[9]

Even the Christian Mary Delaney, a cleric's wife, was prepared to comment spitefully on the death of the noted beauty, Lady Coventry, one of the famous Gunning sisters, in 1760:

[8] *The Wedgwood Letters*, ed. Ann Finer and George Savage (London, 1965), p. 221.
[9] Malcolm Elwin, *The Noels and the Milbankes* (London, 1967), pp. 39–40.

What a wretched end Lady Coventry makes after her short-lived reign of beauty! Not contented with the *extraordinary share* Providence had bestowed on her, she presumptuously and vainly sought to mend it, and by that means they say she has destroyed her life; for Dr Taylor says the white she made use of for her face and neck was rank poison.[10]

Character assassination in diaries was commonplace, with scurrilous rumours and factual details often intertwined; Farington noted, for example, that John Hunter had treated the painter Morland for a venereal infection,[11] and that Monro had diagnosed a 'hectic fever' afflicting Hoppner the artist.[12]

Letters were generally more informative than diaries about illness when the writer wished to explain its course to a distant correspondent, and they also identify medical practitioners more positively than the private diary, where entries such as 'Dr W' are regrettably common, intended to inform only the writer rather than the historian two centuries later. Not all correspondents, however, chose to burden their friends or relatives with their own health problems; an example of such restraint was the poet William Shenstone, who referred to his extensive correspondence as 'the history of my mind' but was also very reticent about his own symptoms, noting only that 'Evil and capricious health (the particulars of which would make a detail of no importance) destroys all my punctuality'.[13] He was always prepared to exchange medical gossip about others, however. The disadvantages of letters for the historian are twofold: firstly, usually only one side of a correspondence survives, and secondly they lack the daily, regular element of the diary as a record of health, suffering or treatment. Many patients continued to keep up their diary entries when they felt too ill to write letters. Memoirs and autobiographies, clearly intended for publication, are an entirely different source for medical history.

The psychology of the diarist and the writer of letters is very different, although clearly diarists can also be correspondents. The typical diarist tended to be orderly, meticulous and painstaking, preferring diary volumes of the same size, colour and format, even, as in the cases of Nicholas Blundell of Little Crosby, Lancashire, and

[10] *The Life and Correspondence of Mrs Delaney*, ed. Lady Llanover (6 vols., London, 1862), vol. 3, p. 584.
[11] *The Diary of Joseph Farington*, ed. Kenneth Garlick and Angus Macintyre (Newhaven and London, 1978–), vol. 3, pp. 907–8.
[12] *Ibid.*, vol. 4, p. 1568.
[13] *The Letters of William Shenstone*, ed. Marjorie Williams (Oxford, 1939), p. 401.

Joseph Farington, keeping rough working notebooks as a first draft and then neat versions of the final journal. The exceptionally committed diarists (Pepys and Farington) had special cabinets made to contain their volumes.

Personal motives for keeping a diary

Although many kinds of people were letter writers, those only barely literate corresponded in a factual, brief style, with few observations or comments. However, eighteenth century diarists were above a basic literacy level and had certain characteristics in common: they were noticeably age, sex and class specific. The majority of eighteenth century diaries surviving were kept by adult males of middle or superior social class. There were exceptions, but of over 500 English provincial diarists recently surveyed for the period 1700–99,[14] only forty were women and a further three young girls; boys' diaries appear rarely to have been kept or not to have survived. The high proportion of male diarists can be attributed fairly obviously to known literacy levels of the period and to the fact that men were primarily engaged in politics, business, public affairs or professional careers for which a personal diary was an asset. Even the occasional humble craftsman, such as Joseph Hill, a wigmaker of Stratford-upon-Avon, kept a diary in which he recorded customers' accounts, their head measurements and the mileage he travelled in visiting their houses.[15] Women were not usually occupied in public or professional life and either managing a household, if she were affluent, or performing domestic tasks gave little uncommitted time for diary-keeping. The exceptional woman, such as Abigail Gawthern of Nottingham, did write a journal, however. As most diaries were essentially personal, the opportunity of writing privately, as in the gentleman's study, was not possible for all and, of course, the poorer diarist, even if literate, would be deterred by the cost of buying the raw materials of ink, pen and paper. Diaries are more common for the later than the earlier eighteenth century, for the practical reasons of wider literacy and a greater chance of the diary's survival. The spectrum of diary-keepers widened considerably when travel was involved, perhaps because more leisure time was available

---

[14] The author carried out a survey of MS diaries in English provincial record offices in 1983.

[15] Shakespeare Birthplace Trust Records Office, Stratford-upon-Avon, PR 117. Even in a diary as modest as this, the writer noted a local surgeon's dissection of a murderess's body and a child's death from smallpox.

and novel scenes were witnessed, but also because a travel diary was commonly read by others than the writer on his return home.

Motives for diary-writing varied greatly. Many diarists began to keep journals as a simple record of work in progress which then expanded; for example, Joseph Farington noted in detail the various stages of his sketches and paintings but gradually extended his account into a wide-ranging social and political diary, with much medical content. Medical details about the writer in a diary were never uniformly distributed, since diarists unless hypochondriacs tended to need medical attention more at certain periods of their lives, especially old age. Information about other people, however, could be evenly recorded. Some diarists noted anniversaries of medical events (Samuel Pepys' lithotomy is a well-known example) and also incidents that occurred many years before of which the writer was reminded. Thus in 1820 a Somerset rector, John Skinner, when visiting Oxford, described an event he recalled from his undergraduate days twenty-seven years before in 1793:

I walked slowly along this same road after having lost part of one of my fingers by the bursting of a gun whilst snipe shooting at Iffley, my companion, Stackhouse, having gone to tell the surgeon, Grosvenor, to attend my arrival in my room.[16]

The practitioner he summoned was John Grosvenor, M.C.S., a surgeon at the Radcliffe Infirmary.[17]

Whether or not diaries were meant to be read by others than the writer also varied considerably; clearly Pepys intended posterity to enjoy his cryptic volumes, but not have them read by household servants and certainly not by his wife, for he left the shorthand code-book with his manuscript bequest for others to decipher after his death. Some manuscripts retain their secrets still. For example, John Coggs, a London printer's apprentice in the early eighteenth century, wrote his commonplace book in three different ways. He wrote in clear (for such events as buying new clothes or travelling on his master's business) and also in simple anagrams, easy to read after a few minutes but not at a casual glance. This basic code he used to record details of his master's family life (when his master and mistress had a 'horrid fauling out' and 'he did not go to her hall night') or when he and his fellow apprentice broke the law by smashing a neighbouring

[16] *Journal of a Somerset Rector, 1803–34*, ed. Howard and Peter Coombs (Oxford, 1984), p. 51.
[17] *Medical Register*, ed. Samuel Foart Simmons (London, 1783), pp. 19, 102.

tradesman's windows, stealing meat or wine, and by gambling. However, there was a third category of information written entirely in shorthand, possibly one invented by Coggs himself, for it matches none of the known eighteenth century systems. The content of these entries, perhaps his sexual escapades, remains a mystery nearly three centuries later.[18] Some women's diaries recorded, by symbols, the writer's menstruation patterns, although very few diaries and letters included sexual information; the exceptions were husbands' comments noting a return to sleeping with their wives after childbirth (Nicholas Blundell, for example) and the entries of boastful but anxious womanisers such as Boswell and Byron. It is possible that more such accounts were originally written but were destroyed as indiscreet.

Other diaries were intended to be read quite openly by the writer's family, such as that of Richard Kay of Bury, kept while he was a surgeon's apprentice in the 1730s as a work and case book, but also as a record of his spiritual experiences and containing nothing of a confidential nature. It is possible that the desire for secrecy by the diarist also encouraged the fairly small format that most writers chose; certainly many printed diaries were advertised in the eighteenth century for particular categories of journal keepers, for example the Lady's Almanack at one shilling. The need to carry the diary in a coat pocket must also have accounted for the usually small size of both printed and self-dated volumes, but the larger, even folio-size journal suggests private storage facilities at home. Not until the nineteenth century, when diary keeping became an acknowledged genteel pastime for the under-occupied, were larger, printed journals commonly sold in stationers' shops. In this period diary writing was so common that it featured in a popular novel, *The Moonstone*, in 1868.

For the purpose of this survey only diaries that are either in English record offices or in print (if privately owned) are considered; those still in private hands in family papers have been omitted because of difficulty of access. The diaries kept by medical practitioners have also largely been excluded, although there are some of considerable interest for this period, since they were apparently little concerned with patients' responses to medical attention. The nineteenth century in fact saw a number of diaries being published, many by county record societies, and others that were edited by descendants of the diarists.[19]

---

[18] Bodleian Library, Oxford, MS Eng misc. f. 78.
[19] Diary selections have been published by various county record societies, for example: *Six North Country Diaries*, ed. J. C. Hodgson (Surtees Soc., 118,

Unfortunately both categories suffered from heavy editing, to remove material then thought to be of little interest (such as comments on the weather), tedious, repetitive or embarrassing. As the editor's subjective judgement was paramount in such publications, medical information suffered by omission in most of these categories; length of the original material was also a problem. Such famous examples as Pepys or Parson Woodforde have suffered from Victorian editors, but so also have less well-known diarists such as Farington, Blundell or, from an earlier period, Ralph Josselin. In the 1920s Farington's diaries (1793–1821) were published in eight large volumes, but much interesting material removed;[20] they are currently being republished in their entirety and may finally extend to twice that length. Blundell's 'great diurnal' had extracts published in 1895 but omitting most of the details of how he managed his Lancashire estate; its publication in three substantial volumes by the Record Society of Lancashire and Cheshire, begun in 1968, illustrates the wealth of medical and other material that selective editing can hide.[21] However, editing by the diarist's descendants is usually of a more radical nature, with editors particularly anxious in the Victorian period to remove any references that appeared discreditable. The most drastic censorship, though, was the excision of parts of letters or whole pages of diaries in the nineteenth century. Thus Lady Bessborough's letters have sentences and paragraphs cut out that, from the sense of the manuscript, appear to have referred to her illegitimate children. Some diaries known about in the nineteenth century have since been lost: for example, the *Book*

1910); *Some Bedfordshire Diaries* (Beds. Hist. Rec. Soc., 40, 1959); *Yorkshire Diaries and Autobiographies in the Seventeenth and Eighteenth Centuries*, ed. C. Jackson (Surtees Soc., LXV, 1865) and *Yorkshire Diaries and Autobiographies in the Seventeenth and Eighteenth Centuries*, ed. C. Jackson and S. Margerison (Surtees Soc., LXVIII, 1883). Family papers generally comprise only correspondence, but occasionally diaries are also included, as in *Papers and Diaries of a York Family, 1764–1839*, ed. Mrs Edwin Gray (London, 1927) and *The Francis Letters*, ed. Beata Francis and E. Keary (2 vols., London, 1901). It is impossible to tell without reading it what a volume contains, as most older works are very badly indexed, listing only well-known personalities, often omitting medical practitioners and invariably lacking a subject index; sometimes there is no index at all.

20 *The Farington Diary, 1793–1821*, ed. James Greig (8 vols., London, 1922–8).

21 *The Great Diurnal of Nicholas Blundell*, ed. J. J. Bagley (Rec. Soc. of Lancs. and Cheshire, 114, 1968–72), 3 vols. Blundell also kept a 'Prescription & Recipe Book' which has not been published. Similarly, editions of Josselin's diary prior to Alan Macfarlane's of 1976 omitted much medical and religious detail.

of Remarks kept by William Storr of Seaton Park, Yorks., had been missing since the 1880s although extracts were published in the *Yorkshire Archaeological Journal* in 1882. Quite unexpectedly it reappeared in December 1983, a welcome addition to the genre with its notes on the weather, remedies and farming activities in the early eighteenth century.[22]

The medical content of diaries and correspondence

Apart from personal medical information, diaries, commonplace books and letters of the eighteenth century can often also provide quite unexpected details of medical interest that did not involve the writer but were of sufficient note to be recorded. Thus monster or multiple births, great longevity and epidemics in distant counties were frequently recorded. From such random comment we learn that there was an outbreak of smallpox at Bicester, Oxfordshire, in 1759, for Parson Woodforde mentioned his aunt's death there as a victim,[23] and Philip Doddridge, a Northampton divine, corresponded in worried tones when the disease occurred at Worcester in 1730.[24] The local outbreak of national epidemics other than smallpox could also be recorded, and is sometimes the only reliable reference for the historian: for example at Alnwick, Northumberland, on 15 June 1782 'the influenza [was] very general in town and county but not fatal'.[25]

Certain medical conditions and treatments were very commonly recorded, particularly gout and visits to spas, usually by the complaining sufferer who hated the diet, hydrotherapy, lodgings, entertainments, other patients and the medical practitioner in equal proportions. The affluent patient with gout presumably had time to engage in lengthy correspondence if his friends were sympathetic; the occasional writer, such as Richard Radcliffe in 1780, could express annoyance and wry humour at his condition:

I wish that plaguy disorder would observe a little more propriety in its attacks, and confine itself to its own circle – the Bishops, Deans, and Canons of this realm. What the plague has it to do with curates and schoolmasters, without indeed it be a forerunner of dignity and preferment.[26]

22 Borthwick Institute of Historical Research, York, M.D. 112.
23 *The Diary of a Country Parson: the Rev. James Woodforde, 1758–1802*, ed. John Beresford (Oxford, 1978), p. 3.
24 *Calendar of the Correspondence of Philip Doddridge, D.D., 1701–51*, ed. Geoffrey F. Nuttall (Nhants. Rec. Soc., XXIX, 1979), p. 61.
25 *N. Country Diaries*, p. 242.
26 *The Letters of Richard Radcliffe and John James of Queen's College, Oxford, 1755–83*, ed. Margaret Evans (Oxford Hist. Soc., IX, 1887), p. 106.

Many elderly writers if healthy were grateful for their long life and proud of surviving, a fitting attitude in a century that valued the tontine. In 1776 one correspondent commented that 'in most respects I am as well as one in ye 65th year of his age may reasonably hope to be, — and do not yet avail myself of ye use of Spectacles'.[27] He lived to be 78. From the evidence of diaries and correspondence, patients' responses to illness varied greatly, but a strongly fatalistic strand runs through much of this eighteenth century material, as well as a stoicism towards personal suffering almost incomprehensible to the modern reader. Some writers, such as Mrs Mary Delaney, especially seemed to relish medical detail in the voluminous correspondence of a long life (1700–88); others note particular events of medical interest. In 1809 Faith Gray recorded in her diary that 'the operation (by Mr Wm. Hey) was completed. It began at 11 and was finished at 12';[28] her sister's death, apparently from cancer, was noted two months later. Farington too was particularly interested in medical detail; in 1799 his diary carried an entry about an acquaintance, Dr Halls, who

underwent an operation which lasted an hour probing to search the bladder for a stone which Mr Cline has decided to have formed a Sack in the Bladder, of course no attempt can be made to dislodge it — sometimes the stone falls out of the *Sack* and then it becomes a common case.[29]

Perhaps diarists recorded the time taken by medical practitioners as an indication of the patient's serious condition; in 1721 one correspondent wrote that Sir Hans Sloane had spent over half an hour on the 'thoro enquiry' of a patient, with a hopeful diagnosis of relief from 'a complication of ailments that [were] making their advances against her precious health'.[30]

Few writers railed at the hazards of childbirth, although Lady Stafford in 1793 sharply referred in a letter to the arrival of her daughter's new baby: 'This is the third child in 21 months; that is too much for the strongest constitution'.[31] Most patients, however, appear resigned to years of truly chronic ill-health, so that in the 1780s Dorothy Yorke, writing of her 'new Companion, the Gout', added that 'Nothing better have I to expect at my time of life, monstrous

27 *Greene*, p. 109.
28 *York Family*, p. 200.
29 *Farington*, vol. 4, p. 1144.
30 *Verney Letters of the Eighteenth Century from the MSS at Claydon House*, ed. Margaret Maria, Lady Verney (2 vols., London, 1930), vol. 2, p. 91.
31 *Lord Granville Leveson Gower, Private Correspondence, 1781–1821*, ed. Castalia, Countess Granville (2 vols., London, 1916), vol. 1, p. 71.

deal of pain I have endured from my foot, now easy but very weak'.[32]
Remarkably few patients seemed displeased with their medical attendant,
although some were critical of his restraints on their behaviour; in 1776
Nicholas Cresswell obviously resented being confined to his room with
a cold and commented that 'The Doctor scolds me and brings me more
of his Damnd nostrums'.[33] Patients were reluctant to accept medical
advice that meant changing their style of life to a more spartan one;
in 1784 Sir Ralph Milbanke lay 'in bed very late, which Bainbridge
says is excessively bad for him — but he is quite angry to be desired
to rise earlier or to ride'.[34] It was always easier to persuade a patient
to accept some courses of action than others, as Joseph Greene wrote
to his brother, a Lichfield apothecary, after having consulted a
Warwick practitioner of considerable local repute, Walter Landor,
M.D. (1733–1805):

I have appli'd for medical relief to Dr Lander, & others of ye best reputed
skill in these parts, & after twice blistering & swallowing above a peck of
their nauseous pharmacal apparatus, am become very little better than when
they first began to tamper with me. The pleasantest advice they have given
me, came at last; 'that my solids being much relaxed, I must frequently
mount my horse for exercise; & in my intermediate state, solace my self
plentifully with good old Port'. Peace to their Faculty-Wigs & Canes!
Though they could not restore *my* health, have put me into a charitable
method of drinking theirs.[35]

Uncritical acceptance of medical advice was noted by Lady Mary
Wortley Montagu, who thought the English 'more easily infatuated
than any other people by the hope of a panacea', and that there was
no other 'country in the world where such great fortunes are made
by physicians'.[36] A number of diarists and correspondents in the
eighteenth century, always a minority, were sharply critical of the
medical attention they or their families had received, although the
tombstone remained the most permanent and public form of criticism
of unsuccessful medical attention. Complaints ranged from unacceptable
treatments to wrong diagnoses and were exclusively from upper or
middle class writers, not obliged to express deference and aware that

32 Merlin Waterson, *The Servants' Hall, a Domestic History of Erddig* (London, 1980), p. 52 (from Erddig MSS at Clwyd County Record Office, Hawarden).
33 *More English Diaries*, ed. Arthur Ponsonby (London, 1927), p. 113.
34 Elwin, *Noels*, p. 249; John Bainbridge was a surgeon-apothecary in Durham.
35 *Greene*, p. 136.
36 Cited in Robert Southey, *Letters from England*, ed. Jack Simmons (London, 1951), p. 293.

their own social standing was far above that of their medical practitioner. In this vein Judith, Lady Milbanke, wrote about her husband's treatment in 1780:

Milbanke has had some return of the complaint in his stomach & was far from well with it yesterday; the People here think it is owing to his Stomach being so greatly relaxed by the rough Mercurial medicines he took three Years ago, for which I have long been convinced both Turton & Bromfield deserve to be hanged. The Person we consult here [Harrogate] has put him on a bracing Regimen and has forbid *Slopping, Salt Meat & much Wine.*[37]

When Mary Noel, Judith Milbanke's aunt, wrote of a friend's childbirth experience, with medical attendants who delivered a dead baby by force, she cited London's three leading practitioners, Warren, Ford and Denman, as a 'terrible list'.[38] Some diarists recorded in retrospect their fears that medical attention had actually been wrong, so that, for example, Anthony à Wood accused the practitioner attending his mother in her last illness of

having killed her by laying on a thick prodigious plaister straight on to her flesh...and this was the doctor she loved and doted on so much as so great, learned and well-deserving physician! Whereas no unskilful quack or huswife would have ventured so much as he did...[39]

A number of wrong diagnoses were recorded in diaries, especially when the result was fatal and particularly if the practitioner or patient were well-known. In May 1755 Mrs Delaney wrote to her sister of Lady Gore's unhappy experiences as a patient of Sir Richard Manningham, a famous and fashionable London accoucheur:

The night she came to her mother's house she was so very ill that Sir Richard Manningham was sent for, who declared that her disorder would soon be over, and *left her*! Almost as soon as he had left her, her pains increased; he was sent for again, found her in violent convulsions, and she had a dead child! She was for some days despaired of, but is now in her senses and better, but knew nothing of what had happened. Is not this like some old novel we have read and thought impossible?[40]

In 1794 Thomas Gainsborough's nephew described the circumstances of his uncle's death in London's gossiping artistic circles in terms entirely detrimental to the two eminent practitioners involved. A cold caught at the trial of Warren Hastings caused a tumour to 'inflame' according to the nephew; Gainsborough then

---

[37] Elwin, *Noels*, p. 173.   [38] *Ibid.*, p. 270.
[39] *More English Diaries*, p. 178.   [40] *Delaney*, vol. 3, p. 351.

applied to Dr Heberden who treated it lightly, and said it would pass away with the cold. He applied to John Hunter who advised salt water poultices which greatly increased the inflammation & a suppuration followed. There seems to have been a strange mistake or neglect both in Heberden & Hunter.[41]

How damaging to the practitioner's reputation such stories were it is impossible to estimate, but some accounts of ill-judged medical attention were still circulating years after the event. Thus the circumstances of Sir Joshua Reynolds' death in 1792 were still retailed seven years later by Lady Inchquin, who said that 'Dr Warren, Sir George Baker &c did not penetrate into the cause of his disorder'. Sir Charles Blagdon was more successful than Baker, who one day felt Reynolds' pulse and 'looked in his face and declared him a sound man';[42] when Dr Moseley failed to diagnose measles in the Duke of York in 1797 he was dismissed by the Prince of Wales.[43]

Diarists also recorded dissent between practitioners, in which the senior man usually triumphed by changing the prescribed treatment and by impugning the other man's competence. The London physician, Dr Henry Reynolds, was particularly inclined to contradict the counsel of various apothecaries; in 1794 he changed the ointment prescribed by Mr White and sent the patient to Harrogate. A year later he 'blamed' Mr Lewis, another apothecary, for telling a patient that she had 'water in her chest',[44] and throughout the Lovelace papers his dictatorial manner towards even his most aristocratic patients can be seen. A number of women patients, especially in pregnancy, were clearly afraid of their medical advisers; in her first pregnancy Harriet, Countess Granville, wrote to her sister, 'I fear Farquhar and Croft as I do viper and vixen and shall expire of fright at being left at their mercy',[45] although Farquhar had already attended her aunt, the Duchess of Devonshire.

Occasionally, a medical mishap occasioned a wryly humorous response from a writer; thus in 1716 when Lady Sutherland was dying 'by having an Artery cutt in blooding', the correspondent, Sir Thomas Cave, added 'we might better have spared him' (her husband).[46] Many patients recorded distaste or distrust of the medication they were given; Dr Matthew Baillie's snakeroot was 'nauseous' to one patient,[47] while

[41] *Farington*, vol. 1, p. 256.   [42] *Ibid.*, vol. 4, p. 1295.
[43] *Ibid.*, vol. 3, p. 805.   [44] *Ibid.*, vol. 1, pp. 194, 417.
[45] Cited in Betty Askwith, *Piety and Wit* (London, 1982), p. 73, from original material in the Castle Howard MSS.
[46] *Verney*, vol. 2, p. 31.   [47] *Francis Letters*, vol. 2, p. 513.

Samuel Johnson, having 'no confidence in rural pharmacy', insisted that no diacodium he could find would 'admit comparison' with that of Robert Holder, a Strand apothecary.[48] Sometimes the diarist recorded a mistaken prescription or over-prescribing; in 1731 Alderman Battison in Bedfordshire 'lay very ill under the Care then of Dr Godfrey, but he had been some time under Dr Wells' care, whose opiates, as they thought, did him much harm'.[49] Another critical diarist, Nicholas Blundell, noted how, in 1710, he had 'discoursed with Dr Smithson about his ordering too much lodinum for Mr Lancaster'.[50] Some writers said that a wrong prescription had actually been given, so that in 1780 Mrs Davison had just recovered from a serious illness which 'was greatly increased by an ignorant Apothecary giving her a wrong medicine when she was first taken'.[51] Some patients were especially suspicious of the medical treatment they were given and wrote scathingly to their friends. In 1791 Lady Wentworth was prevailed upon by her husband to

take a prescription of Dr Vaughan's which she says makes her worse. Indeed I don't think it does her any good, but Lord W. is so fond of his Esculapius that he thinks he must always be right.[52]

The same correspondent wrote of a friend, Mrs Biscoe, that 'Dr Denman thinks she will miscarry. She has been blooded & lays on a couch, so if she is not ill, they will make her so'.[53] Sometimes a writer recorded a medical opinion that was to prove particularly unfortunate when he or she died soon afterwards, often after considerable suffering. Thus on 30 November 1781 Sophia Curzon in London wrote to her aunt, Mary Noel, of her condition:

I can now inform you of Dr Ford's opinions about me...He has been with me this morning & he almost certainly confirms my suspicions which were that my child has been dead some time. He won't say that he is certain of it but that it is *most* probable. But he assures me I shall continue very well until the time & then he says I shall be in no more danger than if the child was alive & shall recover afterwards faster than usual. I told him that if he apprehended I should be particularly ill I beg'd he would say so, as I should let you know as I was certain you would come to me, but he said I had

[48] *The Letters of Samuel Johnson*, ed. R. W. Chapman (3 vols., Oxford, 1952), vol. 3, p. 194.
[49] *The Diary of Benjamin Rogers, Rector of Carlton, 1720–71*, ed. C. F. Linnell (Beds. Hist. Rec. Soc., xxx, 1949), p. 26.
[50] *Blundell*, vol. 1, p. 257.   [51] Elwin, *Noels*, p. 159.
[52] *Ibid.*, p. 399.   [53] *Ibid.*

nothing to alarm me or fret me but the not having a live child. He desires
I will go on just as usual & said he would call on me to see how I went
on...I confess it has been much on my mind lately and I cannot help feeling
more frighten'd than usual [she already had two children, born in 1779 and
1781]. Thank God I did not stay to be confin'd in the Country. I hope with
a proper trust in God I shall be able to go on through this affair...[54]

By January 1782 she was very ill and consulted Dr John Turton, but
wrote that she wished he

would take more effectual means to recover me as the medicines don't seem
to have effect enough but Ford & Turton seem'd to me to be like all other
Doctors to be of a different opinion & as Ford mentioned Bath I think Turton
will be for sending me to Tonbridge...[55]

Six months later, at the age of 24, Sophia Curzon was dead.

Medical terminology of patients and practitioners

Patients' language in correspondence was usually euphemistic, even
between close relatives when greater frankness might have been
expected. Medical terminology was only rarely used, and almost
exclusively by men who, like Johnson and Farington, moved in
medical circles. Women's gynaecological problems particularly attracted
euphemisms, even between women correspondents themselves, and
always when the practitioner himself was advising. One woman wrote
of her hoped-for pregnancy to an aunt in 1777:

I sent for Fox as soon as I came here...he thinks my illness is owing to
impoverished Blood & a Nervous Habit, but he is at present rather cautious
about giving me much Medicine, as there is a possibility that there may be
a reason for being careful, it being just eight weeks today since any appearance
of a certain affair. You & I who are acquainted with the irregularity of my
Constitution shall not flatter ourselves much from this circumstance, but was
I to hurt myself by any imprudence I should be miserable ever after –
therefore am resolved to bear with patience any disagreable (tho' not
alarming) complaints a short time rather than run any risques...[56]

The approach of menstruation in a 13-year-old girl was described by
Dr Reynolds as 'the onset of a certain period' that caused her
indisposition,[57] while in 1797 one diarist commented that there were
double the number of female lunatics than males in asylums 'partly
owing to *constitutional causes*'.[58] Relief at not being pregnant again was

[54] *Ibid.*, p. 185.   [55] *Ibid.*, pp. 188–9.
[56] *Ibid.*, pp. 77–8; John Fox was a surgeon-apothecary at Leicester.
[57] *Ibid.*, p. 415.   [58] *Farington*, vol. 3, p. 888.

recorded by one correspondent writing to her sister of the arrival of 'a most welcome visitor'.[59] The change from eighteenth to nineteenth century anatomical terminology in aristocratic society at least is exemplified in two comments. In 1777 Elizabeth Noel wrote to her aunt

My Br[other]'s disorder was an Abscess upon his Bum, wch after ten days confinement to his bed, was without any danger cut by Kirkland, who said he might perhaps be able to Hunt before the Winter was over...[60]

Four decades later, when Georgiana, Duchess of Bedford, noticed a young guest wearing a gown cut very low at the back, she shrieked, 'My dear, when do you mean to favour us with a sight of your bottom?' The female correspondent added the comment in a letter to her sister, 'I am ashamed of having written it'.[61] Euphemisms referring to male patients were in an equally narrow range; Boswell's inability to keep silent about his sexual adventures ensured a contemporary's comment that 'his excesses have brought his constitution to a crisis which has alarmed him much' which would, though not explicit, be widely understood.[62]

The level of medical confidentiality within certain narrow social circles in the eighteenth century was low, and senior practitioners seem to have disclosed details about prominent patients they had treated to other patients, who then exchanged this piece of gossip for other information. Even third-hand gossip was passed on to and about equals or superiors, although rarely to those much further down the social hierarchy than the writer. Thus Addington's treating Chatham's gout or Sir George Baker's attention to the Princess Elizabeth were reported by Mrs Delaney to her various correspondents.[63] When, in 1793, Gibbon, the historian, was in 'a very indifferent state of health at Bath, Dr Milman told Mr Lysons he thought recovery doubtful', an opinion Lysons passed on to his friend, Farington;[64] Gibbon died the next year. In some cases medical confidentiality was broken merely by recording that a well-known practitioner, famed for particular skills, was treating a patient – as, for example, when Edmund Burke was attended by Dr Francis Willis in 1795.[65]

59 Askwith, *Piety*, p. 104.
60 Elwin, *Noels*, p. 76; Kirkland was presumably Thomas Kirkland of Ashby de la Zouch.
61 Askwith, *Piety*, pp. 124–5.   62 *Farington*, vol. 2, p. 330.
63 *Delaney*, vol. 5, p. 269, and vol. 6, p. 315.
64 *Farington*, vol. 1, p. 71.   65 *Ibid.*, vol. 2, p. 291.

Patients' estimation of practitioners

Medical practitioners were themselves likely to be the subject of gossip in the eighteenth century, some of it clearly untrue; it was, of course, easy to condemn anyone as alcoholic, illegitimate, insane or of democratic sympathies. Humble origins or ambitious marriages regularly occasioned comment, whether of medical practitioners or not, so that when Dr Clarke became a physician at the London Dispensary, having trained at Edinburgh, contemporaries recalled his illegitimate status as the son of an apothecary in Crutched Friars, London, and Mrs A., with whom the apothecary lived.[66] Even a man as eminent as Sir Lucas Pepys was said to be suffering from an 'imbecility of mind' when ill,[67] while Dr Salt of Bath was so afflicted with 'a Hypochondriack disorder as to be obliged to relinquish his profession' in 1800. Unseemly medical wrangles about public appointments also caused gossip, for example in 1798 between Dr Batty and Mr Lewis, who both sought the post of surgeon at the Lying-in Hospital.[68] Perhaps the most detailed character sketch of a contemporary medical practitioner in an eighteenth century diary was that describing the abilities and faults of William Cruickshank, who died in 1800:

[he had] of late been much addicted to drinking & of late Ale in large quantities. He was a man of a very nervous habit & very passionate...He died in a fit, as they say, of something like appoplexy. He was of late in habits of expence and was reducing his fortune which is now supposed to be £3000. He married a Sister of Nicol, the bookseller, from whom He has been long separated & He has till lately kept a mistress. Out of his profession He was thought to have only moderate abilities, but was very skilful as a Surgeon. He suffered much from fanciful apprehensions. If he failed of performing a Cure even where it cd. not be expected, He was apt to suspect that people reflected on him. Ideas of this kind afflicted him much & were carried very far.[69]

Undoubtedly medical affluence and incomes caused gossip, especially in London, exactly as did the earnings of other prosperous men, such as fashionable artists or architects. Annual incomes were discussed, and physicians said to be 'worth' particular sums or individual fees cited. Other marks of prosperity on the eighteenth century yardstick were also noted: that Dr Reynolds allowed his son £300 a year in 1798,[70]

[66] *Ibid.*, vol. 4, p. 1338.
[67] *Ibid.*, vol. 3, p. 96, and vol. 4, p. 1422.   [68] *Ibid.*, vol. 3, pp. 964–70.
[69] *Ibid.*, vol. 4, p. 1412.   [70] *Ibid.*, vol. 3, p. 1021.

or that in 1774 the coach belonging to Dr Macnamara at Margate was 'splendid' and 'very pretty indeed', with 'Copper Plate Pannels and Painted Blush Colour'.[71] Rumours of medical incomes varied. Reynolds in 1779 was said to make £6,000 a year,[72] while Richard Mead was reputed to have earned some £5,000 a year for three decades, but because he 'lived handsomely' left only about £50,000 at his death in 1754; in 1797 Richard Warren died worth £170,000.[73] Far more modest incomes, however, were generally earned in eighteenth century medicine; in the provinces incomes were much lower for most practitioners, with the exception of some well-reputed men of large practice in cathedral cities and county towns who had secured all the affluent local patients to attend. One diarist was sufficiently interested in medical incomes to record a conversation he had had with two young Norfolk physicians in 1795, each of whom practised at Fakenham where £400 a year was possible for a man aged 28.[74] Complaints about medical fees were surprisingly few, although Fanny Burney wondered if it were not more economical to spend money on fuel bills than on the apothecary.[75] In 1721 one Buckinghamshire lady wrote to her husband of her dissatisfaction at the recent costly medical attention she and her children had received. Dr Cheshire, of whom she complained, she had recently praised as a 'very civil ingenuous man' before he presented his bill:

the doctor said he woud give me no more physick, so I have dispatcht him, he had seven ginues of me and I gave his man a crown, and I have paid Mr Turner's bill for all the things that I and the children had so I thank God I've got all of under 10 pd. and I daresay if I had gon to London it would have cost me fivety.[76]

Large professional incomes could cause criticism in times of epidemic, and Mrs Lybbe Powys noted in her diary that

---

[71] *Francis Letters*, vol. 1, p. 213; in 1716 Blundell had described a practitioner's coach as 'large and handsome...drawn with only one horse' (vol. 2, p. 173).
[72] *Farington*, vol. 3, p. 712.
[73] *Ibid.*, vol. 4, p. 1244.
[74] *Ibid.*, vol. 3, p. 380.
[75] *The Famous Miss Burney*, ed. Barbara G. Shrank and David J. Supino (New York, 1976), p. 266.
[76] *Verney*, vol. 2, p. 84; Mr Turner was the local apothecary. She noted that Cheshire had qualified nine years ago and was a Balliol College, Oxford, man. Further down the social scale a Sussex tradesman in 1760 resented the half guinea paid for a visit from a local physician, who could charge as he pleased and 'not be culpable according to any human law' (*Thomas Turner, the Diary of a Georgian Shopkeeper*, ed. G. H. Jennings (Oxford, 1979), p. 47).

When the influenza was so violent this spring at Bath, Dr Parry visited 120 patients in two days; and Mr Crook, the apothecary, only wished he could have a lease of the same influenza for eight years — he should not desire a better fortune.[77]

From the evidence of family and estate account books the largest medical fees in the eighteenth century were understandably paid for lunatics under residential care, a point noted by one contemporary attorney, perhaps with envy, in 1733:

we are ready to be Devour'd by the mad Doctors for Mony. Dr Monroe alone demanding for himself and assistants about £130 tho we think not a Qur. could be due or deserved.[78]

In spite of the fees they paid, not all patients were sensible and obedient; Lady Newdigate wrote how she had abused Dr Richard Jebb's advice and taken a dangerous dose of nine opium pills,[79] while Horace Walpole erroneously swallowed an emetic, 'designed for one of the maids', instead of the hartshorn he was regularly prescribed for fever.[80] Patients also experimented with each other's medicines, Blundell taking 'a dose of physick: twas part of what was ordered by Dr Lancaster for my wife' but without any apparent ill-effects.[81]

In attempting to understand the eighteenth century patient's view of the medical practitioner, perhaps the most interesting part of both diaries and correspondence, especially the latter, is when the practitioner's own words to or about the patient are quoted verbatim, and in this respect letters are more informative than journals, since presumably the diarist remembered what he or she was told. The flavour of the practitioner's words can occasionally seem to cross two centuries when reported by a skilful correspondent such as Josiah Wedgwood, who in 1772 wrote to his friend, Thomas Bentley, describing his wife's pregnancy and medical attention:

23 August: [her] sickness and Vomiting, with all the unfavourable symptoms are returned, and as Doctor Darwin, who attended her yesterday, apprehends an inflamation of the Liver, and she is so extremely weak and emaciated, I am really alarmed for her safety, and in great distress... Mr Bent had all along assured me, what indeed seemed very probable, that Mrs Ws was a

---

77 *Passages from the Diary of Mrs Lybbe Powys, 1756–1808*, ed. Emily J. Climenson (London, 1899), p. 352.

78 *Verney*, vol. 2, p. 84.

79 Lady Newdigate-Newdegate, *The Cheverels of Cheverel Manor* (London, 1898), pp. 45–6.

80 *Berry*, vol. 1, p. 317.   81 *Blundell*, vol. 2, p. 62.

Breeding case only, and no danger at all attending it, but upon her relapse I sent for Docter Darwin, who is very clear in his opinion of the inflamation, and from his questions to her I believe he apprehends a schirrus to be the cause of it, but he would not tell me any farther particulars, only that she was very ill, but that she had this in her favour, that *Breeding* and *Liver cases* were often very much alike, and he would come and see her again in two or three days, when I shall be very happy if I can give you a better account of the health of my Dear Girl...

7 September: Mrs Wedgwood had an extreme bad night, and miscarried this morning. Her situation is attended with much danger. Mr Bent says her case is the most singular one he had Ever known and nothing but the greatest attention in nursing and keeping everything quiet about her can save her life...[82]

As transport was difficult and even the wealthy and their physicians were unable to travel in very bad weather, patients resorted to consultation and prescriptions by post. Unfortunately, relatively few patients' letters have survived, although they are known to have existed in quantity from the evidence of contemporary probate inventories.[83] Physicians' letters to patients have more frequently been retained in family papers, especially those of the country gentry, who sought advice from London or county town physicians when they returned to their remote rural seats; some of Erasmus Darwin's letters to his patients, for example, have recently been published.[84] Earlier in the century Sir Hans Sloane corresponded with many families; in 1705 he wrote to Lady Mordaunt an extremely detailed letter of advice for her husband who was apparently recovering from fever, but added a recommendation to her ladyship as well, that 'the pain in [her] back seems to come from the kidneys; for that I know no properer remedy than a little syrup of marshmallows'[85] (Fig. 1). In 1722 he wrote to Lord Fermanagh apologising for not being able to visit Lady Fermanagh, prevented by his own 'hoarseness and cough', but, having prescribed bleeding, blistering, laudanum, Bath waters and wine as well as his

[82] *Wedgwood Letters*, pp. 131, 133–4; James Bent was a surgeon-apothecary in Newcastle-under-Lyne.

[83] When William Johnston, M.D., of Warwick, died in 1725 his trustees commented with feeling that there were 'vast numbers of Letters and various mixt accounts being endless to peruse', including a great many patients' letters which have unhappily not survived. The letters, as waste paper, sold for 10s 6d (Joan Lane, 'The household of a Stuart physician', *Medical History*, xvii (1973), 82–7).

[84] *The Letters of Erasmus Darwin*, ed. Desmond King-Hele (Cambridge, 1981).

[85] Warwick County Record Office, CR 1368/vol. 3, 73.

favourite marshmallows, he promised to call the next day provided
he was informed before 8 o'clock.[86] Occasionally physicians' bills were
more informative than might be expected; Sloane's to Lady Sedley
in 1709 recorded 'my attendance upon and care of her sister Mrs
Newdigate for many months', for which he received twenty-five
guineas.[87] County town physicians also corresponded about their
distant patients, so that, for example, in 1791 Dr Landor of Warwick
wrote an extremely detailed account of his recent treatment and the
medication provided for George Lucy of Charlecote during a 'paralytick
attack', as well as his professional opinion on the patient's ability to
make a will.[88] Practitioners' letters were passed round members of a
patient's family. In November 1760 Mrs Delaney returned to her niece,
Mary, a letter written by Dr Burgh about her sister, Mrs Dewes, living
in Warwickshire;[89] the doctor appears to be Thomas Burgh, M.D.,
of Coventry (d. 1771), who had already treated other county families.[90]
When Mrs Dewes died a few weeks later Dr T. Ford of Bath wrote
a sympathetic but uninformative letter to Mrs Delaney in 1761:

A little before twelve Mrs Dewes complained to Nanny that the pain
increased towards her back, and 'wished I had not been gone'; by her
direction I was sent for. She said, 'You see I have kept my promise with
you' (meaning that she had sent on her growing worse); she was exceedingly
sensible, and took a cup with pennyroyal water in her own hand and helped
herself to it, at about a quarter after twelve. Her speech began to falter, though
she did not attempt to say anything *but what I perfectly understood*. After this
she lay perfectly quiet, and a quarter before one *without a struggle or groan*
passed to a state of infinite happiness.
That God may be your support in this hour of trial, and that you and I resign
this life with the same patience, tranquillity, and dependence on his mercies,
is the prayer of,

Madam,
Your faithful humble servant,
T. Ford.[91]

Most medical advice was authoritarian, and the practitioner usually
'declared', 'pronounced' or was 'of the opinion'. Patients were
invariably 'in the hands of', 'in the care of' or 'under' named
practitioners. Even the most eminent patient was expected to be
obedient to medical instructions; thus Dr Turton 'ordered' the famous

[86] *Verney*, vol. 2, p. 93.   [87] W.C.R.O., CR 136/B. 2507.
[88] W.C.R.O., CR 931/295 and 297.   [89] *Delaney*, vol. 3, p. 615.
[90] C.C.R.O., 105/5/35 and W.C.R.O., CR 136/v. 156.
[91] *Delaney*, vol. 4, p. 629.

judge, Lord Mansfield, to have a change of air and Princess Elizabeth had to obtain Sir George Baker's 'leave to dance' when she was convalescent. Patients, however, usually noted that they 'sent for' or 'ordered' even leading practitioners to attend them. Some patients were unreasonably demanding, others merely inconsiderate; the Honourable Mrs Boscawen wrote in 1782 of a friend, 'ill all day yesterday, but did not send for Dr Ford until night',[92] and even Sir Hans Sloane was 'sent for' to attend a fever patient in 1737.[93] The country gentleman's relationship with a provincial apothecary was clearly similar to that with other local tradesmen, albeit of a superior kind. In 1701, for example, Sir John Mordaunt wrote to his wife, who was in London, of his own ill-health and treatment in the country, with several interesting comments:

I did take ye Powders last night, & ye twitching or rather convulsion in my right hand I writ to you about, returning in ye night & this morning, having ordred Mr Bradshaw to come over, he tooke away seven ounces of blood from me which makes me begin my Letter ye sooner, to give you an Account how I am after these remidies, it is now four of ye Clock, my Powders have wrought three times & I believe have done working, ye first cups of my bloode appear foule & discolour'd, the last is clear and of good colour; I did feare that twitching upon my Nerves & the tingling in my hands & numness in my Fingers, might proceed from want of a due circulacion in my blood, & am now confirm'd in it, for I have had nothing of them since an houre after I was blooded, & thanks be to God I find myself very well...[94]

Diaries and letters also noted when physicians visited patients in their country homes, nicely illustrating the travel problems in eighteenth century England. In 1715 Richard Frewin, an Oxford physician, was expected at Claydon, Buckinghamshire, but as it was January the 'rainy weather prevented him',[95] and when Dr John Wall travelled from Worcester to Halesowen in 1757 to treat Lord Dudley's inflamed leg, he was obliged to 'stay there all night'.[96]

Very occasionally a practitioner refused to attend when summoned although not visiting another patient. One correspondent reported in 1721 that, when his wife had 'hysteric cholic' at midnight a practitioner named only as 'Sir R.B.' [? Sir Richard Blackmore] was sent for, but 'he would not come out of his bed'. Dr Smart 'of the

---

[92] *Ibid.*, vol. 6, pp. 347, 429, 116.   [93] *Verney*, vol. 2, p. 145.
[94] W.C.R.O., CR 1368/vol. 1. John Bradshaw, an apothecary, lived at 1 Jury St, Warwick.
[95] *Verney*, vol. 2, p. 23.   [96] *Shenstone*, p. 462.

Hospital' came until Dr Chamberlain was able to attend this particular patient.[97] Further down the social scale, apothecaries often made several visits in one day or night to an insistent patient (Farington at Bath, suffering with haemorrhoids in 1801, was attended many times by Mr Sloper in the same night).[98]

Even when the practitioner came and gave advice, for many patients actually interpreting the medical opinion was difficult, especially when so ambivalently expressed as that of Mr Evans. His 'nervous' young patient was to go to Harrogate or Cheltenham in the summer to make her 'stout' (strong), but he added that

if it does not all we wish, the fault will be in her natural Constitution, which tho' not a bad one is irritable & he does not think any Course of medicine would alter it, but if injudiciously given might injure her very materially...[99]

The eighteenth century practitioner was obliged in certain cases to give bad news to the patient's family and many writers reported prognoses of despair. For example, Dundas had 'no hopes' of a girl with scarlet fever, while Darwin was able to give the Wedgwood family 'little hope'; in fairness to such eminent practitioners, it should be added that they were often called in only at the last and desperate moments. Some practitioners warned their patients against a course of action for less than obvious reasons; thus Dr Alexander Hunter of York, not wishing to lose an affluent, titled patient, told her that a trip to Lisbon, then a fashionable resort for English consumptives, would induce sea-sickness that might be 'attended with the most fatal consequences'.[100] Only fairly infrequently was medical advice to poor patients recorded, usually because of literacy limitations, but one Coventry weaver, Joseph Gutteridge, who had been a sickly child, recalled

one old physician, a Quaker, named Dr Southam, refusing to prescribe for me, remarking that the money in my case would be wasted. He recommended that which suited my tastes and habits much better, namely, as much exercise in the open air as I could take...[101]

Gutteridge lived to be 83. Other practitioners deliberately kept back

97 *Verney*, vol. 2, p. 81.
98 *Farington*, vol. 4, pp. 1488–9, 1492, 1496–7.
99 Newdegate, *Cheverels*, p. 135. Thomas Evans of Knightsbridge was the family's surgeon–apothecary when they were in London.
100 *Ibid.*, p. 30.
101 *Master and Artisan in Victorian England*, ed. Valerie E. Chancellor (London, 1969), p. 87.

unpleasant information from the patient, so that Charles Hawkins, attending George III in 1788, advised Fanny Burney, Her Majesty's lady-in-waiting, 'but you need not tell that to the Queen'.[102] Lady Newdigate conferred with Mr Evans out of the patient's hearing in 1792 and described the incident to her husband by letter (the young patient, Sally, was suffering from inability to sing in public, a course on which she was being urged by her ambitious patrons):

[Evans] confirms my opinion of its being nervous but speaks of ye Consiquences as being more serious than I had apprehended. He does not absolutely object to her singing or learning to Sing if she can do it without difficulty & as it were in Sport, but on no Consideration must her mind be agitated with hope or fear. He orders her Valerian & to steam her head over Rosemary & says he will see her again in a day or two. I have follow'd him out of ye Room to know his real opinion & he has frighten'd me sadly. He says her Nerves seem to be very delicate & that she has a Scorbutic irritability about her, that must be prevented from fixing there by taking care to keep her in an even tranquil state of Mind; that he has known Girls at her Age with ye Like delicate sensations lose all power of voice, even of speech, have a Paralytic Stroke or become stupify'd from great exertion of Spirits. No doubt these little Tryals before Company have been such to our Dear Girl...[103]

Admiration and regard for a medical practitioner did not apparently depend upon his success or a pessimistic prognosis; when Elizabeth Berry consulted Dr Baillie, 'very rational, kind and sensible', she added that he 'pitied' her complaints but was 'by no means sanguine in his hopes of removing them'.[104] At the time she was corresponding with the great hypochondriac of the period, Horace Walpole (Lord Orford), and she herself lived a further forty-five years; it was, perhaps, part of Baillie's skill that he recognised a patient who did not wish to be told that she was in good health. Walpole himself usually had opinions about his various medical attendants, most of whom he approved. Thus in 1791 he described his surgeon, Mr Watson, as 'all tenderness and attention, and is persuaded today that I shall recover the use of my lèft hand, of which I despaired'; later he referred to Watson as his 'oracle'.[105]

Even unwelcome advice was still followed; in the 1740s when Dr Oliver was treating Mercy Doddridge, her husband, Philip, complained at her long absence in Bath, quoting Oliver's response that he must

[102] *Burney*, p. 211.
[103] Newdegate, *Cheverels*, p. 131.
[104] *Berry*, vol. 2, p. 333.
[105] *Ibid.*, vol. 1, pp. 280, 371.

'consider it as one of the HARD LAWS of NECESSITY which can
be conquered by nothing but SUBMISSION – so I SUBMIT'.[106] The
occasional patient queried the medical advice given and Walpole would
not accept the apothecary's proposed ether treatment 'without
Hewetson', his regular practitioner.[107] Most writers, although dubious
about a practitioner praised by another patient, were usually prepared
to experiment:

I have got Mary to promise she will see Reynolds when in Town, & tho'
I do not expect such things as you attribute to his prescriptions, I shall be
most happy if he can give her better health.[108]

Many patients understandably complained at certain types of uncomfortable treatment:

yᵉ violence of my fall, though attended with but a short duration of Pain
at first, produced a small tumefaction near yᵉ groin on my right side, which,
on shewing it to Mr Pestell of Stratford he pronounced it to be an incipient
Hernia or rupture of an Intestine; and by his advice, I wear at this instant
an elastic steel Truss, which by his means I procured from London: and
though this uncouth bandage keeps yᵉ Peritonaeum from a farther dangerous
descent, yet the wearing it constantly in the daytime, rather bruises yᵉ
Contiguous Parts; and is, at times very troublesome to me...[109]

Only a minority of writers recorded their gratitude to practitioners
in journals or correspondence; however, one diarist noted, even though
her sister had died under medical care, 'The Doctor's kindness and
attention ought never to be forgotten',[110] while another grateful
patient gave the Coventry surgeon, Richard Jones, who had successfully
inoculated her against smallpox in 1751, a 'present of a Handsome silver
Coffy Pot'.[111] An Essex miller appreciated the 'generosity & politeness
of Mr Sharp' in charging him only five guineas when he expected a
bill for four times that amount.[112] Judith Milbanke was enthusiastic
about being treated by Sir John Elliott in 1782 because she attributed
feeling so much better than she was two months ago 'entirely to his
advice'. She wrote in the same year of an attentive but unnamed
apothecary whose efforts 'certainly saved Sophy's life & he sat up with
her all night & nursed her as if she had been his own Child'.[113]

[106] *Doddridge*, p. 177.
[107] *Berry*, vol. 2, p. 13.   [108] Elwin, *Noels*, p. 388.
[109] *Greene*, pp. 149–50; Charles Pestell, a Stratford-upon-Avon surgeon-apothecary, was twice mayor of the borough.
[110] *York Family*, p. 202.   [111] *Doddridge*, p. 350.
[112] Essex County Record Office, diary of John Crosier, Nov. 1779; T/A 387.
[113] Elwin, *Noels*, pp. 201, 206.

Patients undoubtedly advised each other to change medical attendants. Walpole urged Miss Berry in 1795 to consult Sir George Baker,[114] and, when seeking an accoucheur for her niece in 1792, Mary Noel surveyed the leading obstetricians. The decision was an important one, for her niece was aged 40 at the time and about to give birth to her first child (who in 1815 would marry Lord Byron). While admitting that Bainbridge had a good record as an accoucheur, never having lost a mother, she was particularly in favour of Underwood, whom she had 'heard very well spoken of', but had reservations about Denman, to whom she was not 'particularly partial'. Mary Noel then asked Vaughan's advice about Underwood, whom she advocated to her niece, having heard that Richard Warren had recommended him and that he had recently attended Lady Melbourne.[115]

The value of a medical reputation is apparent from the evidence of diaries and letters; as well as accoucheurs, other practitioners had reputations beyond the immediate circle of their own patients, and having treated an aristocratic patient successfully, a man was often able to extend his practice quite considerably, with a cure his best possible advertisement. Thus to treat his eyes Wedgwood deliberately sought Dr Elliott, who had recently attended both the Duchess of Bedford and the Duchess of Norfolk.[116] Although few practitioners were addressed in verse by a leading poet of the day (Cowper's 'Heberden, virtuous and skilful') or immortalised in a lyric ('Robin Adair'), physicians were well or ill reputed generally for their individual skills, their personal qualities and occasionally for their social standing. In many instances the adjective 'eminent' was used (Dr John Wall of Worcester[117] or Dr W. Garrow of Barnet, Hertfordshire[118]) in the mid eighteenth century, although by the early nineteenth century the phrase 'highly spoke of' frequently referred to practitioners,[119] perhaps suggesting a change of values when a patient enquired about a practitioner. Flattering descriptions were randomly given; Dr Charleton of Bath was 'in great reputation' in 1760[120] while Dr Hale of Bishop's Stortford, Hertfordshire, was 'an old physician of great repute' in 1748.[121] A variety of men were praised as 'ingenious' (as having a high intellectual capacity): for example, a new physician, Dr Cheshire, in

---

[114] *Berry*, vol. 1, p. 491.
[115] Elwin, *Noels*, pp. 402–4.
[116] *Wedgwood Letters*, pp. 87–9.
[117] *Shenstone*, p. 467.
[118] *Delaney*, vol. 4, p. 169.
[119] *Journal of a Somerset Rector, 1803–1834, John Skinner*, ed. Howard and Peter Coombs (Oxford, 1984), p. 71.
[120] *Delaney*, vol. 3, p. 625.
[121] *Verney*, vol. 2, p. 242.

Buckinghamshire in 1721, Dr Jones of Hatton Garden, London, in 1734[122] and Dr Quin in Ireland in 1759.[123] News of success in a particular medical skill was passed from one grateful patient to another, so that Dr Hays of Windsor in 1755 had 'particular success with the smallpox'[124] while a physician who prescribed little or seldom – for example, Dr Farrer of Northamptonshire in 1736[125] – was known for his attitude.

Some practitioners were so highly regarded that they were referred to by the nick-name Aesculapius: for instance in 1788 Mr Clark was called 'the Cheltenham Aesculapius' while in 1791 Mr Power was 'our little Aesculapius' when he successfully treated an elderly patient with erysipelas. Practitioners were also valued for their qualities in a successful relationship with patients. Mr Bully (by 1783 a partner in the Reading practice of Messrs Bulley and Ring) was described as 'a very sensible man...he is an enemy to much medicine, & only approves of Red rose leaf tea & elixir of vitriol'[126] for a woman recovering from a miscarriage. Written comments by some appreciative patients suggest a personal relationship with a practitioner. In 1754 Mrs Delaney was 'much concerned for Dr Heberden on the death of his wife; his gentle and affectionate disposition will make him for some time very miserable'. She also referred to the royal surgeon as 'the gentle Hawkins' in 1770. The sorely tried Queen Charlotte described Sir George Baker in 1786 as her friend, whose advice would be 'that of a sensible and feeling man' (with the contemporary usage of 'sensible' to mean 'sensitive').[127]

Sometimes only qualified praise was accorded to even the most eminent men. When Dr Wilkes of Willenhall, Staffordshire, died in 1760 he was 'little lamented but for his judgment in physick. He was without all doubt a good physician but no charity' according to one local correspondent.[128] This is a strange testimony indeed for Richard Wilkes, who had a lifelong concern for the health of the poor in his area, but also a reputation for bluntness ('He told nobility the truth' as his tombstone recorded).[129] Other eminent men were also criticised

---

[122] *Ibid.*, pp. 84, 104.

[123] *Delaney*, vol. 3, p. 558.

[124] *Ibid.*, vol. 2, p. 314.

[125] *Verney*, vol. 2, p. 217.

[126] Elwin, *Noels*, pp. 332, 389, 73.

[127] *Delaney*, vol. 3, p. 308, vol. 4, p. 288, vol. 6, p. 344.

[128] *Shenstone*, p. 307.

[129] Norman W. Tildesley, 'Dr Richard Wilkes of Willenhall, Staffs., an eighteenth century country doctor', *Lichfield and South Staffs. Archaeological and Historical Society Transactions*, VII (1965–6), 1–10.

by their contemporaries; Richard Brocklesby was depicted as a man of 'moderate pretensions', even of false modesty, by one diarist.[130] Sir Lucas Pepys, frequently mentioned by eighteenth century writers and with a reputation as a 'friendly tyrant', was thought an '*unequal match*' in the eyes of the titled family into which he married in 1772, although a 'gentleman by birth, and certainly by education and manners'.[131] Certain diarists, however, utterly condemned a particular practitioner and also recorded the adverse comments of others about the man. Dr Fraser of Bath in the 1790s was criticised for his professional qualifications ('not a Scholar – He was formerly a Surgeon's Mate in the West Indies of America') and for his social standing ('a respectable man, but of a more common sort'), and yet he had been recommended by Pitcairne to a patient who was leaving London to live in Bath.[132] Medical inoculators were also assessed by contemporaries so that in 1786 Judith Milbanke was of the opinion that 'Fox is just as good as Dimsdale indeed almost any Apothecary of Character is equal, as in my mind there is but little skill in the Matter'. Even on arrival in a strange town a medical reputation could be investigated; thus at Scarborough a local physician, Dr Johnson, was 'reckoned very clever' in 1777.[133] Humbler patients too had views and reported reputations current about their contemporaries; one miller in Essex in 1780 described a local practitioner, Dr Malden, as 'noted for his sense and skill in his profession and fam'd likewise for his Epicurean abilities', while in the same county in 1784 William Heatheley of Witham was 'respected for his abilities in his profession, likewise for his mirthful and social turn of mind, but was of too liberal a cast to save money'.[134] The valued family apothecary was perhaps exemplified by Mr Partridge of Nottingham, who had attended the Gawthern family in the town for half a century and who figured prominently in the diary of Abigail Gawthern, not only in a professional capacity but in a personal relationship. Mr Partridge attended her husband's funeral, spent six Christmas days with the family as well as one Easter Sunday, and was mentioned at least nineteen times in her diary. When he died she wrote appreciatively, even affectionately, of his career and character:

20 July 1808: Mr Partridge, apothecary, departed this life, aged 87...a

[130] *Farington*, vol. 3, p. 712.   [131] *Delaney*, vol. 4, pp. 458, 463.
[132] *Farington*, vol. 3, pp. 665, 663.   [133] Elwin, *Noels*, pp. 300, 65.
[134] E.C.R.O., Diary of John Crosier, Sept. 1780 and May 1784; T/A 387.

remarkably sensible man, read a great deal, and had an excellent memory; his opinions of authors were truly just, his ideas of religion the true Christian; though he did not constantly attend the church he did not omit the duties of the sabbath; his political opinions were strongly in favour of our good and gracious king and the love of his country, despising the monarchy of France; he was in his profession an apothecary and made up all his drugs himself, being particular in the choice and goodness of them; he attended me and my family for above fifty years; he left a widow and two daughters...[135]

Only a handful of diaries but many more letters give detailed accounts of medical treatments, sometimes of people other than the correspondents. A diary might contain only a short entry that was full of facts; thus Abigail Gawthern noted an accident to her 2-year-old son in 1788:

Frank had a fall and cut his lips most terribly, Sep 8: obliged to have a silver pin from the Infirmary to run through the underlip to unite it; Mr John Bigsby performed the operation.[136]

Important patients and famous practitioners

Sometimes the illnesses and accidents of famous or titled patients were mentioned by the diarist, even though they were not acquainted; when the Marquis of Tavistock fractured his skull in 1767 a local incumbent, William Cole, recorded in his diary that the patient had been trepanned two or three times and finally sent his servant to Mr Filkes, the apothecary, to make further enquiries and ascertain the truth of the gossip he had heard.[137] Rumours of ill-health could be used in correspondence for the writer's own advantage. Thus one cleric, anxious to secure a more prosperous living, wrote to his patron that one would soon be vacant since a rival incumbent

having been much troubled with severe fits of the Stone, the Paroxysms of which have of late seemingly been every time more dangerous, so that his whole frame is visibly shatter'd, and this at the great age of seventy five or seventy six, as I am now well assur'd by a friend of mine...[138]

[135] *The Diary of Abigail Gawthern, 1751–1810*, ed. Adrian Henstock (Thoroton Soc., xxxiii, 1980), p. 138.
[136] *Ibid.*, p. 47. The Gawthern family had been supporters of the new Nottingham infirmary and attended various fund-raising events. John Bigsby belonged to a medical family and was in practice in Nottingham before the infirmary opened on 12 February 1781; he attended the rest of the Gawthern family.
[137] *The Blecheley Diary of the Rev. William Cole, 1765–7*, ed. F. G. Stokes (London, 1931), pp. 195–6.   [138] *Greene*, p. 90.

The ailing incumbent lived a further five years and the writer for three more decades.

Of all the well-known patients in the eighteenth century the Duchess of Devonshire was perhaps most often mentioned in diaries and letters, not merely because of her medical treatments but because she achieved a certain notoriety among contemporaries for her style of life, unconventional even by the standards of Georgian England. In 1796 Miss Berry was told by letter how

The Duchess of Devonshire has been in great danger of losing her sight by catching cold very indiscreetly. They have saved her eyes by almost strangling her with a handkerchief, and forcing all the blood up into her head, and then bleeding her with leeches.[139]

If this were the version of the Duchess's treatment retailed in society gossip, a more detailed account was written by the Duchess's sister, Lady Bessborough, who went to Devonshire House to attend her 'through a dreadful operation, which she bore with wonderful courage, and I with wretched cowardice'. Later she wrote that her sister was improving slowly, but

it was thought necessary to perform a most painful operation upon her, applying Causticks behind her ears and a blister to the back of her neck for four hours. I never saw anything like the agony she suffer'd, and the exertions I made to hold and soothe her brought my old complaint of spasms with great violence...she seems charmingly well again, but it was shocking to see; only her fortitude and patience really made it something wonderful.[140]

Lady Bessborough was herself ill four years later after a fall downstairs when she banged her head, having only recently given birth to her second illegitimate child. She was clearly terrified of an operation of any kind; her five medical attendants ordered her 'poor head' to be shaved, but she had nightmarish dreams of Everard Home, the surgeon

standing over me with the instrument to open my head. I wak'd quite cold and trembling. He says he must come and see me very often and take off the impression of horror I seem to have of him. But he is quite mistaken, for I like him very much.[141]

For many kinds of cases, but obviously chiefly for prosperous

[139] *Berry*, vol. 2, p. 15. Apart from her large gambling debts, Georgiana, Duchess of Devonshire (1754–1806) occasioned society gossip at the numbers of her lovers, including Charles Grey, later prime minister, by whom she had an illegitimate daughter in 1792.

[140] *Leveson Gower*, vol. 1, pp. 134–7.   [141] *Ibid.*, vol. 1, p. 284.

patients, joint consultations took place; in 1746 Philip Doddridge was treated by both Dr William Oliver of Bath and his Northampton physician, Dr James Stonhouse, while Nicholas Blundell often had two or three practitioners treating him simultaneously. The wealthy hypochondriac or chronically ill patient could consult a number of famous practitioners. For example, Sir George Beaumont was treated for a possible liver condition during a seven-year period (1794–1801) by six different men (Drs Pitcairne, Ewer, Harrington, Saunders and Baillie as well as the surgeon, Henry Cline). Beaumont did not die until 1827. The decision to consult a second practitioner was frequently prompted by the patient and for some cost was a deterrent. Samuel Johnson wrote to his wife, Tetty, in London, in 1740:

If M [   ] does not easily succeed in his endeavours, let him not [?scruple] to call in another surgeon to consult with him. Y[ou may] have two or three visits from Ranby or Shipton, who is [?said] to be the best, for a Guinea, which you need not fear to part with on so pressing an occasion, for I can send you twenty pouns more on Monday.[142]

A substantial group of writers, however, noted a search for a second opinion in the last, hopeless stages of an illness; 'Dr Merrick from Reading and Dr Lee from London' attended a dying woman in 1739,[143] while William Shenstone, anxious for his brother's life in 1751, 'purpos'd to send for Dr Wall from Worster', although Dr Hervey was already in attendance.[144] Sometimes a patient was passed on from one practitioner to another, forever seeking medical relief for his complaint, confiding to his diary his hopes of a new treatment and his despair at not finding a cure. In 1796 Joseph Farington was advised by Dr Fraser at Bath to try Jenner at Cheltenham; five years later his illness was exacerbated by depression at his wife's recent death. In 1801 at Bath he consulted Dr Parry, Dr Salt, Mr Sloper, an apothecary, and Harry Atwood, a surgeon, having earlier sought treatment at Oxford and Stratford-upon-Avon while on his travels.

Farington, no doubt from his own experience, appreciated the 'delicacy' required in seeking an alternative medical opinion from Richard Warren for his friend, Smirke the artist, in 1797:

it would be an affront to a professional man to suppose He would pay more attention on recommendation than where persons trusted to their integrity. – but [Lysons] would speak to Mr Angerstein, whose family Dr Warren

[142] *Johnson Letters*, vol. 1, p. 16.
[143] *Verney*, vol. 2, p. 129.   [144] *Shenstone*, p. 306.

attended much, and perhaps procure a note from him requesting to know when Smirke could wait upon Dr Warren.[145]

The same diarist noted how, in a country area, a joint consultation was arranged:

on the subject of [Miss Fountaine's] complaint Bailey is to meet Dr Marshall of Lynn tomorrow morning at Narford – Bailey is convinced that Her cough &c are symptomatic only, & that an injury of the spinal bones as described by Pott, is the cause. She has another expressive symptom, viz., a weakness & uncertainty in walking. She is abt. 22 years old.[146]

Clearly the greater the patient the more conferring was common; Heberden, Warren and Turton were all consulted in Lord Edward Bentinck's illness in 1768[147] but Johnson was embarrassed that Pepys felt offended when only Heberden and Brocklesby, Johnson's London neighbour, conferred in Johnson's illness of July 1783, and Johnson added the pithy comment that 'to call three had made me ridiculous by the appearance of self importance'.[148]

Diaries and letters suggest that in the eighteenth century a certain amount of antiquated but reassuring professional medical advice was still being quoted and passed from one patient to another long after the practitioner had made his pronouncement or prescribed for an individual patient. One diarist noted in 1796 that John Hunter, who had died three years earlier, was 'of the opinion that a little excess now & then is good for the constitution, it puts the Stomach on a salutary exertion'[149] – a welcome view to many patients. Darwin's prescription of chewed peppercorns for weakness of the bowels and Cadogan's of rhubarb, ginger and magnesia in peppermint water for 'any accidental excess' were quoted long after they were originally prescribed.[150] Novel medical treatments, such as electrification, were also commonly noted, more frequently in letters than diaries, often, it seems, to impress the reader.[151]

Early in the eighteenth century even practitioners of national repute were prepared to travel to provincial centres and attend patients who might never have been able to journey to London. In 1728, Nicholas

---

[145] *Farington*, vol. 3, pp. 794–5.
[146] *Ibid.*, vol. 2, p. 384; John Bailey was a surgeon-apothecary of Swaffham, Norfolk.
[147] *Delaney*, vol. 4, p. 181.   [148] *Johnson Letters*, vol. 3, p. 47.
[149] *Farington*, vol. 3, p. 663.   [150] *Ibid.*, vol. 1, p. 225.
[151] For example, electrification of patients is mentioned in the *Noels* letters (p. 343), the *Wedgwood Letters* (pp. 240–9) and by Shenstone.

Blundell, always anxious about his eyes, tried to find out when Cheselden was expected at Chester and made arrangements to consult him:

15 February: Dr Bromfield made a Viset to Fanny she being under his charge.
22 February: I took a second Doce of Pills according to Dr Cawood's Direcsions. Dr Bromfield came to see Fanny and Ordred a Fomentasion for her, he cut a Wart off her Brest.
23 March: Mr Chisleton, Dr Fernihough &c came to my Lodging. I advised with him about Mally's Eyes and mine & about Fannys Laimnes.[152]

The greatest families living in the provinces could always consult the leading London practitioners, even later in the century it became more common for patients to travel to London; in 1766 when the 13-year-old daughter of Lord Cardigan fell ill in the family's Northamptonshire home, she was attended by both Robert James and Anthony Addington, although to no avail.[153]

It is striking how the great names of eighteenth century medicine so regularly appear in the diaries and correspondence of the period and also how dominant some names were; Erasmus Darwin, the Hunters, Pepys, Sloane and Warren are particularly prominent in this respect. It is easy to understand, even without complete account books surviving, how such men made fortunes out of medicine; they were consulted, recommended and talked about in society to an extent that made prosperity inevitable, especially as they all appear to have worked very long hours indeed. How medical reputations were made or lost by patients' gossip can be seen in the cases of two wealthy patients John Hunter treated a year before his death. In 1792 one correspondent wrote to a mutual friend that

Jack Tempest had an alarming complaint, a swelling in his thigh. Hunter says it is a gathering & must be discharged & the danger is that it may weaken him too much & Old Tempest is very uneasy about it...[154]

In this case the patient died a year later. Also in 1792 Sir Ralph Milbanke wrote that he had recently visited Sir Willoughby Aston who

is confined to his couch in consequence of an operation he has had performed for a Hydrocele. The operation was performed by Tomkins & they say in a bungling manner. He has since had John Hunter and is doing well, but he looks ill & grilled...

---

[152] Blundell, vol. 3, p. 234–7; Fanny, aged 22, and Mally, aged 24, were the diarist's daughters. Dr James Bromfield came from Liverpool and Dr Philip Fernihough from Chester; Cawood was an oculist in Ireland.
[153] Joan Wake, *The Brudenells of Deene* (London, 1953), p. 276.
[154] Elwin, *Noels*, p. 418.

A fortnight later Sir Ralph was able to report that

Sir Willby is about again, but looks shockingly; whether the Surgeon's hand slipp'd or not I cannot tell, but he lost a most alarming quantity of blood, but perhaps if he can recover it he may be the better for it...[155]

In spite or because of surgical intervention by Hunter, Sir Willoughby recovered and survived a further twenty-three years.

Patients' own ideas of why they were ill or well seem to have been curiously unrelated to their education, class or sex. There was a distinct belief in the value of a change of air and, to a lesser extent, in the merits of fresh air, but one correspondent insisted that 'native air is the best physic', and the patient in question certainly seemed to be home-sick as well as ill.[156] Only rarely was regular exercise, perhaps in the form of 'Dr Horse', advocated by contemporary practitioners, who also advised a stringent, self-denying regimen with few hopes of success. Many correspondents noted how reluctant a particular patient was to reform an indulgent way of living, especially in his or her diet. However, some writers attributed their health almost entirely to the regimen that suited their constitution best; in 1795 one man who had eaten 'unwisely' for two days noted in his journal that his health depended 'much' upon his diet, and that he was seldom unwell if he ate 'plain food', but that 'made dishes and sauces' never failed to 'disorder' him.[157] Many writers, of course, were excessively worried at any apparent symptom of ill-health, but the truly phlegmatic approach can be seen in references to those whose health was said to be 'indifferent', which almost invariably meant that their death was imminent. One old-fashioned expression for being in good health was 'pure well', frequently used by Mrs Delaney in her massive correspondence, and the view that one disease 'drove out' another was also recorded by correspondents. The idea that nature should take its course was pronounced early in the century, but the diaries and letters of the period also display an amazing catalogue of bizarre, self-help cures, even from the educated writer. For example, in 1723 one country cleric advocated using moles' feet for his child suffering from convulsions.[158] The eighteenth century, like Pepys, greatly feared damp and cold; Joseph Gutteridge's mother had rheumatic fever from 'going too soon into a newly built house',[159] while William Stout

---

[155] *Ibid.*, p. 521.
[156] *Eaton Letters*, p. 118.   [157] *Farington*, vol. 2, p. 417.
[158] *The Diary of Thomas Naish*, ed. Doreen Slatter (Wilts. Arch. and Nat. Hist. Soc., xx, 1964), p. 79.
[159] *Master and Artisan*, p. 87.

thought he became ill as a result of 'the starve' he got returning from
the Isle of Man to Lancashire[160] ('starved' meaning 'very cold' was
in widespread use in country areas well into the present century).
Writers understandably tried to explain physical symptoms they did
not comprehend in the light of their own recent behaviour or events;
one writer thought she had a nasty headache because of a high wind,[161]
while a diarist noted that his daughter's convulsions had returned when
she saw a mouse in her room.[162] Generally the language in diaries is
remarkably unforced, not intended to convey an impression to the
reader, and an accurate guide to usage as well as meaning in eighteenth
century English.

The value of diaries and correspondence to the medical historian

Diaries and correspondence of the eighteenth century also contain a
mass of interesting details for the medical historian that are randomly
scattered. For example, Malthus had speech difficulties because of a
hare-lip (a problem noted by a fellow guest at a dinner party),[163] while
the death of John Hunter, including its sudden circumstances, was
recorded by a variety of writers.[164] Some medical practitioners had
a close personal relationship with the diarist; Blundell's attendants
regularly dined with his family and shared his sporting pursuits. A
minority of practitioners also helped their patients with non-medical
problems; Darwin found a French ex-prisoner of war to teach the
Wedgwood children[165] and Harry Wallbank, a Buckingham surgeon,
searched for a cookmaid for the Purefoy family, whom he attended.[166]
Even bald and scrappy comments can be valuable but, in spite of their
interest, diaries and correspondence remain for modern researchers a
relatively difficult source to use, if only because of the sheer bulk of
the material that has to be examined for medical comment or details,
for very few writers confine themselves to this area only. The
haphazard, incidental nature of the medical entries ensures a greater
chance of their being reliable; they were recorded in the same way
that weather or crops were noted, rather than, for example, much of
the political comment of the period, when the writer's personal bias

[160] *The Autobiography of William Stout of Lancaster, 1665–1752*, ed. J. D. Marshall
(Manchester, 1967), p. 91.   [161] Newdegate, *Cheverels*, p. 20.
[162] *Blundell*, vol. 3, p. 159.   [163] *Berry*, vol. 2, p. 475.
[164] *Ibid.*, vol. 1, p. 401; Walpole notified Mary Berry of Hunter's death in a letter
and Farington noted it in his diary (vol. 1, p. 71).
[165] *Wedgwood Letters*, p. 247.
[166] *The Purefoy Letters, 1735–53*, ed. L. G. Mitchell (London, 1973), p. 148.

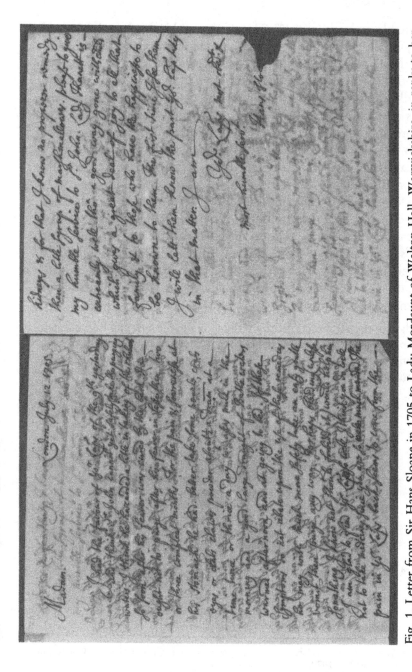

Fig. 1. Letter from Sir Hans Sloane in 1705 to Lady Mordaunt of Walton Hall, Warwickshire, in reply to her report about the health of her husband, Sir John Mordaunt (1650–1721). A partial transcript is printed in Elizabeth Hamilton, *The Mordaunts: An Eighteenth Century Family* (London, 1965), p. 58. (Warwick County Record Office, CR 1368, III, 73.)

is inevitable and apparent.[167] The diarist could also be selective, of course, usually noting the items that seemed of interest at the moment and omitting others; Josselin noted one bastardy case, for example, but seven others were recorded in contemporary local sources. Paleography is usually only a minor problem for the researcher, although most writers used both sides of the paper and shadow reverse writing can therefore make progress slow (Fig. 1). Most diaries were kept in English in the eighteenth century although Latin journals kept by physicians have survived;[168] correspondents such as Johnson occasionally wrote medical details to practitioners in Latin, suitable for the 'gross images of disease'[169] and he deliberately kept his own health diary wholly in Latin for the last months of his life.[170] For greater privacy from casual readers some diarists kept entries on their own and their family's health in Latin. Thomas Gray, the poet, did so,[171] while early in the eighteenth century a retired Sussex barrister, Timothy Burrell, used Latin for recording family disputes as well as for entries about his own health and medication:

Yesterday having wetted my feet by walking out in the dew and having eaten a small piece of new cheese, I have been today tortured with flatulent spasms. By taking two doses of hiera picra the pains in my stomach abated. Thanks to the great God for his mercy towards me.[172]

167 Some diarists were both long-lived and verbose; one Herefordshire gentleman, John Biddulph, left forty-two pocket-books and thirty-four journals for the years 1787–1841 (Hereford County Record Office, G2/IV/J/1–76), while Katharine Plymley of Longnor left 137 volumes in all up to 1837, of which fifty-five cover the years 1791–1800 (Shropshire County Record Office, 1066/1–55); she also kept fourteen travel diaries and six books of 'thoughts' in the same decade. In some country gentry families there seems to have been a tradition of diary keeping. For example, the Spencer Stanhopes of Cannon Hall, Cawthorne, Yorkshire, have left ninety-seven volumes covering the years 1680–1817 and kept by six members of the family; even the reputed illegitimate son of one diarist himself filled twenty-four diaries in the years 1785–1811 (Sheffield City Library, Sp. St. 60630, 60632–3, 60635–6, 60649, 60651).
168 For example, the diary (1737–42) of William Brownrigg, M.D. (1711–1800), who practised in Whitehaven and retired to his family estate near Keswick. His Latin notes include medical cases, although some are in English (Carlisle Public Library, E104). His portrait was painted by William M. Craig in 1794; Farington noted this and his death aged 90.
169 *Johnson Letters*, vol. 3, p. 36.
170 Johnson's *Aegria Ephemeris* was translated into English by Ann McHenry and published in 1979.
171 Review of J. Moultine (ed.), *Gray's Poetical Works*, *Gentleman's Magazine*, XXIV (1845), 229–35.
172 Arthur Ponsonby, *English Diaries: A Review of English Diaries from the Sixteenth to the Twentieth Century* (London, 1923), p. 144.

We know little of the diarists' methods of keeping their journals, except by inference, but surviving records show that some clearly kept rough jottings, often on loose leaves, which they later re-wrote in a more finished form. An exception was William Jones, who kept a slate and pencil by his bed-side, ready stringed and pegged, to permit him to write 'at perhaps far too early an hour to rise...any thought or reflections which present themselves'[173] which were later entered in his journal. Some diarists attempted to summarize the year's events in December (Blundell, Jessop[174] and Mydelton[175] all did so), noting an epidemic or harvest failure in a region, but the majority did not. The risk of a bogus eighteenth century diary is slight, although that of Anne Hughes provides a salutary warning to all researchers and illustrates the vital importance of checking a printed against a manuscript source whenever possible.[176]

Although diarists do not set out to record their own attitudes to their medical attention, this is frequently implicit in their comments and even in the length of entries on the subject of health. The patient's attitude to the medical practitioner depended almost wholly upon his or her own social standing as the recipient of that attention. Even famous London practitioners, treating the great county families, displayed an extravagant deference, at least in their correspondence, typical of the age, while the same great families, such as the Milbankes, were highly critical of their treatment. Middle class patients were far more likely to write with gratitude of their medical practitioners. Upper and middle class patients clearly recognised the distinctions between the different categories of practitioners, and at least when they wrote did not, as has been suggested,[177] indiscriminately use the term 'Doctor' for a surgeon or an apothecary when they meant a physician. Thus the accounts of one Midland gentry family noted for medical attention in 1696–7

---

[173] *The Diary of the Revd William Jones, 1777–1821*, ed. O. F. Christie (London, 1929), p. 128.

[174] *The Diary of Arthur Jessop*, ed. C. E. Whiting (Yorks. Arch. Soc. Rec. Series, CXVII, 1952), pp. 24, 33, 37.

[175] Ponsonby, *More English Diaries*, p. 117.

[176] *The Diary of a Farmer's Wife, 1796–7*, compiled by Suzanne Beedell (London, 1965). The recent televising and reprinting of this 'diary' have exposed it as modern fiction in diary form. If genuine, it would have been very valuable as a countrywoman's journal. It lacks essential features of the authentic diary and local research has never, for obvious reasons, been able to identify the people and places in the border area of Herefordshire–Monmouthshire.

[177] Geoffrey Holmes, *Augustan England: Professions, State and Society, 1680–1730* (London, 1982), pp. 167–9.

Mr Edwards for letting the Infant Wightwick's blood	5s 0d
Dr Johnson for a visit to the Infant Wightwick	£1 0s 0d
Mr Bradshaw apothecary for things formerly delivered by direction of Dr Johnson for the use of the s^d Wightwick.[178]	4s 6d

Diarists' own unspoken estimations of a practitioner's status may be seen in the social events they shared when the patient had the initiative as host. Nicholas Blundell gambled, ate and drank with all his local practitioners and visited Vauxhall Gardens with a surgeon, Mr Medcalf, who treated Blundell after a coach accident,[179] while Abigail Gawthern entertained most of Nottingham's medical fraternity on various occasions and was acutely aware of their status differences. Patients higher and lower in the social order did not enjoy such familiarity with practitioners. Among poorer patients, however, any man in any kind of medical occupation, even the quack, was dignified with the title of 'Doctor'. The accounts of the Overseers of the Poor particularly illustrate this deference by title, so that any practitioner attending the parish paupers was usually cited as 'Dr'[180] even though trained by apprenticeship as a surgeon, apothecary or surgeon-apothecary, or totally unqualified. Although some men were clearly engaged in practice of a general nature – preparing medicine, delivering babies and carrying out surgical procedures – they were still seen by their more educated patients in the eighteenth century as having distinct skills in different spheres.[181]

From the journals and letters of the eighteenth century, with all their limitations, it is possible to gain a curiously immediate sense of the period, and its attitudes to health, disease and death. The practitioner's part in the horrors and amusements of daily life, attending his patients, is perhaps an underexplored aspect of medical history, as is the patient's

[178] K. T. Swanzy, *The Offchurch Story* (Abingdon, 1968), p. 125. 'The Infant Wightwick' was the 16-year-old John Wightwick Knightley, preparing to enter Oxford; 'Mr Edwards' was William Edwards, a Kenilworth surgeon; 'Dr Johnson' was William Johnston, M.D., of Warwick (1643–1725), a very well-known physician (see note 83); and 'Mr Bradshaw' was the same John Bradshaw consulted by Sir John Mordaunt (see note 94).

[179] *Blundell*, vol. 3, p. 116.

[180] Joan Lane, 'The early history of general practice, 1700–1850: sources and methods', *The Society for the Social History of Medicine Bulletin*, xxx (1982), 19–21.

[181] Irvine Loudon, 'Two thousand medical men in 1847', *The Society for the Social History of Medicine Bulletin*, xxxiii (1983), 4–8, deals with the nineteenth century general practitioner and his emergence.

response to his attention. The correspondents and especially the diarists of the period display a wide variety of reactions to medical attention, from the hypochondriac to the stoical, to add a few more pieces to the jig-saw puzzle that is the English eighteenth century. One of the diarists himself expressed his personal reasons for keeping a voluminous diary that can hardly be bettered:

This work of mine may seem to some to be very useless, I confess several things that are set down are of no consequence, yet considering the uncertainty both of the things I shal afterwards have a desire to know, or the day of the month which may be necessary for me to give account of, it is not improper to be something particular, considering the trouble is so small and the advantage that I have already found by it has been very great and has abundantly over balanced my Troble.[182]

I should like to thank a number of archivists and librarians for individual assistance during my preliminary research on diaries. Responses to my enquiries were, with only two exceptions, more than helpful; I am particularly grateful for their goodwill and patience to Dr Robert Bearman, Shakespeare Birthplace Trust Records Office; Mrs M. T. Halford, Shropshire County Record Office; Miss S. Hubbard, Hereford County Record Office; Miss Monica Ory and Mr Richard Chamberlain-Brothers, Warwick County Record Office; Mr Robin Price, Wellcome Institute Library, London; Mrs Margaret Turner, Sheffield City Library; Miss Sue Wallington, University of Warwick Library; Mr C. C. Webb, Borthwick Institute, York; Mr E. R. Wilkinson, Carlisle Public Library.

Bibliography

William Matthews, *British Diaries: An Annotated Bibliography of British Diaries Written between 1442 and 1942* (Berkeley and Los Angeles, 1950). Matthews lists 240 eighteenth century diaries, printed and MS, all, except those privately owned, in the national record repositories and large public libraries, apart from twenty in local record offices.

Linda A. Pollock, *Forgotten Children* (Cambridge, 1983) cites 107 British diaries of the eighteenth century, of which only sixty-six were actually kept in the century. Of these sixty-six only two are MSS. Some published editions she quotes have been superseded by full, modern versions of the text: for example, Josselin's and Clegg's diaries.

Arthur Ponsonby, *English Diaries: A Review of English Diaries from the Sixteenth to*

[182] *Blundell*, vol. 1, p. 13.

the Twentieth Century (London, 1923) covers 117 diaries, of which twenty-nine are of the eighteenth century, some now very well known.

Arthur Ponsonby, *More English Diaries: Further Reviews of Diaries from the Sixteenth to the Twentieth Century* (London, 1927) with nine of eighteenth century date.

Arthur Ponsonby, *Scottish and Irish Diaries from the Sixteenth to the Nineteenth Century* (London, 1927); only four Scottish diaries are of the eighteenth century.

Lawrence Stone, *The Family, Sex and Marriage in England, 1500–1800* (London, 1977) uses fourteen printed English diaries for the eighteenth century.

Bibliography of British History, 1714–89, ed. S. Pargellis and D. J. Medley (Oxford, 1951) lists diaries among correspondence, journals, memoirs and biographies (pp. 248–64), but diaries are also located in many other sections, for example, in Nonconformity.

Bibliography of British History, 1789–1851, ed. Lucy M. Brown and Ian R. Christie (Oxford, 1969) is similarly arranged.

9

Prescribing the rules of health: Self-help and advice in the late eighteenth century

GINNIE SMITH

The two classic divisions of European medical science are those of prevention and cure; and if we wish to look at the normally healthy individual in historical perspective we are speaking the language and regime of prevention. By far the larger part of individual health care is taken up by routine private maintenance, compared with which any curative intervention is an occasional public crisis. But the very nature of a multitude of low-level, dispersed acts has meant that the processes of prevention have not been as 'visible' to historians as the processes of cure.[1] Investigation is further hampered by the fact that prevention has very rarely been of prime professional interest; preventive medicine was not even truly called 'medicine' as such. Medical historians have regarded therapeutics in general as 'an awkward piece of business'; and prevention in particular as a 'murky bog of routinism'.[2] Prevention, moreover, is and was barely newsworthy, being a passive or negative operation; in comparison, the combative techniques and reported statistics, the public and private cost of illness, are relatively accessible to the historian. Demographers and structuralist medical historians have taken disease beyond the supposedly inflated claims of curative medicine – 'the emphasis on disease has great possibilities for it gets outside the narrow field of clinical medicine as practised by doctors'.[3] The full range of preventive or survival

---

[1] For a perceptive sociological analysis of the invisibility of self-care, see S. Levin, A. Katz and E. Holst (eds.), *Self-Care: Lay Initiatives in Health* (London, 1977), esp. ch. 2, 'The social nature of self-care'.

[2] C. Rosenberg, 'The therapeutic revolution', in C. Rosenberg and Morris J. Vogel (eds.), *The Therapeutic Revolution: Essays in the Social History of American Medicine* (Pennsylvania, 1979), pp. 3–26, p. 3.

[3] J. Woodward and D. Richards, 'Towards a social history of medicine', in *idem* (eds.), *Health Care and Popular Medicine in Nineteenth Century England* (London, 1977), pp. 15–55, p. 18.

techniques, however, has not so far caught the attention either of demographers or of historians.[4]

From the individual's point of view, 'good health' historically speaking may not have represented any choice at all, but may have been considered to be a matter of good luck, fate or reward. But for individuals who sought some means of rational and prudential control for reasons of simple survival or personal enlightenment, there were the medical advice books. These vernacular works were written ostensibly for the lay individual, and until recently have been considered as an antiquated source of old wives' tales and quaint remedies, well outside or at best on the fringe of orthodox medicine. For a large number of people they could well have been a far more familiar source of information than the personal advice of the trained physician. Some early recognition of their importance has been given by German historians; and more recently, by scholars in the United States.[5] By contrast, British sources have scarcely been touched. There are partial studies, but there is no comprehensive account of popular medical works – which include in large proportion the specific subdivision or genre of hygienic preventive medicine known as 'regimen'.[6]

Advice books and regimens

One of the most obvious facts relating to the medical advice books is that they are published in English, and were on the face of it accessible to all those who could actually read – not just those who could read

[4] The fertility-led model of population growth does not accord hygiene the same significance it had with the mortality-led model; but E. A. Wrigley and R. S. Schofield, *The Population History of England, 1541–1871* (London, 1981), p. 484, leave open the question of behaviouralism in family and household units, with its possible influence on differential mortality rates. P. E. Razzell drew attention to empirical hygienic behaviour in 'An interpretation of the modern rise of population in Europe: a critique', *Population Studies*, xxviii (1974), 5–17.

[5] See C. Rosenberg and M. R. Vogel (eds.), 'The Therapeutic Revolution', *op. cit.* (ref. 2); Guenter Risse, Ronald L. Numbers and J. Waltzer Leavitt (eds.), *Medicine without Doctors: Home Health Care in American History* (New York, 1977); J. Waltzer Leavitt and Ronald L. Numbers (eds.), *Sickness and Health in America: Readings in the History of Medicine and Public Health* (Wisconsin, 1978).

[6] The early modern period has been investigated by Paul Slack, 'Mirrors of health and treasures of poor men: the use of vernacular medical literature in Tudor England', in Charles Webster (ed.), *Health, Medicine and Mortality in the Sixteenth Century* (Cambridge, 1979), pp. 237–73. See also Charles Webster, *The Great Instauration: Science, Medicine and Reform 1626–1660* (London, 1975), pp. 264–7.

Latin. But what were the limitations on their use, apart from general literacy? We need above all to know how many of these types of work were in circulation at any one time; but unfortunately information on the quantities of vernacular medical works published is at present minimal. It is more precise for the lesser number of works published before 1700, than for the increasing quantities published between 1700 and 1800. With the benefit of the *Short Title Catalogue*, Paul Slack has estimated a total of 153 medical titles (with 392 known editions) between 1486 and 1604. He estimates that in 1604 there would have been one in use for every twenty people.[7] He acknowledges, however, that this must be a minimum estimate on the basis of those works which have actually survived. Between 1600 and 1800 total quantities become much less clear, since no equivalent exercise has been carried out on the recently established eighteenth century *Short Title Catalogue*.[8] There is for instance no information at present on medical works as a percentage of all eighteenth century publications, that is comparable with Slack's estimate of medical works as 3 per cent of all titles before 1604; or on vernacular medical works as a percentage of all medical publications in the same period. Given the number of works still unknown, it is impossible to make similar useful estimates of the number of editions, or the number of copies potentially available per head of population.[9] The best we can suggest is that vernacular medical works were an expanding market in the eighteenth century.

The most complete catalogue of preventive works for the period 1600–1800 is Sir John Sinclair's *Code of Health and Longevity*.[10] As its title indicates, it was a specialised compilation of works on general health, which omits the herbals, plague tracts and works on anatomy and surgery that are also found in the pre-eighteenth century *Short Title Catalogue*.[11] It was, moreover, a personal selection, including only

---

[7] Slack, 'Mirrors of health', pp. 239–40.

[8] See M. Crump and M. Harris (eds.), *Searching the Eighteenth Century, Papers Presented at the Symposium on the Eighteenth Century Short Title Catalogue in July 1982* (London, 1983).

[9] Slack, 'Mirrors of health', p. 239. Using an estimate of 1,000 copies per edition, he concludes that there would have been 400,000 copies of printed works in circulation between 1486 and 1604 of which 166,000 would still have been in use at the end of the century. The number of publications was increasing towards the end of the century.

[10] Sir John Sinclair, *The Code of Health and Longevity: or, a Concise View of the Principles Calculated for the Preservation of Health and the Attainment of Long Life* (4 vols., Edinburgh, 1807–8).

[11] Slack, 'Mirrors of health', p. 243. See Table 1 for his full classification of subject types found.

publications of 'real note and merit'.[12] Matching Slack with Sinclair we may compare Slack's total of ninety-seven titles between 1486 and 1604 with Sinclair's total of fifty-four works between 1600 and 1700, and 211 works between 1700 and 1800. The approximate total for 1600–1800 can be pushed to 310 titles with the inclusion of works from Richard Reece's short essay, the 'History of Popular Medicine', and miscellaneous references derived from the works themselves, and other bibliographic sources.[13] However, even an unconfirmed increase of 33 per cent in the British literature indicates a significant market expansion. By 1770 there was a large reservoir of these works in existence. Despite the probable loss of many ephemeral or unbound works, many older works from the early eighteenth century and beyond still had shelf-life alongside the rapidly increasing numbers of modern medical advice books, by then appearing annually.[14]

Though there are no figures which could be used to give an accurate account of the scale of publication, bibliographic evidence from the vernacular works as a whole does suggest the importance of the regimen 'type'. It was certainly a genre comparable to the better-known herbals; and apparently also one which could have had its roots in the 'little' as well as the 'great' tradition.[15] Slack provides evidence of the significant part books of regimen played in the early vernacular medical book market before 1600. They were in fact the most 'popular' works not only in terms of new titles, but also in numbers of editions, in price, and in their handy pocket size. They were closely followed, but not exceeded in number, by the collections of receipts which historians have traditionally regarded as representative of popular medicine. 'Regimens' also changed little in character, and had

---

[12] Sinclair, *Code of Health and Longevity*, vol. 2, pp. 301–3; 185–7.

[13] See Appendix 1, 'Approximate distribution of all titles 1600–1800. General health and longevity'. R. Reece's bibliography is contained in *A Practical Dictionary of Domestic Medicine* (London, 1808). Other sources were R. Watt's *Bibliotheca Britannica* (Edinburgh, 1824); E. J. Waring's *Bibliotheca Therapeutica* (London, 1878); the Wellcome Collection; miscellaneous volumes in the British Library. No full check on these or other extant library holdings has been made pre-1770. The nineteenth century bibliographies cited titles – with or without the date of publication, or authorship. Appendix 1 is therefore a stop-gap measure pending a fuller bibliographic review. A modern bibliography on balneology is Charles Mullett's, 'Public baths and health in England, sixteenth to eighteenth century', *Bulletin for the History of Medicine*, Suppl. 5 (1946).

[14] Slack estimates a shelf-life of thirty years; but good binding and the value placed on bound works could have doubled this, barring fire or accident.

[15] See P. Burke, *Popular Culture in Early Modern Europe* (London, 1978).

a longer publishing life than other specialised genres.[16] Conventionality combined with sustained demand suggests a powerful vernacular tradition; but Slack nonetheless argues that the readership of vernacular works was confined to 'a relatively small elite of practitioners and laymen'. Contemporary claims for a popular readership 'need not be taken at face value. If writers seem to have felt the need to justify opening the secrets of the "noble science" of physic to the multitude, a large part of this was a calculated appeal for readers'.[17]

Slack's view of the figures leads him to conclude pessimistically that the small total percentage of vernacular medical works in the publishing market up to 1604 must have precluded any 'major social or medical impact'.[18] Although quantitative evidence is undoubtedly important, to be excessively rigorous at this stage is to miss the point: that is, the wealth of metaphysical beliefs and other social practices associated with the regimen tradition, which to a large extent defy quantification. Nor can we assume that the great interest in the preservation of life found amongst the earliest printed medical works, was restricted to one class. A structural assessment of the scale and composition of the readership must rely as much on evidence of content as on necessary but skeletal surveys of production and ownership. One book may pass through many hands; and it may also be transmitted orally. Slack sees these medical works as 'challenging' oral culture, and failing. They were the playthings of the rich, and 'simply gave a few people more to talk about'.[19] The works could have provided only socio-psychological 'reassurance', where they were used at all, since they were scientifically valueless. An alternative view suspends the value judgement on science, and gives more weight to the interaction between oral and literate culture. The printed word certainly had a life of its own, but it may equally well have confirmed and consolidated the pre-existing oral culture. It is unlikely, as Peter Burke has confirmed, that the two cultures were entirely separated, though he suggests that the first noticeable divisions were beginning to take place at some point between the seventeenth and eighteenth centuries.[20] Qualitative evidence suggests that there was an antiquity and continuity of intellectual tradition centred on regimen which would have ensured oral as well as literate dissemination. Moreover,

[16] Slack, 'Mirrors of health', pp. 246–7.
[17] *Ibid.*, pp. 273, 257.   [18] *Ibid.*, p. 240.
[19] *Ibid.*, p. 260. Note Slack's primary interest in sickness, p. 261.
[20] Burke, '*Popular Culture*', pp. 28–30.

certain developments in the therapeutic advice after 1604 cannot in any
light be solely attributable to the academic or 'literate' tradition.
Broadly speaking, each written contribution to the genre that we have
from the late eighteenth century was derived from a specific oral/literate
culture stretching over 300 years, and it is arguable that by 1770 few
sections of the population would have been untouched by some notion
of regimen.

The university contribution to medicine from the seventeenth
century has been extensively discussed under the heading of 'professionalisation' – the development of occupational groups who claimed
authority on the basis of a university education.[21] But 'polite' learning
and self-education amongst the laity are at present less well understood
than the claims of academicism; and it is these problems of 'opposition'
across professional boundaries which lead to a distinction between
'self-help' and 'advice' in the vernacular medical works. Classical
Greek preventive hygiene was one of the five Institutes of formal
medical education, but it was also the one most closely associated with
the interests of the laity, rather than with the essentially curative
function of the physician. Sir John Sinclair recognised this distinction
in 1807, when he stated that it was not his intention to 'meddle' with
the curing of disease. However, the 'preservation of health and the
prevention of disease, is a kind of neutral ground, between the several
branches of medicine, and the common sense and daily observation
of well informed men, and of course is open to everyone'.[22] Prevention
was at the periphery of the physician's professional interests; and there
is a considerable amount of evidence which suggests that regimen was
an intermediate area which was apparently revived in the face of
professional apathy by the moral and practical concerns of the laity.
During the religious struggles of the Protestant Reformation and
subsequent Puritan revolution, Dissenters attacked what they considered
to be a hierarchical monopoly of practice and information. However
the profession at that time had a rather more limited practical and legal
basis, and despite this perceived public concern, other structural
evidence indicates the constraints on professional power.

21 The debate on professionalisation in medical science has been expanding at
great speed since the days of the 'Merton thesis'. See Gary A. Abraham,
'Misunderstanding the Merton thesis', *Isis*, LXXIV (1983), 368–87. See also
S. Shapin and A. Thackray, 'Prosopography as a research tool in the history
of science: the British scientific community 1700–1900', *History of Science*, XII
(1974), 1–28.
22 Sinclair, *Code of Health and Longevity*, vol. 1, p. 170.

The medical advice books themselves suggest a population at many different stages of education, or self-education; and rigid sociological divisions based on the assumption of professional qualification in medicine through formal institutional training can be historically misleading when assessing levels of literacy in earlier periods. In the late eighteenth century, when informal education was arguably at a high point, the level of lay medical erudition derived from private tutoring and self-education could be remarkably high.[23] Those trained physicians who chose to participate in public debate were pragmatically accommodating themselves to lay interests, although there were still those who saw vernacular medical works as an intrusion on hard-won professional privileges. A second issue concerns the Protestant religion, which also undeniably stimulated literacy amongst new groups. On the face of it, religious issues split horizontally along economic class lines; but an individualist belief in the spirit might be strong, where 'class' consciousness was weak. We might therefore reasonably expect to find a quietist readership of medical advice books, concerned with pious domestic or private self-revelation, outside the more visible constituency of democratising or liberalising activists.[24]

Politics and metaphysics apart, medicine was of necessity practised in one form or another by most groups of the population; and professional assertions were meaningless where specialist help was non-existent, insufficient, disliked or economically unobtainable. In the absence of professional assistance, many such groups prescribed for themselves routinely; and either supplied themselves with drugs, skills or other technical aids, or paid for practical services on a limited or selective basis. Advice books must always have been required for use as reference books and practical manuals by part-time practitioners, and

[23] Roy Porter, 'Lay medical knowledge in the eighteenth century: the *Gentleman's Magazine*', *Medical History*, xxix (1985), 138–68.

[24] Quietism was a notable feature of sectarian groups driven under by the Restoration, but as yet little is known of its historical role. But see Jonathan Barry in this volume; and discussions by L. Barrow, 'Anti-establishment healing and spiritualism in England', and J. Pickstone, 'Establishment and dissent in nineteenth century medicine: an exploration of some correspondences between religious and medical belief systems in early industrial England', in W. Sheils (ed.), *The Church and Healing* (Oxford, 1982), pp. 225–48, 165–90; L. M. Beier, 'The creation of the medical fringe', and R. Cooter, 'Interpreting the fringe', in *The Society for the Social History of Medicine Bulletin*, xxix (1981), 29–32, 33–6; Ginnie Smith, 'Thomas Tryon's regimen for women; sectarian health in the seventeenth century', in London Feminist History Group (eds.), *The Sexual Dynamics of History* (London, 1983), pp. 47–65.

can be considered as a simple commercial item of medical equipment, an *aide mémoire* of practical therapeutics. From the individual's point of view the chief bar was time to read and absorb the knowledge, and money to acquire it. Depending on personal condition, the individual could either make time to carry out essential services, or hire them from others on a selective basis, or do without. Thus up until the mid-eighteenth century there were many diverse groups associated with the advice book market, whose requirements ranged from the utopian to the pragmatic; and the potential readership of the late eighteenth century is strongly suggested by the wide range of authors who served them.

The therapeutic system

The problems of interpretation remain. The specificity of regimen makes it necessary to understand the underlying schema in order to gauge what the eighteenth century authors were offering their public. The whole system, or structure, was ultimately derived from Greek medical philosophy and science, and bears a close resemblance to contemporary holistic Chinese folk medicine and other national and regional systems currently being investigated by medical anthropologists. It was dominated by the well-known elemental polarities of hot and cold, moist and dry, sweet and sour; as well as by other customary polarities such as male and female, purity and impurity, infancy and old age, mineral and vegetable.[25] Whether it was as a holistic metaphysical paradigm or as a practical set of rules, the European schema was regarded as authoritative until a very late date.[26] From the limited evidence yet available, we can detect an internal

---

[25] See K. Gould-Martin, 'Hot cold clean poison and dirt: Chinese folk medical categories', *Social Science and Medicine*, xii (1978), 39–46; M. Kay and M. Yoder, 'Hot and cold in women's ethnotherapeutics: the American Mexican West', paper from the Hot and Cold Food and Medical Theory Symposium, Eleventh International Congress of Anthropological and Ethnological Sciences (Vancouver, 1983). For an early view of problems and possibilities see also E. Ackerknecht, 'Natural diseases and rational treatment in primitive medicine', *Bulletin of the History of Medicine*, xix (1946), 467–97. Greek science is being dissected by G. E. R. Lloyd: see *Polarity and Analogy* (Cambridge, 1966), esp. ch. 2, 'Theories based on opposites'; and also, on the permeability of literate Greek science by earlier oral culture, in *Science, Folklore and Ideology: Studies in the Life Sciences in Ancient Greece* (Cambridge, 1983).

[26] L. J. Rather, 'The six things non-natural: a note on the origins and fate of a doctrine and a phrase', *Clio Medica*, iii (1968), 337–47; and Peter Niebyl, 'The non-naturals', *Bulletin for the History of Medicine*, xliii (1971), 486–92.

therapeutic shift between 1500 and 1700 which left its trace on late eighteenth century works. The changing system is evident in the handful of well-known works which to us constitute the landmarks of popular medicine, works as disparate as the *Salerno Regimen Sanitatis*, and those by Elyot, Cornaro, Cheyne, Wesley and Buchan; but its more truly popular outline can be found in scores of lesser-known works.

To a greater or lesser degree these subscribed to a common format, consisting of the 'regimen of the non-naturals'. These six non-naturals corresponded to the six human activities concerning air, diet, sleep, exercise, evacuations and passions of the mind, as laid down by orthodox Greek hygiene. This was commonly reduced to simplified 'correct' procedures for the individual – domestic and personal routine for the time of day, the day, the month, the year. It was further tailored to individual need by age, sex, location, and personal habit and custom (habit meaning, literally, personal constitution; custom meaning 'way of life', i.e. occupations). Therapeutic control related particularly to diet (you are what you eat), to activity (you are what you do) and to control of temperature and moisture (through housing, clothing, bathing, food) according to age and condition. Whatever procedure might be prescribed for the six universals, they were brought into harmony for each individual case by the principle of constant regulation – the 'ordering' of the non-naturals – throughout life. The conservation of energies in a steady progress towards natural old age (longevity) was achieved through temperance, or avoidance of unnatural excess, in any one or all of the non-naturals. The full programme was in general directed towards the healthy or health-conscious individual of mean age; but because of specific 'scientific' conditions, popular advice in practice was also broken down into advice for the old, the young, females, and for special occupations or conditions such as scholars, travellers, sailors, or the sick and conva-lescent (considered 'weak' or vulnerable, as were the young and old). As the seventeenth century *Macbeath Regimen* put it:

there are three aspects of the Regulation of Health. Conservatium, that is, guarding; Preservatium, that is fore-seeing; and Reductivium, that is guiding backwards...Conservatium to the healthy man, it is right. Preservatium to those that are going into unhealth, and to those in debility, it is a duty. And Reductivium to such as one in illness, it is a necessity.[27]

[27] *The Regimen Sanitatis*, trans. H. Cameron Gillies (Glasgow, 1911). A manu-script document written in the early sixteenth century or possibly earlier, for

Nothing occurred until the late nineteenth century to disturb this macro-biological pattern of inter-linked polarised universal elements; but the detailed therapeutic conclusions were nonetheless revised during the early modern period by what amounted to a shift of polarisation within the schema. Following the collapse of the rigorous standards of classical medicine and up to the sixteenth century humanist revival of Greek and Latin works in their pure form, diet and a 'hot' regimen of stimulating meats and drinks dominated the paradigm.[28] A Galenic orthodoxy had been established which gave overwhelming preference to the physiological behaviour of the bodily fluids, and their manipulation through diet (food and drink) and other substances perfected in Arabic drug lore. Hot regimen cleansed and purged inwardly, throwing out excreta, infections and all 'nastinesse', using food and other drugs to regulate the inner functions. Food-taking was the principal feature of Thomas Elyot's enormously popular *Castle of Health*, though it was set nominally within the framework of full regimen. Cornaro took the practice of diet to the extreme of life-long dedication; but his own handbook was preceded by the influential aphorisms of Sanctorius, published in conjunction with his experimental work on the physiology of digestion. By the mid-seventeenth century there is some evidence of growing dissatisfaction with minute dietary ruling – 'such progidy, tediousness, and inconvenience' – and with the simplistic humoral theory that accompanied it.[29]

The vernacular regimen works of the seventeenth century show a re-discovery of the theoretical structure of all six non-naturals which

the MacBeath family, hereditary physicians to the Lords of the Isles and the Kings of Scotland; probably written for the King as client, as well as for family instruction.

[28] O. Temkin, *Galenism: The Rise and Decline of a Medical Philosophy* (Ithaca/London, 1973). See also E. Ackerknecht, *Therapeutics: From the Primitives to the Twentieth Century* (New York/London, 1973); Vivian Nutton (ed.), *Galen: Problems and Prospects. A Collection of Papers Submitted at the 1979 Cambridge Conference* (London, 1981).

[29] Francis Bacon, quoted in Sinclair, *Code of Health and Longevity*, vol. 4, p. 158. From the Wellcome Collection, Thomas Elyot, *Castle of Health, gathered and made by Sir Thomas Elyot knyghte, out of the chiefe Authors of Physyke, where by every man may knowe the state of his own body, the preservation of health, and how to instruct well his physician in sickness that he be not deceived*, 1st edn 1539, nine edns by 1595. Luigi Cornaro, *Discorsi della vita sobria*, first English trans. in Lessius' *Hygiasticon*, by George Herbert in 1636, as *Sure and Certain Methods of Attaining a Long and Healthful life*, 3rd edn 1722, thirty-six edns by 1826; Sanctorius, *Ars...de statica medicina* (Venice, 1614), trans. as *Medicina Statica; or Rules of Health, in Eight Sections of Aphorisms...* (London, 1676).

thereafter were resolved into the pursuance of the neglected theme of 'exercise', linked to what was extensively termed 'cool regimen'. Exercise was the second part of dietetics known as the 'art of activity', or 'athletics', or simply, 'the healthy movements of the body'. 'Cool' regimen emphasised the care of the external solids calling for a 'hardening' of the body on a 'low' diet; it was characterised by the idea of process, or dynamics. The emergence of balneology as a subdivision of the therapy of exercise was directly related to this change. The cooling and hardening of the body in water was analogous to ventilating and cooling the body in cold air; the passions could be cooled as well as heated; cool vegetables were the antithesis to hot meats. Living according to nature in the cool British climate meant employing cool regimen to bring body and environment into harmony.[30] The development of the Hippocratic orthodoxy was gradual and piecemeal, and powerfully influenced by the 'sceptical' teaching of Sydenham, and Boerhaave, established as orthodoxy in the progressive and influential medical school of Edinburgh University. It was signalled in the major advice works from the early eighteenth century such as those by Cheyne, John and George Armstrong, and at the prestigious end of the market, pre-eminently in the clinical practice of John Hunter, John Arbuthnot, William Heberden, and many other metropolitan advocates of 'the healing power of nature'.[31]

More indicative, however, than the work of top London physicians, is the evidence of enthusiasm for cool regimen which came from base-line popular medical writers between about 1670 and 1750 such as Thomas Tryon, John Hancoke and John Wesley. During this period in Britain, medicine had acquired an element of those who vocalised their opposition to orthodoxy and hierarchical status, and anti-professionalism became a creed of public or 'natural rights' versus

---

[30] See John Floyer, *The History of Cold Bathing Ancient and Modern* (London, 1706), Dedication.

[31] G. Cheyne, *An Essay on Health and Long Life* (London, 1724), 4th edn, nine edns by 1725; John Armstrong, *The Art of Preserving Health*, a poem (London, 1744), five edns by 1757. Boerhaave is known as a main proponent of the '*vis medicatrix naturae*', while Sydenham was the hero of British Hippocratists; but therapeutic scepticism was not an isolated phenomenon, and we should be aware of the process of hagiography, or iconography. See for instance L. S. Jacyna on the use made of John Hunter's name, in 'Images of John Hunter in the nineteenth century', *History of Science*, XXI (1983), 85–108. The Edinburgh Boerhaavian model and its domination of the curriculum until the 1770s is fully described by C. J. Lawrence, 'Medicine as culture: Edinburgh and the Scottish Enlightenment' (University of London, Ph.D. thesis, 1984).

private monopoly by an incorporated group claiming customary privileges.[32] While orthodox 'knowledge' was certainly a support to the self-taught and was not necessarily to be 'turned upside down', this did not inhibit the political rights to interpret or 'order' that knowledge, or the right to empirical investigation. Preventive hygienic medicine, embodied in cool regimen, was a platform from which to abuse venal physicians, the monopolist dispensers of unnatural, expensive (and mineral) drugs. The holistic philosophy at the core of preventive hygiene also fitted well with indigenous traditions of herbalism.[33] The 'extraordinary self-taught genius' Thomas Tryon was an outstanding propagandist – the complete list of his works as recorded by Sir John Sinclair totals eighteen titles, all written to promote his revelatory fundamentalist faith in the spiritual purity of cool vegetable regimen. After breaking with the Anabaptists in 1657 he continued his medical studies; while investigating the works of the chemists, 'those marvellous wonders so much talked of and so little known, and not being able to penetrate into nor comprehend them', he went to sleep and dreamed of

The Globe of the Universe, whereon was only written in Capital Golden-letters, REGENERATION; which was to me a clear manifestation, that obedience to God's Laws and Commandments, was the only thing needful to be inquired after; and that there is no other way to obtain the great Mystery and Knowledge of God, his Law, and our Selves; but by Self-Denial, Cleanness, Temperance, and Sobriety; in Words, Imployments, Meats and

[32] Webster, *The Great Instauration* (note 6), esp. pp. 263–73. On natural rights, see Quentin Skinner, *The Foundations of Modern Political Thought*, vol. 2, *The Age of Reformation* (Cambridge, 1978), esp. part 3, 'Calvinism and the theory of revolution', pp. 189–358; D. D. Raphael (ed.), *Political Theory and the Rights of Man* (London, 1967); C. B. Macpherson, *The Political Theory of Possessive Individualism: Hobbes to Locke* (Oxford, 1962). See also E. P. Thompson, *The Making of the English Working Class* (London, 1968); and Christopher Hill, *The World Turned Upside Down: Radical Ideas During the English Revolution* (London, 1975).

[33] Thomas Tryon, *The Way to Health* (London, 1683) includes as Contents, 'of Temperance, of Flesh, of the Seasons of the Year, of Cities, of Fatness, of the Causes of Wars, on English Herbs, of Bugs, of Teeth, of Marriage...'. See also Webster, *The Great Instauration*, pp. 469–71, on husbandry, herbals and Bacon's 'Vegetable Philosophy', though he does not choose to pursue vegetable therapeutics. See also *ibid.*, p. 261, pp. 298–9, on baths and spas. Paracelsian chemistry is accounted the main substitute for the 'heathen' Galen's humoral physiology, *ibid.*, pp. 282–8. See more recently F. Delaporte, *Nature's Second Kingdom: Explorations of Vegetality in the Eighteenth Century*, trans. Arthur Goldhammer (Cambridge, Mass., 1982).

Drinks; all which unites our souls to God, and our Neighbours; and keeps our Bodies in Health, and our minds in serenity; rendering us unpolluted Temples, for the Holy Spirit of God to communicate with.[34]

He took to drinking water only, eating vegetables and conforming to 'an abstemious self-denying life'. Tryon's Voice of Wisdom was benevolent, and paternalistic – it would 'inform man, in all the particulars of his life which is right and the contrary. It will teach him what food and drinks are most profitable... when to speak... what words are proper... what garments are most useful... as also of houses, furniture, beds, labour, and exercise, and in a word, all circumstances belonging to the inward and outward man'.[35] The ascetic life laid down in his sectarian Rules for a 'Society of Clean and Innocent Livers' ensured that the body was physically cleansed of all gross matter – of fat and filth – through a vegetable regimen which cleansed inwardly. Both the outward and inward man was cleansed by plenty of cool fresh air, bathing, and exercise in rural surrounding, with simple clean clothes, rooms, and bedding. The effect he found was that he was 'more nimble, brisk, eesie, and lightsome'.[36]

John Hancoke's *Febrifugum Magnum* (1722) was a radical tract on cold water as a universal preventive and healer which had a renowned popular success not only for its therapeutic powers, but as a blast against the physicians.[37] The early radicalism of balneology led early twentieth century hydrotherapists, perhaps justifiably, to complain bitterly at the damage done to the orthodox professional status of water treatments at this crucial period at the turn of the century, by John Hancoke in particular.[38] John Wesley's handbook *Primitive Physic* (1747) was a miscellany of radical initiatives, starting with a philosophical commitment to natural holism, and then firmly by-passing all theory (including regimen) with a deliberately unstructured compilation of

[34] Thomas Tryon, *Memoirs* (London, 1705), pp. 40–1.
[35] *Ibid.*, pp. 35–7.
[36] *Ibid.*, pp. 26–7; see also Smith, 'Thomas Tryon's regimen for women' (note 24).
[37] John Hancoke, *Febrifugum Magnum*, 6th edn (London, 1723). See pp. 10–11 for his rejection of the Mechanick Account of medicine; and on p. 18: 'I have looked into many Physic books both Ancient and Modern, but cannot find the least hint of my notion, and so can produce no Authorities'. First edition 1722, eight editions by 1726.
[38] S. Baruch, *The Principles and Practice of Hydrotherapy* (New York, 1899), pp. 421–2, where he comments, 'with natural aversion, English physicians neglected a remedy which had thus been lauded into popularity'.

radical empiric remedies.[39] They included the enthusiastic endorsement of cold water therapy, which Wesley recommended as a drink, in the humoral tradition, and as a bodily application in the style of what was rapidly becoming known as 'Modern Medicine'. By the third quarter of the eighteenth century 'Modern Medicine' had sublimated a radical enthusiasm for cool regimen into a moderate or liberal hypothesis of hygienic treatment. Medical scepticism, enshrined in the '*vis medicatrix naturae*', promoted the 'cool' antiseptic use of food, water and air, and the regular exercise of the faculties.

The works, 1770–1820

Certain occupational patterns emerge from a sample of sixty-two titles published between 1770 and 1820.[40] There are problems of identification, but occupation has initially been inferred from the use of formal titles or the implication (stated or otherwise) of normal employment. In those cases where the authors remain anonymous, it is recognised that the attribution of public status was a personal decision; the non-use of a title, or reticence about normal occupation, was a precise choice which allowed the author to hide or mask his intentions. In a similar sense, there is no way of knowing how many authors used pseudonyms. On paper, twenty-six authors were stated M.D.s or held public positions, while seven implied that they were full-time general practitioners (one woman practitioner and midwife actually used the doctorate title twice, once reversed as D.M.). Six authors unambiguously stated they were surgeons; five were chemists, pharmacists or purveyors of drugs; and three more obviously dealt in drugs, but did not directly associate themselves with the trade. The old distinction between purveyors of mineral and purveyors of herbal drugs was still upheld by these authors. Eight were 'lay' authors identifiable by title (Sir, Esq., Mrs, Rev.) or by occupation (sailor, businessman, housewife or housekeeper, hairdresser, commercial writers); two were unclassifiable but could have been 'genteel'; and

[39] John Wesley, *Primitive Physic* (London, 1747); thirty-five edns to 1842. The best and simplest account of Wesley's therapeutic intentions is A. W. Hill, *John Wesley Amongst the Physicians* (London, 1958). Wesley's influence has been variously discussed by Sir George Newman in *Health and Social Evolution* (London, 1931); and by G. S. Rousseau, 'John Wesley's *Primitive Physic*', *Harvard Library Bulletin*, XVI (1968), 242–56.

[40] There is an additional group of authors who wrote advice for public institutions – regimen for camps, ships, cities, schools and hospitals. They are not included in this sample, though they certainly affected an unknown number of individuals at their place of work and, sporadically, in their own homes. This sample relates to domestic medicine only.

five were anonymous but included writers on behalf of two public baths owners, one auto-didact, one editor of Cornaro, and an eighteenth century editor of *Aristotle's Works*.

Identified lay authors made up less than a third of the sample, which was dominated by the accredited physicians. However, lay aims and methods often merged indistinguishably with those of the surgeons and chemists. Surgeons and chemists were clearly 'marginal men' able to serve either lay or professional interests as they chose.[41] Laymen, surgeons and chemists together balanced the contributions of the physicians and general practitioners, though they did not invest so much money in their publications. Lay and 'semi-professional' works were more likely to be slim, small, cheap, and of the earlier 'miscellaneous' (or almanac) format. Authors with an 'interest', or ambition, wrote longer, more heavily structured works, of higher price and larger size. The average price of a family advice book ranged from six shillings to half a guinea and above for the most detailed works (such as Buchan's *Domestic Medicine*). Information could also be purchased through sixpenny series of weekly or monthly issues of works, and penny and twopenny tracts. The impression is that there had been a reduction in the proportion of lay works compared with Slack's period of 1486–1604, and that their prestige had waned; but there were still notable exceptions to this trend (Sir John Sinclair's volume being one). Whatever the multifarious occupations of the authors were, medical scepticism along a wide front certainly contributed to the strong revival of the advice book market in the 1770s, and strongly sustained it up to *c.* 1810.[42]

Public scepticism: self-help and dissent. It is more appropriate to look first at the lower end of the market, since for these books it is not only

[41] See Ian Inkster, 'Marginal men: aspects of the social role of the medical community in Sheffield 1790–1850', in J. Woodward and D. Richards (eds.), *Health Care and Popular Medicine in Nineteenth Century England* (London, 1977), pp. 128–63, on the problems of marginal status and survival amongst full-time medical practitioners. But see more recently Irvine Loudon on the emergence of the general practitioner 'during the second and third decades of the nineteenth century', p. 4 in 'Two thousand medical men in 1847', *The Society for the Social History of Medicine Bulletin*, XXXIII (1983), 4–8; and also Geoffrey Holmes, *Augustan England: Professions, State, and Society 1680–1730* (London, 1982).

[42] See the general survey by Isabel Rivers, *Books and their Readers in the Eighteenth Century* (Leicester, 1982). Judged by the Wellcome Collection, the Napoleonic Wars marked a significant drop in output, which begins to recover from the 1820s. This is partially confirmed by other bibliographic sources.

likely that their total bulk exceeded the more expensive productions, but they are less well known to us. Works in this cheaper or lower-status part of the market were strongly intent on self-help. Mrs Cole, Mr Astley, Peter Crosthwaite, the Rev. W. Wilson, John Corry, Ebenezer Sibly, John Trusler, and four anonymous works all assumed some measure of self-sufficiency in health care. As the *Domestic Pharmacopoeia* put it:

If every man ought, through motives of self-preservation and defence, to be his own lawyer, his own broker, his own brewer, etc.... for a still stronger reason ought he to be, as far as his other pursuits will enable him, his own physician.[43]

Or as John Trusler wrote in *The Physical Friend*: 'By an occasional resort to this book, many a tormenting and expensive sickness may be prevented'.[44] For patent medicine salesman Samuel Solomon, the dictate of temperance

has those particular advantages above all other means of health, that it may be practised by all ranks and conditions, at any season or in any place. It is a kind of regimen into which every man may put himself, without interruption of business, expense of money, or loss of time.[45]

Prevention was prudent common-sense, saving time, money and personal anguish; most domestic 'regulations' or customs were based on this survival principle.[46] It was also prudent not to put yourself into the hands of strangers, or to take too many unnecessary risks, such as using unknown potions. As W. Smith, the discreet salesman of a Tonic Tincture, told the young full-time practitioner bluntly in 1774,

people in general dislike physicians as such, and abominate the very thought of swallowing medicine. This arises from an inherent notion, strongly confirmed by observation, that physicians are of less service than they are willing to have it believed, and that medicines do sometimes more hurt than good.[47]

Public scepticism was modified in the case of cool regimen, with or without accompanying drugs. Cool or cold regimen was the main

---

43 [Anon.], *Domestic Pharmacopoeia* (London, 1805), pp. vi–vii.
44 John Trusler, *The Physical Friend* (London, 1776), Preamble.
45 Samuel Solomon, *The Guide to Health* (Stockport, 1801), 52nd edn, pp. 284–5.
46 See Lucinda McCray Beier, in this volume, for the local and personal nature of Ralph Josselin's medical experiences.
47 W. Smith, *Nature Studied with a View to Preserve and Restore Health* (London, 1774), p. 87.

recommendation of most of the advice works in a way which suggests that consensus had been achieved. A small minority of authors, pre-eminently the compiler of the oldest advice book, *Aristotle's Works*, were exclusively concerned with drug receipts and the inner physiology of food taking. With food in general, however, a moderate 'low' diet prevailed, with distinct emphasis on 'cool' vegetables. No one recommended the virtues of hot air, which caused dangerous miasmas and enervation; and only a few authors, later in the period, actively promoted hot or warm water, which was greatly distrusted on account of its weakening or relaxing qualities. There were those who mixed old hot and new cool regimen in succeeding passages, and there were various degrees of attachment to drugs; contradictions abounded, and the choice of therapeutic mix was entirely personal. Mrs M. Cole, Ebenezer Sibly, and the majority of the works, were dutiful admirers of cool fever regimen in the sick room. Astley and another owner of public baths paraded it as an enticement to their customers, suggesting cold bathing both as a pleasure and as an essential accompaniment to health. Hairdresser David Ritchie advised that heat and dryness damaged the hair. Even while preaching cool regimen, essayist John Corry and the Rev. William Wilson, salesman of an anti-arthritic powder, felt bound to debunk the current medical scene.

Corry pugnaciously attacked those who advised flannel next to the skin ('such as Count Rumford'): 'Do these Quacks wish to reintroduce the sweating sickness, once so fatal to Englishmen?' At the same time he satirised the new jargon: 'There is no such thing as "sweat" nowaday; even the coal porter and the butcher's boy "perspire" – elegant creatures!'[48] Corry's admiration of the 'opulent tradesmen' of London could have easily fitted Wilson's view of a *nouveau riche* spending increasingly on health. In 1804 the fashion for natural health was well under way. Wilson jeered at the romantic city dweller who squandered his money on the expense of a country residence; the fatigue of travel; the ruin and neglect of business; and the 'dull amusement' of the 'search for hot and cold water'. He cautioned,

One proposes to cure all diseases by aliment alone... Another is for adding to this, cleanliness, country air, and exercise. No doubt these are of considerable use, but if they can be recommended to prevent or cure diseases, which they can neither prevent nor cure the prescription is a deception... All figures and hyperbole are improper, however they may shine as beauties in

[48] John Corry, *The Detector of Quackery* (London, 1802), pp. 80, 110.

poetry and romance... Of all your acquaintances, who have set out in search of the temple of health, how few have returned?[49]

The cost of the simplest hygienic precautions, however, were, as authors constantly reminded their readers, not dependent on the great expense of time or money but on the strength of personal conviction. Simple food, simple exercise, simple air, simple medicines, and the author's book (modestly priced) were sufficient. At the other extreme, as now, hygienic health care could be an item of fashionable expenditure, stretched as far as the purse allowed.

Either as a way to save money, or as a way to spend it, new cool regimen was a popular success; but others upheld the moral cause. An enlightened and evangelical attitude towards medical knowledge was taken by the gentleman statistician Sir John Sinclair. He embarked on his four-volume *Code of Health and Longevity* in order to provide an exhaustive reference book on preventive medicine (he was one of the few to call it Hygiene) in the manner of Enlightenment philosophes. The old theme of longevity was nothing less than the achievement of moral and physical improvement of the human species, jointly achieved through universal knowledge. Thus he looked for 'the fullest information... of the most recent doctrine of the most intelligent men on the Continent',[50] and the full bibliography of 'British and Foreign Authors' was designed to stimulate the public debate, and public medical education. In contrast to European theoreticians such as Haller, Francke or Hallé, Sinclair was more confident collecting the empirical bibliographic evidence than he was with theoretical interpretation. Comparing Hallé's plan of the new Hygiene from the *Encylopédie méthodique*, which he translated and added as an appendix to his own, he said 'the former seems, on the whole, to be best calculated for a scientific, the latter for a popular work. Indeed, in the plan adopted by Hallé, there are too many divisions and subdivisions for a treatise intended for the use of the bulk of mankind' – adding conscientiously, 'of that, however, the reader will be better enabled to judge by examining both treatises'.[51]

[49] Rev. William Wilson, *The Philosophy of Physic: or the Natural History of Diseases and their Cure. Being an Attempt to Deliver the Art of Healing from Barbarism and Superstition and from the Jargon and Pedantry of the Schools* (Dublin, 1804), pp. xix–xx. An extended satirisation of health expenditure combined with rising social expectations – the move to the suburbs – is contained in John Trusler's *The Way to Be Rich and Respectable* (London, 1796).

[50] Sinclair, *Code of Health and Longevity* (note 10), vol. 3, p. 261.

[51] *Ibid.*, vol. 3, p. 261. See also W. Coleman, 'Health and hygiene in the *Encyclopédie*: a medical doctrine for the bourgeoisie', *Journal of the History of*

Self-taught sailor Peter Crosthwaite was as earnest about his science as about his faith. He had a clear idea of the modern science of regimen, and laid out all the most recent and progressive work on the non-naturals, with particular attention to hygienic prophylaxis on board ship. He firmly believed in his own right to contribute to the store of empirical knowledge:

The useful observations I have made on the dispositions, custom, etc. of mankind in different parts of the world; the experience I have gained by being attentive to the causes of various changes produced in my own constitution, and my having studied the nature and properties of the human structure...have enabled me to write this book.[52]

His practical contribution was a full description of the Indian technique of body-washing, and hygienic advice on fever regimen to his fellow-sailors. But his primary aim was to recommend the use of cold water in all its forms, and his scientific 'proof' was supplementary to an inherently religious perspective. The sub-title to the work encapsulated his views on cold water, and the indivisibility of the material flesh and the psychic spirit:

shewing how the Health, both of Body and Mind, may be preserved, and even revived by the mild and attenuating Power of a most valuable and cheap medicine. Its singular and most excellent property is to subdue the FLESH to the will of the SPIRIT; by which happy means, Mankind may enjoy a State of Temperance instead of Intemperance, and a State of Virtue instead of Vice. The continued use of this Medicine eradicates most diseases, and is seriously recommended to the People of this Island.[53]

The non-naturals of the mind and body were traditionally controlled by temperance; and temperate morality was a constant ingredient in other lower-status works, ranging from the ascetic dietary view of the 1770 edition of Cornaro, to the simple statement of E. Bullman, a full-time woman practitioner: 'To conclude, those who live philosophically, temperately, religiously, and wisely, seldom want a physician.'[54] Solid but genuine convictions on temperate regimen can be found in Samuel Solomon, and more passionately in another proprietary author, Joshua Webster (with his anonymous editor).

Medicine, xxix (1974), 399–421; and L. J. Jordanova, 'Earth science and environmental medicine: the synthesis of the late Enlightenment', in L. J. Jordanova and R. Porter (eds.), *Images of the Earth: Essays in the History of the Environmental Sciences* (Chalfont St Giles, 1979), pp. 119–46.

[52] Peter Crosthwaite, *The Ensign of Peace* (London, 1775), Advertisement.

[53] *Ibid.*, Preamble.

[54] E. Bullman, *The Family Physician* (London, 1789), Preface.

Webster's 'English Diet Drink' was a herbal or vegetable preparation;
Webster put his faith in vegetables, and vegetarianism. He demanded
that physicians should follow the example of John Wesley (who had
become vegetarian in middle age), and

> revert to the simplicity and nature of the origins of the medical art; they
> should turn their attention from Minerals, Metals, etc., and seek the Goddess
> of Health in her native abode – The Vegetable Kingdom.[55]

Webster exhibited a fundamentalist preoccupation with one element,
in this case earth-bound vegetality, which was similar to Crosthwaite's
belief in water as a universal healer; or Ebenezer Sibly's preoccupation
with the universal spirit of the air, gases, and the occult aether.
Minerals, artifice, mystery and speculation versus vegetables, nature,
truth and empiricism were seventeenth century themes, and Webster,
Crosthwaite and Sibly were clearly heirs to the radical tradition.
Webster did not mention 'Old Tryon' but he did invoke more recent
heroes such as Wesley, and Benjamin Franklin. Sibly and Crosthwaite
referred discreetly to ancient philosophers and divines, but chose to
refer directly to the scientific moderns, and progressives.

  In most cases the sales of preparations were quite unselfconscious,
and Solomon, James Graham, and probably Webster printed dirt cheap
for advertising purposes, with both books and tracts. The religious tract
was taken as a model, and tract readers were clearly an audience – one
author going out of his way to attract Baptists (he was the owner of
a new suite of floating river baths).[56] As a group, however, they sold
their products in close association with the works, and would frequently not 'guarantee' success unless a 'course' of regimen accompanied the preparation. Solomon's massive and enormously popular
Guide to Health was also an essential Guide to the Balm of Gilead, which
he sold mail-order in crates of six bottles. Certainly the apothecary who
sold it in the shop would have had a copy, which could have been
used as a general manual by his customers. Although regimen can be
seen as a sound business precaution, the advice given tended to limit
the overall number of drugs used – except for the specific preparation
so generously on sale. Webster simply echoed the ancient belief that
drug-taking was irrational and usually excessive when he commented
that 'Mankind have since the dawn of what is called "medical

55 Joshua Webster, *Practical Observations on the Preservation of Health* (London,
   1804), p. xxiii.
56 [Anon.], *The Efficacy of Bathing in the Promotion and Preservation of Health,
   Vigour, Beauty, and Long Life* (London, 1778), pp. 3, 7.

knowledge" been absolutely drug-enamoured, and unaccountably attached to prescripts' – but he was not going to question the use of a universal healer and preventive.[57] Obviously most drugs salesmen did not write manuals, but those that did frequently took a flexible moral line which authenticated but did not disturb trade. Such were E. Senate (The Balm of Mecca) who dealt with sexual diseases and no doubt feared that moral inculcations might frighten away the customers; and W. Smith (a Tonic Tincture) who seems to have concluded that temperate morality was not relevant for a practitioner with ambitions amongst the military.[58]

Vegetality, radicalism and religion were outrageously combined in the holistic regimen of James Graham, an extreme example of this trait amongst the chemists and commercial salesmen. Graham was the most notable enthusiast for all radical approaches, and his career was dominated by his semi-mystic universalist beliefs. Graham threw up an orthodox medical education and eventually became a Behmenist – 'the divinely illuminated Jacob Behmen' – and derived his notorious therapies from an ascetic view of cool vegetable regimen and the power of the elements. The earth-bathing, water-bathing, sun-bathing, and breathing of the electrical aether were exaggerated variations on holistic cool regimen, and were to be used as an accompaniment to a changed moral life-style. In *The Guardian of Health, Long-Life, and Happiness: or Dr Graham's General Directions as to Regimen* (1790) Graham opened with the comment 'I consider regimen, or your general manner of living and conducting yourselves, to be of far greater consequence to...bodily health and firmness, and of mental contentment, serenity, and cheerfulness, than loads of harsh, nauseous, and unnatural medicines from doctors and apothecaries'.[59] And for those asking advice about Graham's 'medicines, regimens, and external applications' by letter, they should understand that

It will be unreasonable for Dr Graham's Patients to expect a complete and lasting cure, or even great alleviation of their peculiar maladies, unless they keep their body and limbs most perfectly clean with very frequent washings – breathe fresh open air day and night, – be simple in the quality and moderate in the quantity of their food and drink – and totally give up using

---

[57] Webster, *Practical Observations*, p. xvi.

[58] E. Senate, *The Medical Monitor* (London, 1810); W. Smith, *Nature Studied* (note 47).

[59] James Graham, *The Guardian of Health, Long-life, and Happiness: or Dr Graham's General Directions as to Regimen, etc. To which are added, the Christian's Universal* (Newcastle-upon-Tyne, 1790), p. 1.

the deadly poisons and canker worms of estates, called foreign Tea and Coffee, Red Port Wine, Spiritous Liquors, Tobacco and Snuff, gaming and late hours, and all sinful, unnatural, and excessive indulgence of the animal appetites, and of the diabolical and degrading mental passions. On practising the above rules…depends the very perfection of bodily health, strength, and happiness.[60]

Graham's constant references to coolness, cleanliness, and frequent washings with 'cold living water' were ritualistic, puritanical incantations against hot regimen and associated evils. The Prayer for his Christian Universal Church, which had as its aim 'to unite every affinity that there is between the elements and man…between man and everything that there is in the universe',[61] called for a life of 'temperance and moderation, in perfect purity, cleanness, and self-denial of body, internal and external'.[62] Sexual chastity and physical purity together made up a religiously orientated 'pollution theory', through which 'cleanness' would bring the spiritual and physical body materially closer to God – Tryon's 'unpolluted Temples, for the Holy Spirit of God to communicate with'.[63] Pollution theory associated with a fundamentalist puritanism can be found in Tryon, and to a lesser extent in Peter Crosthwaite. Graham's practice was built not only on the desire to promote a hygienic universalist Christendom, but also on the necessity to sanitise and thus consecrate the sexual act; people came in their hundreds to the Temple of Health to hear about good clean sex (pure propagation).[64] Graham's opinions on prevailing hygienic standards (and moral laxity) were uncompromising, and his advice was also rigorous: people must always bathe or wash 'their face, neck, hands, feet, and private parts – ESPECIALLY THE LATTER, with pure COLD water…every night and morning'.[65] His own

[60] James Graham, *A Short Treatise on the All-Cleansing, All-Healing, and All-Invigorating Qualities of the Simple Earth* (Newcastle, 1790), p. 18.

[61] James Graham, *The Guardian Goddess of Health: or the Whole Art of Preserving and Curing Diseases and Enjoying Peace and Happiness of Body and Mind…Precepts for the Preservation and Exaltation of Personal Beauty and Loveliness* (London, 1780), p. 11.

[62] Graham, *The Guardian of Health*, p. 12.

[63] Mary Douglas, *Purity and Danger* (London, 1966) and *Natural Symbols: Explorations in Cosmology* (London, 1978 edn). See also Thomas Tryon, *Memoirs* (note 34) on the veiling of women, and other purity rules; quoted in G. Smith, 'Thomas Tryon's regimen for women' (note 24), pp. 63–4.

[64] Roy Porter, 'Sex and the singular man: the seminal ideas of James Graham', *Studies in Voltaire and the Eighteenth Century* (1984), 1–24.

[65] Graham, *The Guardian Goddess of Health*, p. 4.

physical repulsion to dirt, and to the unenlightened foetid masses, was unrestrained:

> so indeed the people in general seem to delight in stench, and in personal dirt and filthiness, both internally and externally; which they take care to cover, keep in, and to add to, by very close doors, windows, beds, and carriages, and by carrying such loads of clothes day and night, as really convert them into beasts of burthen – into moving dunghills, nurseries of vermin, or into filthy Infirmaries for all manner of diseases to thrive in, and to be propagated in; and though they seldom wash their public, and NEVER their PRIVATE parts, they fancy that they either are, or will be thought clean, by putting on clean linen.[66]

Carriage owners and frivolous wasters were his target; they were also his fashionable clientele. He offered them moral beauty – 'the delights that shine in poetry and romance' – or just 'Beauty'. A more traditional aid to pure beauty were the cosmetics sold by Solomon: such as his 'Abstergent Lotion' (probably a soap wash) which restored the skin 'to a degree of fairness and purity beyond the powers of description'. Instead of 'distressing pimples', a 'Beautiful Comlexion, and a healthful Appearance, are the admiration of all who behold them, the pride of all who possess them, and the envy of all who want them'.[67] Graham and Solomon sold high and low; Crosthwaite, on the other hand, took the poor as his parish. Less disingenuously than Graham, Crosthwaite sustained a radical attack on 'the vicious…the governing part of the world… who…canonize vice disguised in her ornaments and apparel'. Their wives were the owners of tall head-dresses 'such as have often been found pestered with live animals…How strange it is that people who pride themselves in making an outward shew of cleanliness, should keep their bodies dirty within, and have a filthy skin?'[68] Revulsion against the upper orders was part of his strategy – the honest, hard-working labourer and tradesman had a duty to lead a hygienic moral reform of which 'the vicious' were incapable. In the light of his experience in India, he judged the practical requirement of cleanliness to be minimal: a bowl of water and a towel. Moral laxity, not cost, was the bar to cleanliness. More pragmatically, however, he

---

[66] Graham, *A Short Treatise…on the Simple Earth*, p. 12.
[67] Solomon, *Guide to Health* (note 45), Advertisement. On the practice of cosmetics, see Margaret Pelling, 'Appearance and reality: barber surgeons, the body, and disease in early modern London', in L. Beier and R. Finlay (eds.), *The Making of the Metropolis* (forthcoming).
[68] Crosthwaite, *Ensign of Peace* (note 52), pp. 36–7, p. 96.

understood that washing techniques themselves were foreign to the British, and had to be inculcated before the custom or habit took root:

In India...the natives think Europeans an dirty people, because they do not wash...and were the practise of frequent washing to become pretty common in Europe, I must needs think, that in this present generation, such as practised it, would perhaps look on them who neglected it, as unnaturally bemired and weakened by weltering in their own dirt.[69]

Professional reformers. Moving in towards the full-time professional, there are noticeable changes in the character of the works. These authors sold their services rather than products, and for this a display of education was required. The transfer of medical education to the public became an internal professional issue, seen in terms of greater emphasis on professional care and control. This was the 'advice' which pre-supposed, in its most extreme and restrictive form, a deference and dependence on specialised knowledge, whereby the book itself provided an extension of rather than a substitute for expert attendance. This was the view of James Mackittrick Adair, in a work intended for 'men of sense' – the 'type of gentleman who reads Newton and Blackstone's Commentaries'.[70]

Nothing but a knowlege of the first principles of an art will ever enable us to understand any part of it. Regimen is a very important branch of medicine, and cannot be understood, unless by those who are previously conversant with the structure and functions of the body. This consideration suggested to me the propriety of giving some outline of the Natural History of the Human Body, so far as was necessary to illustrate the principles of regimen; as it was conceived that the chief reason why invalids are less disposed to submit to regimen, is their not understanding the grounds of the prescription.[71]

Adair commented contritely on his earlier more forthright 'Essay on Regimen' that there had been 'some criticism that medical reasoning was lacking'; a fate that also attended William Buchan and Disney Alexander.

Hardliners on professional privilege in the professional group included W. Moss (surgeon), R. White (M.D.), Thomas Beddoes and James Parkinson. Both Moss and White represented specialist

[69] *Ibid.*, p. 125.
[70] James Mackittrick Adair, *Philosophical and Medical Sketch of the Natural History of the Human Body and Mind...intended for those who are, or are not, of the Medical Profession* (Bath, 1787), p. x.   [71] *Ibid.*, pp. vii–viii.

professional interests: Moss in child care, White in balneology. White produced the classic plea of the licensed water-doctor – that the process of bathing was fraught with dangers, and that the patient was 'earnestly recommended...that they would first apply for advice, to some experienced person of the Faculty'. He wrote his advice book specifically to 'correct the propensity which people of all ranks have discovered towards sea-bathing'.[72] Moss's professional objections were more subtle. Male professional opposition to female doctoring and health care in the home had been gathering support well before the 1780s;[73] and there are several indications in the works that the mastery of the new regimen was at issue between male and female professionals. In 1806 Walker Keighley (M.D.) wrote *A New System of Family Medicine* on behalf of the British Ladies Institution, with regimen as the centrepiece, expressly to 'unite all the parts of medical and chirurgical knowledge that are strictly necessary, to make an intelligent female equally well prepared for the extraordinary case, as the most general medical man'. The patronesses were alarmed at the decline in female nursing, and pointed to the example of orderly management in aristocratic households, where 'females of the highest rank, enjoying every luxury, wisely restrict their children in the important particulars of diet and regimen'.[74]

But twenty-five years earlier in 1781, William Moss's *Essay on the Management and Nursing of Children* was a respected work in a relatively new specialised advice field; his progenitors were William Cadogan (1748) and the child clinician George Armstrong (1769), brother of the natural health poet John Armstrong.[75] Moss stressed (as had Armstrong) that the non-naturals had 'not been so minutely investigated...nor have the discoveries, made thereon, been improved upon

[72] Robert White, *Use and Abuse of Sea Water, Impartially Considered* (Bury, 1779), p. 9.

[73] When midwife Elizabeth Nihell complained about their professional intrusion, and their 'cloud of hard words and scientific jargon': *Treatise on the Art of Midwifery* (London, 1760), pp. 158–9. Quoted in Jean Donnison, *Midwives and Medical Men: A History of Inter-Professional Rivalries and Women's Rights* (New York, 1977), p. 33.

[74] Walker Keighley, *A New System of Family Medicine* (London, 1806), p. ix, p. 186.

[75] George Armstrong, *An Essay on the Diseases most fatal to Infants. To which are added Rules to be observed in the Nursing of Children*, 1st edn (London, 1767); a small pamphlet by William Cadogan, *An Essay upon Nursing, and the Management of Children, from their Birth to Three Years of Age. By a Physician* (London, 1748), was an early attack on old (female) hot regimen; it had gone to eight editions by 1764.

or so generally applied to practise'. Moss made it quite clear that the problem and necessary area of child-care reform lay with the customary female control of the non-naturals – customary but not taught. He continued:

In the inquiry into this omission, it will appear that they (the non-naturals) have always been considered as situations that necessarily fall within the sphere of domestic control and superintendancy; and custom, that grand arbiter whose decision on appeal is seldom solicited, continues to enforce the opinion, and preclude all other aids, except on urgent occasion. The nursing of infants, and lying-in women, no doubt comes within this limitation so far as concerns the executive part; but it does not follow from thence, that the direction of it is to be considered in the same light.[76]

As in balneology, the recommendations for the new-style nursing demanded a 'nice and exact attention and judicious regulation' of all the hygienic non-naturals. Children should 'be gradually accustomed to be kept cooler'; firstly by washing them in cold water every morning 'from the birth', and then by exercise and a low diet.[77] A particular point was made of bringing in the father, as parent and family head, to enforce the new regulations. The use of drugs – a highly contentious point in child care as not being customary – was not ruled out.

A more discreet professionalism prevailed amongst other works, also from specialists, such as those by George Armstrong, Hugh Downman, Christian Struve, W. Logan, William Falconer. Armstrong, Struve and Falconer in particular refrained from drawing attention in their advice books to the professional role; they did not have to, it was there in their minute and conscientious attention to experimental detail. This did not apply to the popular works of Thomas Beddoes, experimenter and natural philosopher, who not only could not abide 'female doctresses', quacks, or ignorant physicians, but more interestingly was very imprecise in his recommendations for 'Hygeian' physiology amongst the middle classes. Beddoes regarded regimen as outdated humoral nonsense, and preferred to draw up his own programme of physiological education, rigorously derived from the work of the scientific elite with which he was associated.[78] Though the science of

[76] W. Moss, *Essay on the Management and Nursing of Children* (London, 1781), pp. vii–viii.

[77] *Ibid.*, p. 129.

[78] See S. Schaffer, 'Priestley's questions: a historiographic survey', *History of Science*, xxii (1984), 151–83; especially on Priestley's relationship with pneumatic medicine; T. Beddoes, *Hygeia* (Bristol, 1802).

physiology was 'unhappily not enough understood for the purposes of minute medical enquiry', Beddoes the educationalist saw no reason why 'future generations should, like the past, be abandoned to their fate'. A similarly elitist view of scientific standards can be found in an admirer of pneumatic medicine, James Parkinson, who wrote a cautionary advice book, *Medical Admonitions*, designed to show that science should not be interfered with; as it clearly was, by the 'too-frequent practise of domestic quackery... with the help of the family medicine chest, and a treatise on domestic medicine'.[79]

Less professional tension, and greater simplicity of language, seemed to prevail amongst the general practitioners than it did amongst the specialists; and it was from the ranks of general practitioners that internal criticism of the profession came. Muted criticism is apparent in unambitious early works by physicians and general practitioners such as Hugh Smith, William Smith and S. Freeman (1770, 1774, 1780). They indicated their market clearly. They were for 'families living distant from a good practitioner', for 'salesmen', 'masters of small ships', estate owners and colonial settlers; and 'for those who cannot afford to purchase more expensive treatises'. The main object of their therapeutic interest was regimen, with simple drugs; or as Hugh Smith noted

good nursing is a part which has either been too much neglected, or mistaken; nevertheless it is of first consequence in the cure of diseases, and the preserving of delicate and feeble constitutions.[80]

Both Hugh Smith and William Smith leant towards milder herbalism in conjunction with regimen; so too did William Meyrick (surgeon) who wrote a herbal and James Johnson (surgeon) who had resorted to vegetarianism in the tropics.

The most provocative and successful attack on the dangers of professional monopoly and the need for a shift in therapy had been mounted earlier, by William Buchan in 1769. His *Domestic Medicine* was a model for liberal reforming advice books after that date – such as those by George Wallis, Walker Keighley and T. F. Churchill (1793, 1806, 1808). Buchan believed in a therapeutic reform of excessive drugging practices; and with meticulous instructions and enlightened philosophical observations he attempted to give professional credibility to hygienic prophylaxis, or nursing, which he regarded as a neglected

[79] James Parkinson, *Medical Admonitions* (London, 1801).
[80] Hugh Smith, *The Family Physician*, 8th edn (London, 177?), p. ix.

subject. It involved an ethical reconsideration on the part of both the patient and the doctor with regard to self-help, and advice:

In the treatment of disease, I have been particularly attentive to regimen. The generality of people lay too much stress upon Medicine, and trust too little to their own endeavours...physicians, as well as other people, are too little attentive to this matter. This part of Medicine is evidently founded in Nature, and is in every way consistent with Reason and common sense. Had men been more attentive to it, and less solicitous in hunting after secret remedies, Medicine had never become an object of ridicule.[81]

To Buchan, preventive medicine was 'the first idea of Medicine' and well worth the life-long crusade:

There still remains much to be done on this subject, and it does not appear to me how any man could better employ his time or his talents, than in eradicating hurtful prejudices, and diffusing useful knowledge among the people.[82]

Buchan was strongly attacked by the profession (for instance by Adair, and James Parkinson, who wished to 'correct' Buchan) for revealing trade secrets without sufficient – or indeed any – cautions. Most frequently he was attacked on academic or scientific grounds; he was content to note simply in 1803 that the 'many prejudices' against his belief in preventive medicine were 'now overcome'.[83]

The political and moral principles that inspired his work were central to his influence and lasted long after his followers and imitators thought fit to re-assess his deliberately casual attitude to scientific theory. The moral belief in popular medical education took hold in certain professional circles, with doctors turning authors – such as William Turnbull writing for magazines, and Disney Alexander printing his 'plain directions for plain people' in pamphlet form for maximum distribution. Educationalists such as T. F. Churchill were more circumspect in their aims, believing in the 'new science' rather than common-sense and elementary principles alone. As he put it, in 1808:

Medical knowledge, like most other sciences, has within a few years, acquired very large and increasing degrees of improvement; and general circulation

[81] William Buchan, *Domestic Medicine*, 7th edn (London, 1781), p. xiii. See C. Lawrence, 'William Buchan: medicine laid open', *Medical History*, XIX (1975), 20–35, on the publication and philosophy of *Domestic Medicine*.
[82] William Buchan, *Buchan Enlarged. Domestic Medicine, etc....* (Dunbar, 1818 edn), p. xiii.
[83] William Buchan, *Advice to Mothers* (London, 1803), p. 139.

of that knowledge, among all classes and ranks of people, is a circumstance very much to be desired and encouraged by every person of feeling and liberality. Were this more properly and universally attended to than it is at present, it would infallibly have the effect of drawing aside that veil of mystery and chicanery, with which it has long been obscured.[84]

Churchill, Richard Reece and Walker Keighley might count as radicals amongst this early turn-of-the-century group of popular physiologists. There are hints that Churchill derived his radicalism from Quaker/ Evangelical roots; as also did George Wallis. Both dealt with a more refined religiosity than the enthusiastic fundamentalism of Graham, or the Wesleyanism of Webster. Old Dissenting beliefs were present nevertheless in their distaste for medical orthodoxy, their commitment to self-sufficiency, and in their concern for the family group.[85] Richard Reece, on the other hand, was a radical who disdained the religious prop, in favour of a perfectly rational science.

Reece, like Sinclair, was a bibliophile, and compiled a *Practical Dictionary of Domestic Medicine* prefaced by a short history of popular medicine. Reece's works had a strong political edge, sharpened by the failure of his own early medical ambitions; and he was quite convinced that a fully scientific future was there to be grasped by the aspiring lower rank practitioner. Prevention was only one part of this future, and he did not share the moral disdain of an earlier generation for the excesses of theory. He criticised Buchan for being 'scientifically supine' and the medical establishment for being bankrupt of ideas – unlike the cadre of popular medical writers. He loftily condemned

the trading physicians who exclaim violently against Domestic writers...In a profession so destitute of real science as that of medicine, it is to be expected that jealousy and illiberality will prevail. Hence it is common for medical men to speak in terms of contempt of works of domestic medicine.[86]

He dealt with modern physiology, chemistry, domestic medicine and medical police in a comprehensive round-up of progressive therapies. He included directly and indirectly both the Edinburgh and the European 'schools' of preventive medicine; but it was also typical of him that he was an early enthusiast for the unconventional shower bath

---

[84] T. F. Churchill, *New Practical Family Physician* (London, 1808), Preface. (Issued in twenty parts.)

[85] Similar to the staunch Quaker family advice books of a later author, J. Harrison Curtis, *Observations on the Preservation of Health* (London, 1837, 1842). See also note 24.

[86] Richard Reece, *The Medical Guide* (London, 1811), pp. v–ix.

and the even more unconventional air-bath – both described in severely practical detail. Naked air-bathing for short periods was 'a species of bath that certainly deserves a fair trial'.[87]

By far the most articulate of the new breed of scientifically orientated domestic medical writers was A. F. M. Willich. He was also outstandingly successful; he sold out two editions of his *Lectures on Diet and Regimen* in the first year of publication, 1799, and went into a third in 1800. Little is known of him, other than that he was an emigré from a German state who had a practice in Paddington; his work suggests he was an oculist. Willich was an active and well-informed propagandist, co-editor of the *Medical and Physical Journal* in 1799–1801 and a regular public lecturer, until his early death. He well understood the case against the profession:

In our times...we trust as much, if not more to ourselves, than to the physician, and we cannot conceive him to be perfectly free from the systems of the schools, from self-interest, or professional motives...[88]

But in his view, scepticism had gone too far. Some of its manifestations, where the doctor 'can neither discover nor comply with the peculiar system of health adopted by his patient', made the honest and necessary practice of medicine 'problematical'. He recommended a middle way; self-care in compliance with advanced vitalist theories of European physiology.

The *Lectures* were subtitled 'the most rational means of preserving health and prolonging life; together with physical and chemical explanations, calculated chiefly for the use of Families'. The book was clear enough for the use of families; but it was also of sufficient density to serve as a reference work for physicians on some of the most recent development of European physiology. In particular it transcribed the work of C. F. Hufeland on the dietary science of 'macrobiotics'; translated and incorporated the asthenology of Christian Struve; and drew on European vitalist experimenters and clinicians such as Hahnemann, Macard, Sömmering and Unzer. Reputable early British sources were not excluded – Priestley, Fothergill, Vaughan, Armstrong and, more recently, Falconer and Adams. Underlying the mass of 'evidence' and therapeutic recommendations, however, was an undiluted belief in universalism, or holism, or vitalism. In the pedigree of academic physiology, 'vitalism' originated in the mystic beliefs of

---

[87] *Ibid.*; no page number, see under 'Cold'.
[88] A. F. M. Willich, *Lectures on Diet and Regimen*, 2nd edn (London, 1799), pp. 26–7.

Georg Stahl and the healing powers of the soul; later in the eighteenth century this primal link between man and the cosmos was modified, and developed, so that 'vital' beliefs proliferated and became incorporated into the body of physiological thought under the metaphor of 'organisation'. In Britain, Karl Figlio and others have suggested, a radical 'immanent' vitalism opposed a conservative or orthodox 'transcendental' vitalism over the issue of where the power of God lay – within or above the mechanics of nature. It has been noted that while physiological properties 'were precisely specified in the technical sense, they were obviously infused with all the shades of meaning attached to ideas of life'.[89] The precise place of God in medicine was an open-ended metaphysical debate which A. F. M. Willich had no need to invoke. There was the self-evident glory of the 'organisation' itself, the processes of growth and decay in man and in all species of plants and animals. Without straining the analogy, the physiological and functional interpretation of living matter could be set beside the ancient 'chain of being' so beloved of classic religious theology:

If we reflect upon the admirable uniformity which prevails throughout the works of nature, both in production and dissolution of matter, we find she moves in a circle; that the smallest particle of matter, though invisible to our eyes, is usefully employed by her restless activity; and that death itself, or the destruction of forms and figures, is no more than a careful decomposition, and a designed regeneration of individual parts, in a manner no less skilful than surprising. We further observe, that in the immense variety of things, in the inconceivable waste of elementary particles, there nevertheless prevails the strictest oeconomy; that nothing is produced in vain, nothing consumed without a cause. We clearly perceive that all Nature is united by indissoluble ties; that everything exists for the sake of another, and that no-one can subsist without its concomitant. Hence we justly conclude, that man

---

[89] L. S. Jacyna, 'Immanence or transcendence: theories of life and organisation in Britain, 1790–1833', *Isis*, LXXIV (1983), 311–29; T. Lenoir, 'The Göttingen School and the development of transcendental naturphilosophie in the romantic era', *Studies in the History of Biology*, V (1981), 111–205; R. D. French, 'Some problems and sources in the foundations of modern physiology in Great Britain', *History of Science*, X (1971), 28–55; J. Goodfield-Toulmin, 'Some aspects of English physiology: 1780–1840', *Journal of the History of Biology*, II (1969), 283–320; see also J. Schiller, 'Queries, answers and unsolved problems in eighteenth century biology', *History of Science*, XII (1974), 184–99, p. 192 on 'confusing terminology' that raises 'misleading problems of semantics that require a thorough study'. Quotation from Karl Figlio, 'The metaphor of organisation: an historiographic perspective on the bio-medical sciences of the early nineteenth century', *History of Science*, XII (1976), 17–53, p. 18.

himself is not an insulated being, but that he is a necessary link in the great chain, which connects the universe.[90]

In its practical form European physiology constituted a science of nursing. It was complete physiological 'management', always a key word in regimen, and no less so in the care and maintenance of perfectly synchronised, holistic physical functions. The essential physiological processes were comprised in skin temperature and physical management (washing); airing and oxygenation; exercise; and to no lesser extent in the arrangements for food and clothing. The repeated use of phrases such as 'proper conduct', 'gradual culture', 'constant habit' and 'steady and equal progress' invoked the techniques of low-level management throughout the carefully distinguished phases of life from birth to death. It also accorded with the sthenic/asthenic principles of moderated nervous stimulation, then currently popular in European clinical practice, which provided a new measurement of the temperature mean between extremes.[91]

What then was new? It may be argued that a physiological paradigm was simply added to existing layers of classical thought; and that the intellectual change was not so much substantive as linguistic. The commitment to hygienic cool regimen was framed essentially as an appeal to natural laws, rules, and order: forethought versus impulse, rationality versus animal instinct, organisation versus chaos. In the acid words of one author, 'Eat, drink, and be merry, is all they aim at: and they do not care how soon their souls shall be required of them'.[92] The emerging scientific order can be seen not in any substantive changes in the acknowledged moral and physical therapeutic system – which was still very much a matter of personal choice or persuasion – but in the professional methods of quantification, precision and re-classification. The absolute division between religious and scientific

[90] A. F. M. Willich, *Lectures*, pp. 28–9. See also W. F. Bynum, 'The great chain of being after forty years: an appraisal', *History of Science*, xiii (1975), 1–20.

[91] The sthenic 'barometer' was a popular device for conveying this in the form of an image, and was also used by later anti-alcohol Temperance propagandists. See G. Gruman, 'The rise and fall of prolongevity hygiene, 1558–1833', *Bulletin for the History of Medicine*, xxxv (1961), 226–7, on C. Hufeland's admiration of Cornaro and theoretical use of a finite quantity of 'vital power'; especially in *The Art of Prolonging Life*, 1st translation (London, 1797). This expensively produced work had a limited circulation, though it was laid out as a popular advice book. But see also Francis Bacon on the conservation of 'vital spirits' in *The Historie of Life and Death. With observations Naturall and Experimental for the Prolonging of Life* (London, 1638 edn).

[92] Anon. editor of Cornaro, *Sure Methods of Obtaining a Long and Healthful Life* (Edinburgh, 1770 edn), p. viii.

belief, however, was only a vaguely discerned possibility; lay and professional practitioners still shared the far broader common ground of religious faith; which made all men equal before God and the Truth, but some more equal than others.

Three very simple questions arise from a preliminary survey of medical advice books pertaining to the genre of regimen: who read them, what was in them, and what did they do? All three questions revolve around a consideration of the works as medical belief systems and as simple artefacts, and both types of historical evidence will be required to disinter this particular body of writings. The evidence of content tends to support the idea that these works were nurtured by a broad popular base, especially if humoral regimen and later non-natural regimen are considered together, rather than separately, as is normally the case. Bibliographic evidence suggests that the works were part of a lively commercial market exhibiting a wide range of differently priced and styled works – so that we are not talking of an elite readership only, but one which potentially stretched down to all but the very poorest, including the various 'middling ranks'. It was moreover a mixed lay and professional readership, reflecting a widespread concern with prevention on moral and functional grounds. Furthermore, the precepts or 'advice' which the books handed out were in a real sense part of the common language of daily life, dealing as they did with the management of the body and its immediate (and extended) environment. Rapid reading suggests that an actual cult of the body was associated with Puritanism, whereas the earlier mediaeval practices were more functional; but this distinction must rest on further evidence of the therapies themselves, so many of which – balneology, cosmetics, frictions and massage, sports and gymnastics, dietetics, herbalism and pharmacy – have only been partially introduced into medical history.

To what extent did the language of science, and its interpretation by physicians and others, influence the economic and social choices involved in city, town and village planning, house planning, gardens, clothing, food, toiletries, games and pastimes? In order to investigate regimen, medical historians will have to take into consideration all the artefacts connected with the domestic household and local community; or to put it another way, the scattered information on medical activities from diaries, letters, novels, and about such things as soap, sewers and spas, cannot be coherently investigated without an understanding of regimen. The running debate in the 1950s and 1960s about the standard

282   *Ginnie Smith*

of living in early industrial England stalled for want of so-called hard evidence; but even quantitative demographic work will founder in its turn if it cannot be related to qualitative evidence surrounding 'the civilising process'. Medical advice books are not an exclusive source of information on the manners, customs and habits of health behaviour, and as Norbert Elias has convincingly shown, social and aesthetic considerations were designed to display the successful life of comfort and pleasure.[93] Less convincingly, he suggests that manners 'preceded' any medical 'scientific theory', whereas it appears that health accompanied wealth and happiness as the goal or philosophy of self-improvement and 'civility'. Future research will undoubtedly put the etiquette books, domestic manuals and medical advice books side by side.

[93] Norbert Elias, *The Civilising Process: The History of Manners* (Oxford, 1978 edn).

Appendix

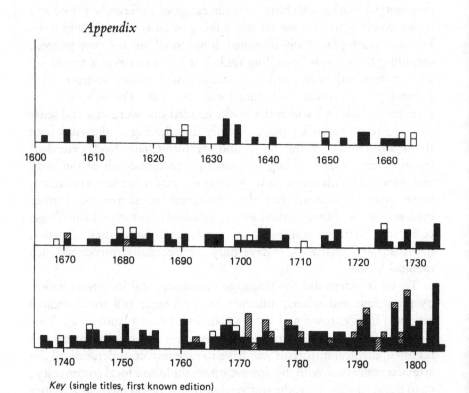

Key (single titles, first known edition)
■ Sinclair   □ R. Reece   ▨ Others

Approximate distribution of all titles 1600–1800 on general health and longevity, including J. Sinclair's totals per year 1600–1804.

10

Laymen, doctors and medical knowledge in the
eighteenth century: The evidence of the
Gentleman's Magazine

ROY PORTER

I

For the nineteenth century the history of English medicine has long
since ceased to be written as though it were simply the annals of heroic
doctors and epoch-making breakthroughs. That old warhorse, the epic
of medical progress, featuring *The Revolution in Victorian Medicine* and
the consequent deliverance (as two recent popular books put it) from
The Age of Agony to *The Age of Miracles*,[1] has for some time now been
comprehensively challenged by a variety of alternative ways of seeing.

For example, complementing Ackerknecht's work, the late Michel
Foucault argued that *The Birth of the Clinic* spelt a revolution in
'medical gaze', with the new normative and technological order of
the hospital entailing fresh diagnostic epistemologies and disease
representations, all generating vast medical power.[2] Paralleling and to

[1] A. J. Youngson, *The Scientific Revolution in Victorian Medicine* (London, 1976);
G. Williams, *The Age of Agony* (London, 1975), and *idem, The Age of Miracles*
(London, 1981) – the former covers the eighteenth, the latter the nineteenth
century.

[2] For surveys of this literature on the social constitution of medicine, see
P. Wright and A. Treacher (eds.), *The Problem of Medical Knowledge*
(Edinburgh, 1982); J. Woodward and D. Richards, 'Towards a social history
of medicine', in *idem* (eds.), *Health Care and Popular Medicine in Nineteenth
Century England* (London, 1977), pp. 15–55; M. Pelling, 'Medicine since
1500', in P. Corsi and P. Weindling (eds.), *Information Sources in the History
of Science and Medicine* (London, 1983), pp. 379–410; Charles Webster, 'The
historiography of medicine', in *ibid.*, pp. 29–43; M. MacDonald, 'Anthropological perspectives on the history of science and medicine', in *ibid.*, pp.
81–98; and L. J. Jordanova, 'The social sciences and history of science and
medicine', in *ibid.*, pp. 81–98. For the order of the clinic see M. Foucault, *The
Birth of the Clinic* (English trans., London, 1973); *idem, Madness and Civilisation*
(English trans., London, 1967); *idem, Discipline and Punish* (English trans.,
London, 1977); E. H. Ackerknecht, *Medicine at the Paris Hospital, 1794–1848*
(Baltimore, 1967).

some degree overlapping with Foucault, many medical sociologists
have trained their spotlight on professionalization as the great dynamo
of medical transformation.[3] Their timely attention to professional
ambitions further reminds us that the Victorian age saw the rise of the
public health movement, and other critical encounters in medicine's
equivocal relations with the state;[4] and this in turn has implications
for what one school of investigators has dubbed the 'medicalization
of life' – a concept often linked with polemical exposés of the
'disabling professions' and 'the expropriation of health', and with a
radical desire to demystify medicine's allegedly hegemonic role as a
secular and naturalizing instrument of 'social control'.[5] Of course, as
'medicalization' proceeded and orthodoxy sandbagged its citadel in
the Victorian age, 'alternative' medical therapies became steadily more
marginalized; and awareness of this polarization has informed recent
explorations of radical and plebeian medicine.[6] All these conceptual
frameworks and patterns of interpretation, which probe the social
construction of medical knowledge and its multifarious functions as
modes of *savoir-pouvoir*, beget their own internal difficulties, of course,
and most remain deeply controversial. The point is, however, that for
the nineteenth century we at least have a rich choice of mappings to
guide our thinking and research.

[3] See for example S. Holloway, 'Medical education in England, 1830–1858: a
sociological analysis', *History*, LXIX (1964), 299–344; M. J. Peterson, *The
Medical Profession in Mid-Victorian London* (Berkeley, 1978); I. Waddington,
'General practitioners and consultants in early nineteenth century England:
the sociology of an intra-professional conflict', in J. Woodward and
D. Richards (eds.), *Health Care* (note 2), pp. 164–88; N. Parry and J. Parry,
The Rise of the Medical Profession: A Study of Collective Social Mobility
(London, 1976).

[4] E.g., D. Fraser, *The Evolution of the British Welfare State* (London, 1973).

[5] P. Goubert (ed.), *La Médicalisation de la Société Française 1770–1830* (Waterloo,
Ontario, 1982); I. Illich, *Limits to Medicine* (London, 1976); idem (ed.),
Disabling Professions (London, 1977); S. Cohen and A. Scull (eds.), *Social
Control and the State* (Oxford, 1983). For a feminist perspective see
V. Kniebiehler and C. Fouquet, *La Femme et les Médecins* (Paris, 1983).

[6] E.g., L. Barrow, 'Anti-establishment healing and spiritualism in England', in
W. Sheils (ed.), *The Church and Healing* (Oxford, 1982), pp. 225–48;
J. Pickstone, 'Establishment and dissent in nineteenth century medicine: an
exploration of some correspondences between religious and medical belief
systems in early industrial England', in *ibid.*, pp. 165–190; R. Cooter,
'Deploying "pseudo-science": then and now', in M. P. Hanen, M. J. Osler
and R. C. Weyant (eds.), *Science, Pseudo-Science and Society* (Waterloo,
Ontario, 1980), pp. 237–72; R. Wallis and P. Morley (eds.), *Marginal Medicine*
(London, 1976).

Not so for the previous age! It is of course noteworthy in itself that far less *research* has been directed at the Georgian period than its successor (or, for that matter, its predecessor), so that the last volume which approximates to being a general survey, Arnold Chaplin's often undervalued *Medicine in England During the Reign of George III*, is now sixty-six years old.[7] And one consequence of this is that many critical developments specific to the century, such as the emergence of London as a towering medical teaching centre, still await proper investigation.[8] But above all, there have been surprisingly few attempts to *characterize* medical activity in Georgian England, to forge an explanatory vocabulary and working models. Being under-interpreted, the Georgian age is often assumed to be either uneventful or dull; indeed, some of the best medical history devoted to the seventeenth or nineteenth centuries paints Georgian medicine in broad caricature strokes, as though it were of interest – though not *great* interest – only as coda or overture. The real watersheds are generally seen as occurring before or after the eighteenth century, with for example the Scientific Revolution, or the emergence of the family doctor in the early nineteenth century, or the coming of medical registration in 1858. In Foucault's *Birth of the Clinic* a decisive rupture is postulated cordoning off the modern 'age of the clinic' from the pre-French Revolutionary past, rendering close characterization of hospital medicine in the earlier period otiose; such a weighting is ironically perpetuated in Gelfand's riposte, for his stress on the pre-1794 'gestation' of the clinic – the evolutionary rather than the revolutionary model – nevertheless keeps the eyes ultimately trained firmly towards the nineteenth century.[9]

In a similar way, eighteenth century developments are often viewed not in their own right but as harbingers of things to come: the 'roots' of sanitary reform, or the 'founders' of 'moral therapy' in psychiatry.

---

[7] A. Chaplin, *Medicine in England During the Reign of George III* (London, 1919). There is a more recent general survey of Western medicine as a whole: L. S. King, *The Medical World of the Eighteenth Century* (Chicago, 1958).

[8] Though see T. Gelfand, 'Invite the philosopher as well as the charitable: hospital teaching as private enterprise in the Hunters' London', and W. F. Bynum, 'Physicians, careers and hospitals in eighteenth century London', both in W. F. Bynum and Roy Porter (eds.), *William Hunter and the Eighteenth Century Medical World* (Cambridge, 1985), 105–28, 129–52.

[9] T. Gelfand, 'Gestation of the clinic', *Medical History*, xxv (1981), 169–80; but see the essay by O. Keel, 'The politics of health and the institutionalization of clinical practices in Europe in the second half of the eighteenth century', in Bynum and Porter, *William Hunter* (note 8), 207–58.

John Hunter, for instance, is regularly cast as the 'father' of scientific surgery.[10] And this clairvoyant history encourages the anachronistic tendency of back-projecting later developments into the Georgian period. Thus it is noteworthy that the rather little sociologically informed analysis of eighteenth century medical change which has been published – for example Waddington's elucidation of infighting between the different professional strata – tends to mobilize concepts, such as 'professionalization' and 'marginality', transferred from *modern* medical sociology and probably inappropriate for earlier stages of medical practice.[11] In general, however, historians of eighteenth century medicine have avoided entanglements with models. For example, Holmes' recent stimulating portrayal of medicine as a boom profession in the Augustan age keeps the empirical nose close to the grindstone, avoiding all engagement with the sociology of the professions.[12]

The striking exception to this picture of the eighteenth century medical world as unfocussed and rather chaotic, still awaiting conceptual mapping, has been the interpretation advanced by Nicholas Jewson. His two brief articles, 'Medical knowledge and the patronage system in eighteenth century England' and, more substantially if slightly less relevantly, 'The disappearance of the sick man from medical cosmology 1770–1870',[13] constitute easily the most challenging attempt until now to provide a thematic reading of the Georgian medical milieu. In socio-cultural terms, Jewson contends, the key to Georgian medicine

[10] See, e.g., J. F. Fulton, 'The Warrington Academy (1757–1786) and its influence upon medicine and science', *Bulletin of the History of Medicine*, I (1933), 50–80; L. S. Jacyna, 'Images of John Hunter in the nineteenth century', *History of Science*, XXI (1983), 85–108; D. Leigh, *The Historical Development of British Psychiatry* (Oxford, 1961).

[11] I. Waddington, 'The struggle to reform the Royal College of Physicians, 1767–1771: a sociological analysis', *Medical History*, XVII (1973), 107–26; I. Inkster, 'Marginal men: aspects of the social role of the medical community in Sheffield, 1790–1850', in Woodward and Richards, *Health Care* (note 2), pp. 128–63; M. Durey, 'Medical elites, the general practitioner and patient power in Britain during the cholera epidemic of 1831–2', in I. Inkster and J. Morrell (eds.), *Metropolis and Province: Science in British Culture 1780–1850* (London, 1983), pp. 257–78.

[12] G. Holmes, *Augustan England: Professions, State, and Society 1680–1730* (London, 1982); compare J. F. Kett, 'Provincial medical practice in England, 1730–1815', *Journal of the History of Medicine*, XIX (1964), 17–29.

[13] N. Jewson, 'Medical knowledge and the patronage system in eighteenth century England', *Sociology*, VIII (1974), 369–85; *idem*, 'The disappearance of the sick man from medical cosmology 1770–1870', *Sociology*, X (1976), 225–44.

lies in the way that physicians moved in the force-field of lay patronage, influenced by the power and tied to the purse strings of rich patients. After the privileged and protected institutional position they held under the Stuarts had been sapped, and before they regained great corporate strength in Victorian times, buttressed by legislation and the policing powers of the state, successful physicians – like other professional men – were perforce the clients of the great.[14] For authority and status, reward and advancement, doctors looked not to collective professional paths to glory, but to the personal favour of grandees. Moreover, in this *ancien régime* fabric of deference and dependence, he who paid the piper called the knowledge tune. In matters of clinical knowledge and judgement relating to diagnosis, prognosis, regimen and therapy, practitioners learnt to kowtow, argues Jewson, to the expectations of polite society. Such intellectual deference, even ingratiation, was the less resistible because in those days before laboratory medicine, medical knowledge was necessarily a currency common to both doctors and patients rather than being the practitioner's esoteric monopoly, a '*savoir*' guaranteeing 'professional dominance'. Before 'scientific medicine', before diagnostic technology, cell science, pathology and the germ theory of disease, sickness, argues Jewson, inhered in the experience of the whole person – body and mind – and it was largely for the patient to specify his 'complaint', for the physician had, as yet, no privileged access to it. Maladies were still thought of as essentially constitutional and individual, explicated in terms of the scientifically moribund but stubbornly resilient holistic humoral tradition.[15] Hence the clinical encounter might be largely stage-managed by the patient; it certainly required negotiation and consensus between physician and the sick person. Medical knowledge

---

[14] For the Stuart situation, I am much indebted to the forthcoming book of H. J. Cook, *Politics, the New Philosophy, and the Failure of the Old Regime in Stuart London*. For Georgian clientage, see J. Brewer, 'Commercialization and politics', in N. McKendrick, J. Brewer and J. H. Plumb, *The Birth of a Consumer Society* (London, 1982), pp. 197–264; E. P. Thompson, 'Patrician society, plebeian culture', *Journal of Social History*, VIII (1974), 382–405; Roy Porter, *English Society in the Eighteenth Century* (Harmondsworth, 1982), ch. 2; H. Perkin, *The Origins of Modern English Society* (London, 1969).

[15] See C. M. Mullett, 'The lay outlook on medicine in England, *circa* 1800–1850', *Bulletin of the History of Medicine*, XXV (1951), 168–84; C. Rosenberg, 'The therapeutic revolution', in C. Rosenberg and M. Vogel (eds.), *The Therapeutic Revolution* (Philadelphia, 1979), pp. 3–26. The essays in this present volume by Jonathan Barry and Ginnie Smith offer major elucidations of the medical world of the eighteenth century laity.

was not yet a terrifying, esoteric specialism, the monopoly of medics, but rather part of a common, open, intellectual culture, to be weighed in the balance before the tribunal of the educated and opinion-makers in society at large.

Jewson's schema has the great merit of escaping the contagions of anachronism and teleology. This he achieves largely because his *aperçus* about the social relations of medicine are taken not from today's medical sociology, but from a well-authenticated model of a different theatre of eighteenth century inter-personal relations: Sir Lewis Namier's analysis of the structure of high politics in the age of George III.[16] For Namier, Hanoverian politics had to be viewed not through the anachronistic and moralistic lenses of the Victorian two-party system, but in terms of personal exercise of political power through patronage and oligarchic connection, dominated by the interests of grandee clans. For Jewson, the Georgian medical world is similarly to be decoded not in terms of later science and pro-fessionalism, but through individual power networks.

Jewson does not disguise the fact that he finds the Georgian medical order outlandish, a clog to the advance of medicine's healing powers: part of his aim is indeed to explain why eighteenth century medicine allegedly remained so stagnant. Nevertheless, his vision is stimulating and packs the promise of explanatory power. For it is a coherent and plausible 'anthropological' reconstruction of an alien medical milieu, its social relations and belief systems, one distinctive from our own in being lay- rather than expert-oriented, and giving the patient a major role in negotiating his own health and medical treatment.

It is odd, then, that Jewson's work seems to have stimulated almost no serious scholarly response. It has not been challenged, but neither has it proved the spur to subsequent research. Nor has Jewson himself followed it up in print, which is a pity because 'Medical knowledge and the patronage system' was presented essentially as an abstract and schematic model with minimal empirical detail. It is not clear for instance how far Jewson sees his account as an accurate and complete map of the Georgian medical order, or essentially as a schematic ideal type. At the very least, Jewson's articles beg questions and leave many loose ends.[17]

[16] L. Namier, *The Structure of Politics at the Accession of George III* (rev. edn., London, 1957). For more general views of the centrality of patronage see D. Jarrett, *The Ingenious Mr Hogarth* (London, 1976); M. Foss, *The Age of Patronage* (London, 1972).

[17] It is not my intention in this paper to undertake a thorough appraisal and critique of Jewson's thesis, though many aspects of his papers invite critical

II

Yet it would be a shame if Jewson's model were abandoned by default, merely for lack of attempts to test and develop it against those everyday realities of Georgian medical relations which Joan Lane explores in her paper in this volume. Admittedly, the historian of Enlightenment medicine does not have at his fingertips that almost embarrassing superabundance of data which deluges his colleague interested in the nineteenth century: the runs of *The Lancet* and the *British Medical Journal*, defining best medical opinion, the cascading pamphlet literature of public campaigns and reform, legislation flooding onto the statute book, and the oceanic proceedings of the professional bodies. These absences may in themselves be suggestive of the ambience of the more informal, less institutionalized eighteenth century medical world. But ample materials do in fact survive, many of them hardly tapped, which will enable us to address those problems of patient/doctor relations, centring on the location and authorization of medical knowledge, raised by Jewson. Not least, alongside the personal and scholarly writings of practitioners, there is no lack of medical diaries, letters and auto-diagnoses penned by sufferers themselves, a literature drawn on by other essays in this volume (in particular, Joan Lane's) and touching directly on Jewson's concerns.[18]

A further valuable source of evidence lies in the appearance during the eighteenth century of medical information, comment and controversy in the press.[19] Only a few studies of the medical content of

discussion. For example, Jewson writes as though his model applies to medical practice as a whole, whereas in fact the 'deference' model probably holds good only for the upper reaches of society. Quite distinct socio-professional relations may apply to patients and practitioners lower down the social scale.

[18] For a general approach see Roy Porter, 'The patient's view: doing medical history from below', *Theory and Society*, XIV (1985), 175–98. See also, for a particular biographical example, B. S. Abeshouse, *A Medical History of Dr Samuel Johnson* (Norwich, N.Y., 1965); [anon.], 'Dr Johnson as a "dabbler in physick"', *Guy's Hospital Gazette*, LXXVI (1962), 321–4; R. W. Sagebiel, 'Medicine in the life and letters of Samuel Johnson', *Ohio State Medical Journal*, LIII (1961), 382–4; Sir H. Rolleston, 'Samuel Johnson's medical experiences', *Annals of Medical History*, n.s., I (1929), 540–52.

[19] G. A. Cranfield, *The Development of the Provincial Newspaper 1700–1760* (Oxford, 1962); R. McK. Wiles, *Freshest Advices* (Columbus, Ohio, 1965); James T. Hillhouse, '*The Grub-Street Journal*': *With Special Reference to its Connection with Alexander Pope, 1730–1737* (Durham, N.C., 1928); G. F. Barwick, 'Some magazines of the eighteenth century', *Transactions of the Bibliographical Society*, X (1908–9), 109–40; R. S. Crane and F. B. Kaye, *A Census of British Newspapers and Periodicals 1622–1800* (Chapel Hill, N.C., 1927); R. T. Milford and D. M. Sutherland, 'A catalogue of English

newspapers have as yet been undertaken, though P. S. Brown has revealed what a vast quantity of advertisements for patent and proprietary medicines were inserted in the Bath newspapers.[20] Half a century ago Fielding Garrison reflected elegantly on medicine as printed in *The Tatler* and *The Spectator*, showing how frequently medical matters popped up in the tea-table fripperies of Addison and Steele.[21] But in general those mausoleums of elite opinion and channels for information exchange have been oddly neglected by medical historians. We do not even have a detailed analysis of the rise of that creature with many heads, the medical periodical – works like the *London Medical Journal* (1781–90) and the *Memoirs of the Medical Society of London* (1787–1805)[22] – still less accounts of the medical content carried by the general periodicals of the time.[23] The main body of this essay, therefore, seeks to fill in one of these lacunae by examining the medical coverage of the leading informative periodical produced for the educated audience, the *Gentleman's Magazine*, in the hope of evaluating Jewson's model, and illuminating how the printed word reflected and shaped patient/doctor relations.[24]

Founded by Edward Cave in 1731, the *Gentleman's Magazine* quickly secured a niche for itself in the jungle of periodical publishing. Appearing monthly, it began essentially as a digest of the political and religious weeklies, but steadily developed a character of its own

newspapers and periodicals in the Bodelian Library, 1622–1800', *Oxford Bibliographical Society Proceedings and Papers*, IV (1934–5), 167–346.

[20] P. S. Brown, 'Medicines advertised in eighteenth century Bath newspapers', *Medical History*, XX (1976), 152–68.

[21] Fielding H. Harrison, 'Medicine in *The Tatler*, *Spectator* and *Guardian*', *Bulletin of the History of Medicine*, II (1934), 477–503.

[22] Fielding H. Garrison, *The Medical and Scientific Periodicals of the 17th and 18th Centuries: With a Revised Catalogue and Check-List* (Baltimore, 1934); W. R. Le Fanu, *British Periodicals of Medicine* (Baltimore, 1938); D. Kronick, *A History of Scientific and Technical Periodicals* (New York, 1962); A. J. Meadows, *Development of Science Publishing in Europe* (Amsterdam, 1980).

[23] Though see Robert Donald Spector, *English Literary Periodicals and the Climate of Opinion during the Seven Years' War* (The Hague, 1966).

[24] C. L. Carlson, *The First Magazine: A History of the 'Gentleman's Magazine'* (Providence, R.I., 1937); A. Pailler, *Edward Cave et le 'Gentleman's Magazine' (1731–54)* (2 vols., Lille, 1975); Edmund Blunden, 'The "Gentleman's Magazine", 1731–1907', in *Votive Tablets: Studies Chiefly Appreciative of English Authors and Books* (London, 1931), pp. 118–31; W. Roberts, 'The Gentleman's Magazine and its rivals', *Athenaeum*, no. 3235 (26 Oct. 1889), 560; idem, 'The history of the Gentleman's Magazine', *Bookworm*, III (1890), 97–101, 129–36, 281–7 and 353–8; and now, more generally, A. Sullivan (ed.), *British Literary Magazines*, vol. 1 (Westport, Conn., 1984).

through whetting and satisfying the public appetite for original informative articles, book reviews, notices of new publications, comment and criticism, and not least by offering a forum for readers' own communications. Unlike the many *Tatler* and *Spectator* lookalikes, the *Gentleman's Magazine* was earnest in tone and factual in content; unlike political magazines, such as *Fogg's* or *The Craftsman*, it aimed to be neutral, comprehensive and judicious, avoiding scurrility and cultivating consensus. The *Gentleman's Magazine* hit on a successful formula. It appealed to the educated man's desire for practical and useful knowledge – in it he could find digests of events, foreign news, Parliamentary reports, records of bankrupts, grain prices, features on improvements in agriculture, machinery and techniques, etc. Yet at the same time it catered for his polite and cultural tastes, his pastimes and avocations, carrying features on books, architecture, the visual arts, literary criticism, popular science, biography, topography, history and antiquities. Conveying information and shaping opinion, the magazine evidently got the mix about right. It was easily the most successful, and the most enduring, periodical of the age, running from 1731 right through to 1907. It commanded a regular sale of several thousand copies, rising at times to over 10,000.[25]

One of the topics prominently featured is medicine. The density of coverage is heavy: not many issues went by without a medical book being reviewed, some medical correspondence appearing, or remedies being touted. The coverage was also regular, month in, month out, for each issue featured health-related items such as the Bills of Mortality, meteorological reports (which routinely discussed epidemics and seasonal afflictions), and an extensive obituary column. Moreover, the medical items spread over a wide range of interests, including hospital reports, biographies of great physicians, requests for practical advice and treatments, case histories, the activities of bodies such as the Medical Society of London,[26] medical poetry (some satirical, some

---

[25] For the reading taste of the educated reader see I. Watt, *The Rise of the Novel* (London, 1957); A. Cruse, *The Englishman and his Books in the Early XIXth Century* (London, 1930); I. Rivers (ed.), *Books and their Readers in Eighteenth Century England* (Leicester, 1982), especially the contribution by G. S. Rousseau, 'Science books and their readers in the eighteenth century', pp. 197–256; A. S. Collins, 'Growth of the reading public during the eighteenth century', *Review of English Studies*, II (1926), 284–94 and 428–38; *idem*, *Authorship in the Days of Johnson: Being a Study of the Relation between Author, Patron Publisher and Public, 1726–1780* (2 vols., London, 1927).

[26] T. Hunt (ed.), *The Medical Society of London 1773–1973* (London, 1972).

uplifting), bulletins on the health of the royal family and other notable personages, and not least great attention to livestock diseases and similar veterinary matters. There are also lists of new medical publications and medical advertisements.[27] Cave and his successors were astute entrepreneurs, with their fingers securely on the pulse of public taste, and we may assume that this weighty attention to medical matters reflected, or created, real consumer demand.

How, then, do these medical articles bear on Jewson's analysis? What do they tell us about the play and sway of power between the public and the physician, or about the generation, ownership, spread and exchange of medical knowledge?

One valuable clue comes from the contributors themselves. Unfortunately, we cannot identify who wrote the bulk of the *Gentleman's Magazine* medical insertions. Many pieces are not only unsigned, but also give no internal clue as to authorship; others are signed only with real or fictitious initials (e.g., 'A.B.' occurs frequently). For such anonymous and initialled items as these, the surviving *Gentleman's Magazine* business files do not often reveal the author's name, and hence his occupation or social standing.[28] Yet the weight of evidence from signed articles, and from those where internal evidence gives clues as to authorship, makes it clear that both laymen and practitioners routinely wrote contributions about health and medicine for the journal. For example, certain medically trained contributors did sign their name, as did, for instance, Joan Coakley Lettsom; some paraded their qualifications (e.g. 'A.B., M.D.'); others, who chose anonymity,

---

[27] James Playstead Wood, *The Story of Advertising* (New York, 1958); J. B. Williams, 'The early history of London advertising', *Nineteenth Century and After*, LXII (1907), 793–800; M. Nevett, *Advertising in Britain: A History* (London, 1982), p. 13; F. Prestbury, *The History and Development of Advertising* (New York, 1929); H. Sampson, *A History of Advertising* (London, 1974). Eighteenth century newspapers are full of quack medical advertisements. By the nineteenth century it could even be a sales gimmick *not* to run them. Cf. this note in the *Tyne Mercury*, 19 May 1812:

> To render the Newspaper still more acceptable to the public, the Editor has determined to dismiss from his columns one considerable source of emolument – he means the disgusting and sickening Advertisements of the poisonous trash known by the name of Quack Medicines...the Editor firmly believing that where one person is cured, the health of thousands is destroyed; and independently of this awful consideration, surely nothing but long custom can have induced those who have the care of young persons to suffer them daily to read the indecent and filthy details with which Advertisements of these Medicines are filled.

(I owe this quotation to Maurice Milne.) For examples of ads in the *Gentleman's Magazine* see IV (1734), 197–8, 224.

[28] J. M. Kuist, *The Nichols File of the 'Gentleman's Magazine'* (Wisconsin, 1982).

discussed medical case-histories in the first person, as only a practitioner would. Still others protected themselves behind an evidently professional pseudonym: 'Physicus', 'Medicus', 'Chirurgus', etc., are all common. *Mutatis mutandis*, the equivalent applies to the laity. Many contributors give their names, or state or hint at their rank or occupation (clergyman, gentleman farmer, traveller, J.P., etc.). Others stay anonymous or pseudonymous ('Poplicola', 'Populus', 'Philalethes', 'Constant Reader', all crop up repeatedly), but in ways that sometimes permit us at least to decipher their social station. Moreover, we know independently that certain contributions were penned by professional writers and journalists (for example, Samuel Johnson's lengthy biographies of Boerhaave, Sydenham, and others, all unsigned).[29]

These hints as to authorship are significant in themselves. Obviously, the mere fact that laymen were writing medical pieces while practitioners were also contributing to a wide-circulation general magazine is in itself an indication that there was some semblance of common medical culture in terms of both production and consumption, supply and demand. This can be confirmed by performing a 'blind experiment' on the anonymous entries. In most cases, I suggest, it is impossible to judge whether they have been written by members of the faculty or by lay authors. This is largely because contributions by lay and medical men alike are typically pitched at comparable levels of assumed medical expertise. And that level is remarkably and impressively well-informed, often involving command and parade of technicalities and a relaxed familiarity with the leading medical authorities. Let me give two instances. In 1751 'R.C.' submitted

An ODE. Written after a Recovery from a Dangerous Dropsy: Inscribed, To the Right Hon. the Lady Anne, Countess Dowager of Coventry.

Beginning

> For health restor'd and lengthen'd days,
>   What thanks to God belong!
> Hear, gracious Lord, my grateful lays,
>   Tho' low, accept the song.

it went on to versify the medical indications of the dropsy from which he had suffered, and explained

[29] L. C. McHenry, Jr, 'Dr Samuel Johnson's medical biographies', *Journal of the History of Medicine and Allied Sciences*, xiv (1959), 298–310; E. R. Atkinson, 'Samuel Johnson's life of Boerhaave', *Journal of Chemical Education*, xix (1942), 103–8.

> To tell the cause *Boerhaave, 'twas thine
>   Whilst I, who try'd the woe,
> Speak what I felt; alas! 'tis mine,
>   The Dire effect to show;

Significantly at this point, the reader is referred to a footnote:

*See Dr Boerhaave's definition of an Anasarca.[30]

Or take a sequence of correspondence from 1749. A letter was printed from 'R.T.' listing the symptoms of distempered cattle. The next issue ran a response asking if

the gentleman who writes from Settle in your Mag. for *April* last, P.150, would acquaint the publick, whether he found the bloody-tinged water, he there speaks of, between the dura and pia mater, or between the pia mater and the brain, seeing they closely adhere.

The gentleman obligingly replied:

The bloody-tinged water there spoke of was found both between the dura and pia mater and also between the pia mater and the brain; and that the Querist may *conceive* rightly *what is meant by vacuities between the pia mater and the brain* and be certain *that they so closely adhere as not to be separated but by suppuration, as he asserts, I must in my turn beg that gentleman will recollect and consult some anatomists,* especially those who have treated more particularly upon the brain and its diseases, such as a WINSLOW, FR. HOFFMAN, WEPFFER, WILLIS, OR VIEUSSENS.

In the next issue, these questions were revolved still further.[31] This dialogue on bovine brains may disconcertingly remind us of Swift's satires upon learned nonsense, but there is no sign that the readership found anatomical discussion at this pitch of technicality or theorizing inappropriate; certainly exchanges of this kind continued throughout the century.

Characteristically, when in 1751 a reader proposed a regular corner for medical correspondence, he foresaw no difficulties arising between the interested amateur, the expert professional, and the free circulation of intellectual property. Readers wanted to know; and it was assumed that polite members of the faculty would be eager to impart their knowledge. The conditions he proposed were liberal: contributors could remain anonymous or pseudonymous if they wished, and could write in English, Latin, French or Italian. That the information might

---

[30] *Gentleman's Magazine*, xx (1751), 326. For the background tradition of learned verse see W. P. Jones, *The Rhetoric of Science* (London, 1966); R. A. Aubin, *Topographical Poetry in Eighteenth Century England* (New York, 1936).

[31] *Gentleman's Magazine*, xix (1749), 150, 249, 457.

be technical posed no problem. 'Nice anatomical disquisitions...[and] chemical experiments on the materia medica' were acceptable, even in their 'most minute circumstances', when such particulars were unavoidable 'in the curing of any disease'. The only restriction was that the information should be strictly factual, empirical and experimental – hypothesis, theory and speculation were ceremonially banned.[32]

This impression of the free flow of sometimes rather high-level medical information is easily confirmed by examining a sample of some of the hundreds of medical books reviewed and extracted in the pages of the magazine. Volumes expounding anatomy and physiology in considerable technical detail were expansively quoted or abstracted if they were thought to be on topics of wide public interest. For instance, the review of Percivall Pott's *Account of the Fistula in Ano* extended over two columns, the writer urging sufferers to read 'this most excellent treatise' because it would assuage unnecessary fears about surgery for the condition.[33] Extensive medical reviewing of this kind almost certainly amounted to more than mere indiscriminate copying or desperate space-filling. And there was a sense of where to draw the line. Indeed, a reviewer would occasionally state that a piece would not be abstracted, specifically because it *was* too technical. For example, the reviewer of James Bent's 'Account of a Woman Enjoying the Use of her Right Arm, after the Head of the *Os Humeri* was Cut Away', deemed that 'as this article cannot be abridged, and would be intelligible only to anatomists, such we must refer to the original'.[34] At no stage was any complaint printed from a reader protesting against the unreasonable plateau of expertise presupposed; rather correspondents uniformly praised the medical contributions to the magazine.[35]

Active and mutual lay/practitioner involvement in issues of health, pitched at a well-informed level, makes itself manifest in the magazine in other ways too. For example, contributors would occasionally explicitly address themselves to both the lay reader and the medical man. The reviewer of J. B. Regnault's *Observations on Pulmonary Consumption* judged of the book that

professional men will find in it a sure guide which has not yet met with any objection, and patients afflicted with a disorder from which spring the most

[32] *Ibid.*, xxi (1751), 308.
[33] *Ibid.*, xxxv (1765), 484, 514.   [34] *Ibid.*, xlv (1775), 29.
[35] See the discussion in Roy Porter, 'Lay medical knowledge in the eighteenth century: the case of the *Gentleman's Magazine*', *Medical History*, xxix (1985), 138–68.

excruciating pains, both of mind and body, a mode of treatment indicated
by nature, improved by art, and confirmed by experience.[36]

And the implication here given that practitioners themselves would
be reading the *Gentleman's Magazine* to keep themselves in the picture
is confirmed elsewhere. Thus the review of a treatise on blindness states
that it deserves to be read by all the faculty.[37] And there are other
pointers to some joint lay/medical involvement in promoting and
disseminating medical knowledge. In the thick of a voluminous
correspondence on medical electricity in 1751, Dr Anthony Floyer –
an assiduous contributor – wrote in with details of a cure wrought
on a boy in Dorchester. To support his claims he appended the
signatures of six witnesses. One was the boy's father; two were
'gentlemen'; and the remaining three formed a microcosm of the
medical hierarchy – Thomas Meech, M.D., Hubert Floyer, surgeon,
and John Sawbridge, apothecary.[38]

Thus medical knowledge enveloped both lay and professional in the
Gentleman's Magazine. Unlike some of the works surveyed by Ginnie
Smith in this volume, it was not a journal aimed at the popularization
of knowledge, didactically simplifying the tablets of medical law.
Neither was it a journal in which doctors taught the people their
medical duties. Rather, free and open exchange of information within
the circle of contributors and readers was the rule.[39]

Within this general framework of reciprocity, however, what were
the precise trade-routes in the economy of knowledge? Many offerings
arose through a build-up of queries and responses over the course of
several issues. As one might expect, in these exchanges it was generally
members of the public who were seeking the information, and medical
correspondents who provided it, or at least medical authority which
was quoted, as in this instance:[40]

[36] *Gentleman's Magazine*, LXXIII (1803), 950–1.
[37] *ibid.*, LXII (1792), 1024.   [38] *Ibid.*, XX (1751), 578.
[39] For the presentation of popularized medical knowledge by medical men to
the public see, for example, C. Lawrence, 'William Buchan: medicine laid
open', *Medical History*, XIX (1975), 20–35; L. J. Jordanova, 'Policing public
health in France 1780–1815', in T. Ogawa (ed.), *Public Health* (Tokyo, 1981),
pp. 12–30; W. Coleman, 'Health and hygiene: a medical doctrine for the
bourgeoisie', *Journal of the History of Medicine*, XXIV (1974), 399–421.
[40] *Gentleman's Magazine*, VII (1738), 184. The question-and-answer format of
publishing was pioneered by John Dunton. See Gilbert D. McEwen, *The
Oracle of the Coffee-House: John Dunton's 'Athenian Mercury'* (The Huntington
Library, 1972).

Mr URBAN,

Please to propose to your learned Correspondents the following material Question, and you'll oblige

Yours, &c.

H.C.

Query, Whether Air enters the Blood, or not; and if it does; How? Sheffield, March 15, 1737.

The reply is worth quoting at length, since it gives a good flavour of how medical knowledge was presented in the magazine, not *ex cathedra*, but openly and experimentally, so readers could see and do for themselves:[41]

Mr URBAN,

In answer to Mr C's Question in your Mag. for April, viz. Whether Air enters the blood; and if it does, How? I am persuaded, he'll think it a Proof that Air enters the Blood, by making the Experiment of a Rat in an Air-Pump. As soon as the Air is drawn off, the Animal dies. But how could this be, if Air does not mix with the Blood: since the Animal might then live without the Assistance of Air? Respiration itself would be unnecessary, except he can prove, that it's needful for some other Purpose, than that of giving the Air Entrance into the Blood, for the Sake of rarifying it, and fitting it for the Circulation thro' the minutest Foramina of Nature. 'Whosoever (says that ingenious Physician and excellent Author, Dr *Robinson) will take nine or ten Ounces of warm human Blood, and place it in a Receiver, as soon as the Air is a little removed by the working of the Air-Pump, you will perceive it to bubble and boil like a Pot, which evidently demonstrates the great Quantity of Air contained in the red Globules of the Blood.' – How it enters the Blood? I shall take Leave, till I see his Objections, to answer this very briefly, by instancing the following Experiment: Syringe warm Water into the Arteria Venosa, and the Wind-pipe will throw out a gross Froth. Since therefore Water can find a Passage, doubtless Air, the Parts of which are infinitely subtiler, immediately mixes with the Blood [etc]

*Theory of Physick, p. 45

The reply continued to expound the experiment in great detail. One wonders whether the author expected readers to rush off and actually perform such experiments. Did they indeed do so?

Yet not all the questions came from laymen, nor all the information from doctors. In 1752, G. Watts, a 'Country Practitioner' from Kent, addressed the editor, applauding the magazine's resolve to 'establish

41 *Gentleman's Magazine*, VIII (1738), 306–7.

a medical correspondence', and under that rubric, seeking advice on how to deliver twins, for

> to speak the truth [we country practitioners] are so ignorant in affairs relating to the obstetrical art that we sometimes, in case of twins, leave one in the uterus, to make its exit into this or that world as it pleases.[42]

Neither, for their part, did laymen feel confined to the role of being advice seekers; they were perfectly confident about giving it as well. By way of qualifications, some flourished their own intellectual credentials, like the 'doctor of divinity' who offered a cancer remedy;[43] others sent in local folk cures;[44] yet others proffered recipes on behalf of coteries of gentlemen (were they meeting in *ad hoc* gentlemen's societies?).[45] And personal experience of suffering backed by the general responsibilities of philanthropy were always authority enough for writing. In 1800, for instance, a 'New Correspondent' submitted some tips on asthma.[46] Though 'no member of the faculty', he was 'anxious to contribute my mite to the relief of my fellow-sufferers', being 'one of the brotherhood' of asthmatics himself. It was indeed standard for readers to profess they were moved by the dictates of humanity. William Chisholme of Chisholme, Roxburgh-shire, explained in a letter that he had long had a 'wen of the steutomatous kind' disfiguring the side of his face. Salt-water bathing had been recommended to him and it had worked: 'I felt it a duty thus to make it public.'[47]

In these market-place exchanges of information, the relations between lay and medical contributors seem generally to have been polite or even cordial. Little resentment against practitioners is voiced, just as, conversely, doctors do not command laymen to stick to their last and keep their noses clear of medical mystery. Just occasionally, however, a jangling note of frustration intrudes. Moved in 1798 to write by a review of Dr Bree's tract on disordered respiration, 'E' submitted his own personal experiences. Suffering from 'pain about the praecordia' and shortness of breath, he had applied to physicians in person and in writing; some had fobbed him off with fancy diagnoses, using pretentious jargon like 'effluvia' and 'nerve'; one had prescribed hemlock; others had deemed his ailment without remedy. Eventually, by trial and error, he had found out for himself that the

[42] *Ibid.*, xii (1752), 172.   [43] *Ibid.*, xviii (1748), 119.
[44] *Ibid.*, lxxiii (1803), 724.   [45] *Ibid.*, lvi (1786), 948.
[46] *Ibid.*, lxix (1800), 639.   [47] *Ibid.*, lxix (1800), 5–6.

only relief lay in keeping very tranquil. Fellow-sufferers might benefit.[48]

Sometimes, however, lay correspondents are not annoyed but rather defensive, in particular when folk remedies are being exposed to the medical glare:[49]

Mr. URBAN   May 28

THE gentlemen of the Faculty would, perhaps, laugh if they were to know who is about to give medical advice, or would bid me stick to my last. Let them laugh, or let them say what they please, so that they will condescend to try my remedy; let them take some poor patient to begin with; they may be very charitable at a cheap rate; and, if they find it succeed there, they may go on to one who will pay liberally for a cure, without caring how simple the means. I can assure those gentlemen, and their patients, that, if it does not cure, it will not kill. That is more, Mr Urban, than be said of all medicines. Providence, ever kind, has put my specifick within the reach of everyone. Under every edge are to be found Clivers (I believe some call it Goose-grass). A large wine-glass full of the juice, obtained by pounding the leaves and stalks in a marble mortar, and taken every morning, will produce a wonderful effect; but perseverance is necessary. Covent-garden will supply any quantity before it will furnish green pease, and at a much cheaper rate. Now is the time.

So much for assertion; now for proof [etc.]

[signed] A.Y.

And once or twice, there is an explosion of anger against the doctors. The year 1749 was a time of deep consternation about cattle disease.

---

[48] *Ibid.*, xxxviii (1798), 296. 'J.W.' wrote in with a parallel instance of bypassing regular treatment in favour of auto-therapy:

Mr URBAN   Kidderm. Mar. 21

A Gentleman of this town of good credit, affirmed last Thursday night in the hearing of many, that, when an electrifying machine was here, 5 or 6 weeks ago, he had a tormenting pain which he apprehends to have been rheumatic, in the smallest joints of the fore finger of his right hand, and had determined next morning to take a surgeon's advice; but going in the evening to see the wonders of electricity, had the curiosity to try its effect upon the pained finger, and for that end, desired a gentlewoman, standing on the cake, to touch with her finger both the joints affected, which she did several times, and he felt its pungency. In consequence of this, he observed the pain to be somewhat abated before he went to bed; that on the morrow it grew much easier; and on the third day his finger was perfectly well, and he continues – Who knows what further experiments and discoveries such an incident may lead to?

I am, Sir, &c.
J.W.

Gentleman's Magazine, xvii (1747), 238. Jonathan Barry has suggested that J.W. may be none other than John Wesley.

[49] *Ibid.*, lxix (1800), 532–3.

Dr Lobb had written on the distemper.[50] Isaac Hallam, of Boston, Lincs., responded with

A TREATISE on the present Diseases among the Horned Cattle, in a Letter to Wm Banks, Esq. of Revesby, in the County of Lincoln; with Remarks on those Accounts which were published by Dr Lobb and Dr Mortimer

in which he flung Horace against the doctor: '*Dicere verum qui vetat?*' Parading his contempt, Hallam alleged that Lobb had no practical experience of cattle, and could indulge only in idle theory and speculation:

The Dr indeed! harangues like an academic school-physician; but as I presume, neither himself nor any other ever experienced the method he describes, so his refined speculative argument, without the sanction of experience to confirm it, is but a vox & praeterea nihil; for tho' he abounds with theory, yet, what can avail his trifling medicines in such an acute, inflammatory fever, when six times the quantity, or more, for a dose, is frequently given in any common disorder? and even Dr Mortimer prescribes eight times as much brimstone, twice or thrice a day, to as little purpose.

I imagine, Sir, that the Dr never attended any one distemper'd beast, consequently never inspected the blood, from whence the diagnostic of a disease is usually taken.[51]

Hallam thus nailed his colours to the mast of experience. Yet he was no anti-intellectual rustic, for he himself went on to recommend treatments taken from Ramazzini, whose ideas had been discussed in the *Gentleman's Magazine* in 1744. But these instances of discord are very much the exception; the medical register of the *Gentleman's Magazine* was generally one of mutual courtesy between laymen and the faculty.

In fact, practitioners got a singularly favourable press. In contrast to the constant barrage of 'dose for the doctor' cynicism and squibs issuing from the literary magazines and from satirists and artists such as Ned Ward, Tobias Smollett and William Hogarth,[52] the sheets of the *Gentleman's Magazine* read almost as panegyric. Samuel Johnson's lengthy biographical memoirs of Boerhaave and Sydenham were for

---

[50] For Dr Theophilus Lobb see *Dictionary of National Biography*.

[51] *Gentleman's Magazine*, xix (1749), 490.

[52] For contemporary critiques of the quackery and imposture of the professions, see C. Probyn, 'Swift and the physicians', *Medical History*, xviii (1974), 249–61; S. La Casce, 'Swift on medical extremism', *Journal of the History of Ideas*, xxxi (1970), 599–606; G. Hatfield, 'Quacks, pettifoggers and parsons: Fielding's case against the learned professions', *Texas Studies in Literature and Language*, ix (1967), 69–83.

example highly sympathetic, in keeping with Johnson's personal reverence for the faculty.[53] And contemporary medical figures of some notoriety who might readily have made sitting targets, even received a few compliments. George Cheyne, for example, butt of mirth in some quarters for his own gourmandizing grossness while evangelizing for a vegetable, seed and milk health-diet, got a celebratory ode:[54]

To Dr CHEYNE of Bath
On Reading of his Works.

> Not all the Gemmy Treasures of the East,
> Nor yet the Spicy Odours of the West;
> Not all the glorious Trophies of the Great;
> Would please so much, or form one Joy compleat,
> Like that I feel, great wondr'ous Genius, when
> I scan th'amazing Beauties of thy Pen;
> Like those true Pleasures eve'ry Sense still meets
> When lost I wander in excess of Sweets.
> 'Tis Magick, Powerful Magick, reigns in this,
> And proves what Sydenham was, bright Cheyne is:
> Great as thy Mind, Immortal Praise, 'tis true,
> And all, save Adoration, is thy Due.
> By thee, how many Thousands live today,
> That else had slumber'd in their Mother Clay! [etc.]

Even the self-styled 'ophthalmiator', 'Chevalier' Taylor – the most preposterously vain of the age's practitioners – won a few kind words:

To Doctor TAYLOR

> REpairer bright of IMpair'd sight
> Best oculist in being...[55]

Occasionally, also, poems were printed dedicated to physicians as *ex voto* offerings, in gratitude for personal cures, as for example these

LINES addressed to DR FRASER, at Bath, by W. HAYWARD WINSTONE, ESQ. on his Recovery from a dangerous illness.

> NEXT to the Almighty's gracious will,
>   Which guides each sick-bed hour,

---

[53] See E. A. Bloom, *Samuel Johnson in Grub Street* (Providence, R.I., 1957); P. Rogers, *Grub Street* (London, 1972).

[54] *Gentleman's Magazine*, III (1733), 205; G. S. Rousseau, 'Medicine and millenarianism: immortal Dr Cheyne', in R. Popkin (ed.), *Millenarianism and Messianism in the Enlightenment* (Berkeley, forthcoming).

[55] *Gentleman's Magazine*, XII (1742), 437.

I owe my life to human skill,
   And Fraser's matchless power.

The Fever seiz'd my shatter'd frame,
   Each limb refus'd my will;
But Fraser came, saw, overcame,
   Each complicated ill.

Oh may Hygeia e'er attend
   Around they genial bed
And all the blessings fate can send,
   On all thy household shed!

That thus, defended from distress
   Of body, as of mind,
You still may tear, while still you bless,
   And renovate Mankind![56]

It is of course possible also to find acid words against the doctors. Occasional strictures were levied against squalid intra-professional rivalry;[57] the pretensions of apothecaries to politeness and erudition were predictably mocked;[58] and the ancient satirical topos of the brotherhood between death and the doctors was given another airing.[59] But the pages of the magazine are entirely free from blanket criticism or abuse of the medical profession, seen as a ramp or monopoly, and no calls were made for its root-and-branch reform.[60] In fact practitioners were hardly viewed as a corporate whole, an organized profession, at all.

Two instances will bring out this point out clearly. It is, first, particularly apparent in the many contributions dealing with quackery. Certainly *Gentleman's Magazine* authors were universally against 'quackery', as they doubtless were against sin.[61] But there was no automatic hostility to the individual practitioners we nowadays so readily identify as the top quack doctors of the times, such as Joanna Stephens, Sally Mapp, Joshua Ward or the Chevalier Taylor. Sally

---

[56] *Ibid.*, LXIX (1800), 373.
[57] *Ibid.*, XXXVII (1767), 517.   [58] *Ibid.*, LXX (1800), 70–1.
[59] *Ibid.*, v (1735), 211.
[60] For some illuminating remarks on the weaknesses of the professional groups in the development of English class society see H. J. Perkin, *The Origins of Modern English Society* (London, 1969), ch. 7.
[61] Obviously the term 'quack' is loaded. For some accounts of 'quacks', see Williams, *Age of Agony* (note 1) ch. 11; E. Jameson, *The Natural History of Quackery* (London, 1961), G. de Francesco, *The Power of the Charlatan* (New Haven, 1939).

Mapp was indeed the recipient of more than one bantering accolade, such as the following:[62]

> YOU Surgeons of London, who puzzle your Pates,
> To ride in your Coaches, and purchase Estates,
> Give over, for Shame, for your Pride has a Fall,
> And Doctress of *Epsom* has out-done you all.
>
> Derry Down, &c.
>
> What signifies Learning, or going to school,
> When a Woman can do, without Reason or Rule,
> What puts you to Nonplus, & baffles your Art;
> For Petticoat Practice has now got the Start.
>
> In Physick, as well as in Fashions, we find,
> The newest has always its Run with Mankind;
> Forgot is the Bustle 'bout Taylor and Ward;
> Now Mapp's all ye Cry, & her Fame's on Record.
>
> Dame Nature has giv'n her a Doctor's Degree
> She gets all ye Patients and pockets the Fee;
> So if you don't instantly prove her a Cheat,
> She'll loll in her Chariot whilst you walk ye Street.
>
> Derry Down, &c.

And the magazine actually gave its editorial blessing to the scheme to raise a public subscription to buy from Mrs Joanna Stephens the secret of her remedy for the stone, publishing lists of, and complimenting, the prominent donors.[63] Other irregular practitioners got a more mixed reception. Bridget Bostock, the Cheshire healer who performed spiritual cures through the agency of spittle, was derided as a throw-back to Popish superstition;[64] and Joshua Ward was treated with suspicion on account of his widely rumoured Jacobite connections, being accused of practising a kind of 'political quackery'.[65] The point, however, is

---

[62] *Gentleman's Magazine*, VI (1736), 618, 747:

SUNDAY 22.

A Lady passing Kent Street in her Chariot towards the Borough, dress'd in a Robe de Chambre, the People gave out she was a certain Woman of Quality from an Electorate in Germany, whereupon a great Mob follow'd and bestow'd on her many bitter Reproaches, till Madam perceiving some Mistake, look'd out and accosted them in this familiar Manner, D__n your Bloods, don't you know me! I am Mrs Mapp the Bone-Setter. Upon which they suddenly chang'd their Revilings into loud Huzza's.

[63] Carlson, *The First Magazine* (note 24), p. 160, discusses this point well.

[64] *Gentleman's Magazine*, XVIII (1748), 448–50.

[65] *Ibid.*, X (1740), 515; M. H. Nicolson, 'Ward's Pill and Drop and men of letters', *Journal of the History of Ideas*, XXIX (1968), 173–96; G. S. Rousseau, 'On ministers and measures', *Etudes Anglaises*, XXXII (1979), 185–91.

that the magazine, and presumably its readership, did not view medical practice in terms of any simple black-and-white divide between practitioners proper and improper, official and marginal, legal and twilight, elite and vulgar; still less did it automatically associate any such categories with what was medically good and bad measured by success and failure rates. Exactly as Jewson's argument would predict, the *Gentleman's Magazine* encouraged the public to judge practitioners for themselves individually, on their own merits, rather than in terms of corporate affiliation. The public would pick and choose as it pleased. The magazine showed no animus against irregular practitioners or practices *per se*. The target of anti-quackery attacks was rather faddism,[66] and, perhaps above all, mystery-mongering, nostrums kept secret contrary to the public interest. Time and again contributors and book-reviewers condemned certain practitioners' habits of puffing proprietary medicines as therapeutic wonders while declining to divulge their ingredients to the public. Such naked self-interest, often sanctimoniously masquerading as philanthropy, raised hackles. Take, for example, the following review from 1767 of *Medical Advice to the consumptive and asthmatick people of England; wherein the present method of treating disorders of the lungs is shewn to be futile and fundamentally wrong, and a new and easy method of cure, proposed* by Philip Stern, M.D.:

The purpose of this advice is to recommend a nostrum invented by the author. It is a solution of certain balsams in a certain chemical liquor, which he says is very volatile, not at all inflammatory, and remarkably antispecific, and antispasmodic...

He conceals his medicine, he says, for no other reason than because if he was to discover it so as that it might be prepared by every apothecary, it would be neglected.

If this answer is thought insufficient, he confesses that he has no better to give. Another, however, tho' not a better, will naturally be suspected. However, it is much to be regretted, that medicines thus offered to the publick are not by appointment of the legislature examined by persons properly qualified to ascertain their inefficacy or utility. That on one hand, a useful discovery might not be disregarded as the imposition of a quack; and on the other, that the weak and credulous might not be defrauded of their money for something that is useless, if not hurtful to their health.[67]

The point, of course, here, as so commonly in the eighteenth century, is that the party guilty of the quack practice of puffing secret nostrums,

---

[66] *Gentleman's Magazine*, v (1735), 10.
[67] *Ibid.*, xxxvii (1767), 316; xxxvii (1767), 34.

was himself an M.D. *Gentleman's Magazine* reviewers and contributors thus perceived the significant divide – as Jewson would lead us to predict – being not between faculty and fringe, but between those practitioners laying their knowledge open and sharing it with the public, and those concealing it for private profit. It is significant that one of the most constructive projects launched in the magazine was to produce a composite list of nostrums, noting where they could be purchased and how much they cost.[68]

The general absence of ingrained tensions between the public and the profession can also be illustrated in a second way, by examining exceptions to this rule. For what becomes apparent is that public suspicion or hostility towards the doctors surfaced only at certain disturbing stress-points, where the laity found itself particularly vulnerable, where lives lay in the doctors' hands. These show up nicely in the magazine. One concerns amputation. There was an anxiety that surgeons were apt to be over-hasty with the knife. Amputations were of course a sadly frequent necessity in the days before antiseptic surgery. Rampant infection and the limitations of operative technique meant that surgeons could count on healing only straightforward wounds or simple fractures; in cases with complications they often felt compelled to resort to the knife. Moreover wounds and broken limbs were themselves all too common in an age of protracted warfare, innumerable riding and carriage spills, and occupational accidents. The magazine ran considerable discussion of how to forestall premature and unnecessary amputation, as for example the warning contained in this review of Henry Yates Carter's 'Case of a Compound Fracture of the Leg':

This narrative affords a striking proof of the necessity there is for great deliberation in cases where amputation may be thought necessary. The poor man who is the subject of it is a collier, sixty years old, who received, from the fall of a bucket down a coal-pit, in which he was at work, a compound fracture of his right leg. The injury, Mr Carter observes, was effected with so much violence, as to occasion an almost complete division of the muscles; so that the foot and lower part of the leg remained hanging only by a small portion of the foleus muscle. As the patient himself refused to be removed to the country infirmary, or to submit to amputation, it became necessary to attempt the cure of the limb at home without an operation; and this was happily effected so that in less than two months he was able to walk with the assistance of crutches. From this and some other similar facts the author

---

[68] *Ibid.*, xviii (1748), 346–50.

concludes that, however necessary and right speedy amputation may be in great hospitals, this ought to be no precedent for country practice, in which much more, he thinks, can be expected from the resources of Nature than many imagine.[69]

There was parallel, but infinitely greater, public disquiet about anatomical dissection, and the suspected involvement of surgeons with 'resurrection men'. Peter Linebaugh's study of the 'Tyburn riot against the surgeons'[70] has highlighted the ferocious resistance of the common people to having their deceased comrades carted off to Surgeons' Hall; and of course Hogarth mirrored public revulsion in the final engraving of his 'Four Stages of Cruelty', suggesting that medical dissection was in fact the logical public *terminus ad quem* of casual, private cruelty. Presumably gentlemen's bones were much less likely to meet such a fate; yet even so the *Gentleman's Magazine* featured scores of scare stories about the illegal procurement of bodies and grave-robbing:[71]

WEDNESDAY 14.

A man going to take up a load of dung in St George's fields, found at the dunghill the bodies of a woman and eight children, cut and mangled in a shocking manner, the handywork, probably, of some young anatomist, who deserves a rigorous punishment for this carelessness and indiscretion.[72]

In such reports, anti-surgeon bitterness commonly erupts as in this letter, deploring levity about grave-robbing, and proposing as a solution that it should be physicians' and surgeons' bones which should be laid open to the knife:

MR URBAN   Oct. 24, 1747.

I HAVE a great veneration for the ashes of the dead, more especially of such, who are interred by the solemn rites of christian burial, and I have often wished that our wise legislators would provide for the repose of mankind as to render it next to impossible to disinter them, after being laid in the bosom of our common parent. The affair which lately happened to the vaults at St Andrew's, Holborn, has particularly affected me, and I never think on

[69] *Ibid.*, LXIX (1794), 448.
[70] See P. Linebaugh, 'The Tyburn riot against the surgeons', in D. Hay *et al.* (eds.), *Albion's Fatal Tree* (London, 1975), pp. 65–118.
[71] *Gentleman's Magazine*, XXXII (1762), 340. See also S. Leblond, 'The anatomists and the resurrectionists in Great Britain', *Canadian Medical Association Journal*, XCIII (1965), 73–8, 113–20; H. Cole, *Things for the Surgeon: A History of the Resurrection Men* (London, 1964).
[72] *Gentleman's Magazine*, XVII (1747), 487.

the relation of the young lady, of Hatton Garden, whose body was taken away by the sexton, the very night of its interment, and sold to a surgeon, without heartily wishing the vile thief might be rewarded with the gallows and afterwards anatomised. I am informed that it is a common practice with these fellows, and their comrades, to steal dead bodies and sell them, which I fear is too true, since, otherwise, the surgeons would never have such plenty of dissections. If there is no law in being for punishing offenders of this kind with death, it is high time that there should be one made.

In conversing with some surgeons about the impiety they are guilty of, by encouraging the theft of dead bodies for their use, I find they make very light on it.

The indignant author went on:

Since this is really the case, and that these gentlemen think cutting, slashing and scraping, a matter of such indifference, I would humbly propose a method whereby they may be very amply supplied with opportunities of improving anatomical knowledge.

First, That Surgeons' Hall should be the public academy or school for the whole faculty of this great metropolis.

Secondly, That all physicians, men and women midwives (for I would not exclude any old woman of the faculty,) surgeons, apothecaries, quacks, tooth-drawers, their pupils, journeymen, apprentices and labourers, shall, as soon as they are dead, be carried to the said hall, and there dissected.

Thirdly, That the bodies of regular-bred physicians, midwives and surgeons, shall be dissected or anatomis'd according to the direction of the will of the deceas'd, whose imprimis shall close with 'and my body I commit to Surgeons' Hall to be decently,' and so forth.

Fourthly, That the bodies of apothecaries, barber-surgeons, quacks, tooth-drawers, pupils, journeymen, apprentices and labourers, shall undergo such operations of dissection and anatomy, as the president, vice-president, & c. shall appoint.

[signed] L.R.[73]

Similar worries also underlay the persistent controversy, coming to a head in the 1780s, about premature burial.[74] The magazine published numerous scare reports of the 'dead', on the brink of being sealed up

[73] *Ibid.*, XVII (1747), 487; XLVII (1777), 529.
[74] See, for the wider European context, J. McManners, *Death and the Enlightenment* (Oxford, 1981); L. J. Jordanova, 'Policing public health' (note 39); P. Ariès, *The Hour of our Death* (London, 1981); H. Dittrick, 'Devices to prevent premature burial', *Journal of the History of Medicine*, III (1948), 161–71; T. K. Marshall, 'Premature burial', *Medical and Legal Journal*, XXXV (1967), 14–24.

in their coffins, awaking from deep coma; and worse still, stories of those actually buried alive:

An Inn-keeper returning from taking a walk with his wife, dropt down suddenly to all appearance dead; the medical persons who were called in declared him to be lifeless. The next day he was inclosed in an oak coffin, and deposited in a chapel till the funeral was to take place. Some of the neighbours hearing a noise in the chapel, ran to the place, and found the poor man bathed in his blood, and really dead, having as it appeared, made most violent but ineffectual efforts to break his coffin.[75]

The problem, a correspondent argued, was two-fold. One aspect was practical – the risk arising from corpses being left, on apparent death, to the female 'layer out', 'an ignorant and unfeeling nurse', all too often allegedly intoxicated.[76] The other was clinical – the problem of the 'uncertainty of the signs of death'.[77] The endeavours of groups such as the Humane Society to overcome this problem were widely reported and applauded in the magazine.[78]

[75] *Gentleman's Magazine*, LXIX (1800), 988; LVI (1786), 1008; XLVII (1777), 422–4. 'R.W.E. reported from West Bromwich (1786, p. 1008) that a workman had accidentally broken open an old coffin in which the position of the body was 'apparently as if struggling after burial':

> It seems not improbable but the body of the unhappy man was buried in a trance and on the best information I could get, it was the body of an old lawyer in the said parish of the name of Whitehouse; and what strengthens my conjecture in the above matter, was the frequent use of large quantities of opiates during his last illness. He died about the year 1764.
> If you think this merits a place in your useful work, it may possibly be the means of preventing others from the too early burial of their friends, after their apparent, if not real decease; as, in my own mind, I have not a doubt but many in a year are buried before all symptoms of life have left them.
> Yours, &c.
>   R.W.E.

[76] *Ibid.*, XLVII (1777), 423.

[77] *Ibid.*, XLVII (1777), 422; XV (1745), 311.

[78] *Ibid.*, XLVII (1777), 423. See also the contribution of J. Boerhadem, *ibid.*, XLVII (1777), 529:

> Mr URBAN
> In confirmation of Mr Hawe's humane cautions against too hastily burying persons apparently dead, I refer him to Turner's 'Remarkable Providences;' a book published in 1697, wherein there is a chapter; concerning 'persons reviving after a supposed death.' From several instances related by him, I have selected the following, which, if your [sic] please, you may insert in your Magazine.

> See more generally L. H. Hawkins, 'The history of resuscitation', *British Journal of Hospital Medicine*, IV (1970), 495–500; J. P. Payne, 'On the resuscitation of the apparently dead: a historical account', *Annals of the Royal College of Surgeons*, XLV (1969), 98–107; P. J. Bishop, *A Short History of the Royal Humane Society* (London, 1974).

These exceptions aside, however, the *Gentleman's Magazine* gives little evidence of deep mistrust or hostility entertained by the public against practitioners, and I would suggest that this accurately mirrors public attitudes. The educated Georgian public did not in general feel itself delivered helplessly into the hands of the doctors. It was only where it did – especially in the case of death, dissection and desecration – that friction was liable to arise.

III

Let us look next from another perspective, that of the doctors. How are we to interpret their participation in the *Gentleman's Magazine*? It should of course be no surprise that they were *readers*, for the eighteenth century practitioner typically wanted to be, and especially to be seen to be, a man of polite culture, taste and learning.[79] But why did they *contribute*? Some answers suggest themselves through examination of their writings. These took various forms. They were, for example, active in responding to specific queries. Thus, following readers' inquiries, flurries of advice appeared in the magazine from time to time recommending treatments for scurvy. Though some responses were apparently from laymen,[80] most came from the doctors.[81] They also took part in controversies. And not least, scores of practitioners sent in advice, remedies and case-histories on their own initiative, such as Dr Cameron of Worcester who expatiated on the properties of bark,[82] or Dr Clifton who ventured a smallpox cure,[83] on top of his recommendations about how to recover fishbones or needles accidentally swallowed.[84] Some became regular correspondents: for example William Rowley,[85] and Dr John Cook who gave readers the benefit of his wisdom on wasp stings,[86] and treatments for worms,[87] alongside his championing of a general family medicine.[88] Similarly Dr Wall

---

[79] See M. Kemp, *Dr William Hunter at the Royal Academy* (Glasgow, 1975), p. 22; G. S. Rousseau, *Tobias Smollett: Essays of Two Decades* (Edinburgh, 1982); idem, 'Literature and medicine: the state of the field', *Isis*, LXXII (1981), 406–24.

[80] *Gentleman's Magazine*, XLVII (1777), 294.

[81] *Ibid.*, LXVIII (1798), 105–8 (by John Sherwen, a practitioner from Enfield).

[82] *Ibid.*, XXI (1751), 543.

[83] *Ibid.*, IX (1739), 270.

[84] *Ibid.*, LIII (1783), 1050.

[85] On Rowley, see C. Sugden, *Our Ophthalmic Heritage* (London, 1967), pp. 153–7. He was a prolific author.

[86] *Gentleman's Magazine*, XXXV (1765), 456.

[87] *Ibid.*, XXXII (1762), 630.

[88] *Ibid.*, XXXV (1765), 208. For Cook see C. F. Mullett, 'John Cook, M.D., physician at large', *Bulletin of the History of Medicine*, V (1946), 498–516.

proffered his expertise on such subjects as smallpox,[89] ulcerated sore throat,[90] and bowel disorders,[91] as well as offering his recipe for longevity.[92]

These contributions suggest that certain practitioners at least saw advantage for themselves in making a broad appeal to the public beyond the confines of their own face-to-face clinical practice. In the great majority of such instances there can have been no expectation of significant immediate financial gain. Few such practitioners were peddling nostrums, or owned patents for medicines. Indeed, many of them divulged recipes which readers could make up at home, or recommend common, easily available, proprietary medicines (Dr Cook, for instance, 'the publick's most ready servant', prescribed Godfrey's Cordial).[93] Neither is it likely that such practitioners published with a view to advancing their esteem, or facilitating their rise, *within* the ranks of the profession. Rather, these insertions were aimed at the public, and it was public favour that determined success or failure for the typical practitioner. For such men, publishing probably served three main purposes. First, as a form of concealed advertising, to bring the practitioner's name, merits and patriotism to the attention of local gentlemen and men of property. Second, as a mode of indirectly publicizing other publications. Even where these were not explicitly mentioned in the magazine, the airing given to the doctor's name might be expected to sell copies – practitioners such as William Rowley were, after all, as Ginnie Smith's essay in this volume shows, tireless authors of medical books and pamphlets. And thirdly, to establish credentials and the reputation for being more than a mere sawbones or shop-keeper apothecary, aiming to win standing as a man of knowledge, science and taste, a citizen in the republic of letters. In all these cases, publishing in the magazine must have been ventured upon chiefly with an eye to renown with the public rather than with the faculty.

This is confirmed by the characteristic bias of the topics practitioners wrote about. In a later age, medical authors typically presented themselves to the public as campaigners. They launched themselves in the press as holy warriors, crusading for improved public health, extended hygiene inspection, higher professional standards, safeguarding the public against charlatans and dangerous drugs, questing for national

---

[89] *Gentleman's Magazine*, XXIV (1754), 370.
[90] *Ibid.*, XXI (1751), 497.   [91] *Ibid.*, XXII (1752), 495.
[92] *Ibid.*, XIII (1743), 279.   [93] *Ibid.*, XXXV (1765), 525.

health efficiency. They aimed to raise the collective authority of the profession, and sometimes to ally the profession with the state.[94] Eighteenth century medical contributors to the *Gentleman's Magazine*, by contrast, had a totally different ethos. Their concerns are almost wholly with the personal wellbeing of individuals rather than with national and corporate issues; they are exercised principally with treating sufferers, offering case-histories, and prescribing remedies. It is directly to the alleviation of sickness that they are speaking; their orientation is not towards the profession, politicians or the state but to the public.

Moreover, the tone of these medical contributions is – almost without exception – sympathetic and accommodating to lay readers. No doctor writing in the magazine claims for the chartered profession exclusive prerogatives over the domain of medicine; perhaps the closest approximation to that was the practitioner who condemned the 'prevailing notion' that a nurse alone was sufficient to look after smallpox cases.[95] Practitioner contributions show no concerted opposition to folk remedies or self-medication, nor are midwives and 'wise women' prominent as bogey figures. Indeed practitioners continued to spell out, without qualm, remedies which would inevitably be lay-administered.

Medical men thus tended to cast themselves as the servants of the public. Dr Cook opened one of his case-histories:[96]

MR URBAN,

Publick utility entirely, and not a mere *scabies scribendi* is the only motive of my writing so often, and which I shall with increasing delight continue to do, as long as I live, and am capable to be any ways serviceable to the poor, and the public. For tho', in truth, I cannot become either a Mead, or a Sydenham, yet I may prove to be an honest COOK; (and honesty is not a commodity to be found everywhere) and not to be the first of the name neither, who has done good service in the profession: Wherefore, I carelessly look down upon all degraders, as surly curs snapping at my shadow. But to the purpose...

Occasionally doctors went further and even appealed to the public as a tribunal or arbitrator in the affairs of the profession. Practitioners

---

94 In nineteenth century England, Thomas Wakley is the obvious example. See C. Brook, *Battling Surgeon* (Glasgow, 1945). But similar attempts to control the public in the name of health were extremely common in late Enlightenment France: cf. L. J. Jordanova, 'Policing public health' (note 39).
95 *Gentleman's Magazine*, XXII (1752), 402.   96 *Ibid.*, XXXV (1765), 524.

who believed themselves maligned in intra-professional disputes not infrequently thus washed their dirty linen in public. For instance a surgeon or man-midwife inserted the following notice in order to redress a slur against his reputation:

THE case of an extra-uterine conception in the last Mag. p 214, was related by a person who never visited the patient, and with such circumstances as are very injurious to the character of the surgeon who attended her. You are therefore desired to publish the following declaration of the patient herself, by which these insinuations are proved to be false.

Yours, & c.   A.B.[97]

William Bromfield and Aylett, the Windsor surgeon-apothecary, fenced with each other over malpractice accusations in the pages of the magazine in 1759;[98] and similarly in 1777 the inveterately bilious John Coakley Lettsom penned an astringent review of Dr George Armstrong's tract on child diseases, insinuating plagiarism,[99] and Armstrong replied, appealing to the candour of the 'reader' against the 'wrangling' of his fellow practitioner.[100] Clearly public esteem in some ways counted for more than keeping professional ranks closed.

IV

A pilot survey like this barely scratches the surface, skimming about 70,000 printed pages over a span of some seventy years. There are obviously grave dangers of reading too much into (or out of) the contents and tone of one single magazine: there were many other contemporary organs, mainly somewhat down-market, which, if examined, might tell different stories.[101] Moreover, this analysis of the printed page has not even been able to raise, let alone resolve, the fundamental and tricky questions of how these articles were penned or even read.[102] It would be possible in certain cases to discover more about the context in which they were written, for the careers of a few of the authors are familiar. But it would be a forlorn hope to expect to discover with any precision the impact they had on the reading public. Moreover, I have here treated a seventy-year span of the

[97] *Ibid.*, xx (1751), 244.   [98] *Ibid.*, xxix (1759), 561.
[99] *Ibid.*, xlvii (1777), 416.   [100] *Ibid.*, xlvii (1777), 633.
[101] Analysis of the *London Magazine* (founded in 1732) would prove similarly fruitful.
[102] For some discussion of the problems of authorship and readership of medical advice literature see Roy Porter, 'Spreading carnal knowledge or selling dirt cheap? Nicholas Venette's *Conjugal Love* in the eighteenth century', *Journal of European Studies*, xiv (1984), 233–55..

magazine as though it formed a homogeneous unity, which did not significantly change over time; and I have had to attribute to the journal some degree of editorial coherence and purpose – whereas one might argue that the *Gentleman's Magazine* amounted to nothing more than space-filling, scissors-and-paste, hack journalism. I have also presupposed the genuineness of the letters published in its pages – possibly a questionable assumption, since it is clear that in many eighteenth century literary periodicals, as in quack bills, similar letters and testimonials were in-house fabrications.

Remembering these qualifications, it appears to me that the *Gentleman's Magazine* medical contributions bear out to a quite impressive degree, both in their content and in their unspoken assumptions, the core features of Jewson's hypothesis. These entries confirm that in the Georgian era sophisticated medical awareness was not the exclusive preserve of the faculty; it involved a common language, which was shared, debated, criticized, and promoted by medics and polite laymen alike. The weight of the medical entries suggests that the literate laity were not just passive uncomprehending recipients of medical treatment, for they could be expected to possess considerable medical familiarity, and hence be in a position to exercise some therapeutic judgement.[103] Moreover, in the process of the diffusion and even augmentation of medical information in Georgian England, the laity were participants as well as recipients. And not least, these contributions point to a degree of mutual interest between practitioners and laymen; there is little evidence of exclusive professional demarcations or jealous rivalry. Practitioners were seeking a role within the theatre of lay medicine, rather than trying to exclude the public from its performance. Medical knowledge was publicly displayed; indeed it was to the advantage of medical men to display their knowledge in the community market-place.[104]

---

[103] For the eighteenth century audience for scientific knowledge see S. Schaffer, 'Natural philosophy and public spectacle in the eighteenth century', *History of Science*, XXI (1983), 1–43; *idem*, 'Natural philosophy', in G. S. Rousseau and Roy Porter (eds.), *The Ferment of Knowledge* (Cambridge, 1980), pp. 53–92; for 'mere' popularization see J. R. Millburn, *Benjamin Martin, Author, Instrument Maker and 'Country-Showman'* (Leyden, 1976).

[104] Discussions of the 'amateur tradition' in English scientific and medical knowledge are illuminating here. See, e.g., M. Berman, '"Hegemony" and the amateur tradition in British science', *Journal of Social History*, VIII (1975), 30–50; Steven Shapin and Arnold Thackray, 'Prosopography as a research tool in history of science. The British scientific community 1700–1900', *History of Science*, XII (1974), 1–28.

Many of these points will be obvious enough. But they certainly help to substantiate core features of Jewson's account of a shared world of medical knowledge in which the laity could participate, even if Jewson's reading must still be taken as a working hypothesis, or as a point of departure, in need of much further refinement and delineation. Of course, moreover, this paper makes no pretence to arrive at or infer the actual experiences and behaviour of sick people. But it may go some way towards showing how a medical culture was disseminated, which provided the facts, assumptions and language within which the Georgian laity met their illnesses, their doctors, and their fate.

I wish to acknowledge my gratitude to the Wellcome Trust for granting me subventions in the summers of 1982 and 1983 to provide research assistance with the task of combing through the *Gentleman's Magazine* and classifying its contents. I also wish to thank Stephen Marriage and Fi Godlee who carried out that work with admirable intelligence, efficiency and good spirits, and Jonathan Barry, Irvine Loudon and W. F. Bynum in particular for their stimulating criticisms of earlier drafts of this paper.

11

The colonisation of traditional Arabic medicine

GHADA KARMI

I

The fifth Abbasid caliph, Harun al-Rashid, had three wives whose beauty, grace and wit were legendary. At the same time, he also had a short, fat, ugly cook named Murjana. One day, while this Murjana was out in the fields, she came across the body of a dead horse surrounded by wild animals. To her surprise, however, not a single animal would come near the carcass. Murjana decided to investigate. When she reached the body, she found a charm hanging about its neck which she removed forthwith and hung about her own neck. No sooner had she done this than the wild beasts sprang onto the horse and began to devour it. When she reached the palace, her beauty amazed all who saw her, not least the caliph who became so enamoured that he married her at once, neglecting all his other wives. Not long after, poor Murjana sickened and died. The caliph was inconsolable. However, the woman who was washing the body before burial came across the charm. She instantly donned it and was, in her turn, transformed such that, when Harun saw her, he forgot all about Murjana and married her on the spot.[1]

This unhistorical but colourful story formed the substance of a favourite Arabic charm widely used throughout the Levant by the peasants during the early part of this century. It was written on paper and wrapped in cloth and, when worn around the neck, it was supposed to confer the same sort of luck on its wearer as befell Murjana and her successor. Amulets, charms, talismans and incantations formed important ingredients of the traditional medicine of the Levant. Taufik Canaan, a Palestinian doctor working in the 1920s, studied the popular medical practices in the villages of Palestine and found that magic and

[1] T. Canaan, 'Demons as an aetiological factor in popular medicine', al-Kullieh, Beirut (April, 1912), 11–12.

superstition were rife as causal explanations and cures for many diseases, especially those of the nervous system.[2] The atmosphere was said to be full of invisible evil spirits (*jinn*) whose entry into the body caused disease and distress. Fifty years on, in the villages of Syria and Jordan, magic and superstition are still important components of popular medicine, with this difference: many ancient superstitions had, by the 1970s, acquired more of a religious guise and were increasingly explained and justified in terms of Islam, a tendency which is in line with the recent Islamic revivalism in the Middle East. This has led to a mixing of the two traditions and therefore to a variety of curious practices and beliefs. For example, I came across a traditional Syrian treatment for sciatica (which, incidentally, was often diagnosed on perfectly reasonable clinical and anatomical grounds). This involved the burning of a wild herb named 'the sciatica plant' (Arabic, *'irq al-nisa*) at sun-rise on a Wednesday morning while Quranic verses were read over it. That it should be a Wednesday morning was apparently crucial for the success of the operation. The patient did not have to be present and would be cured wherever he was. Despite the Quranic verses, the ancient pre-Islamic roots of this ritual are not difficult to unravel: the Palestinian peasants of Canaan believed that on Wednesday nights the evil spirits were abroad, filling their water-skins;[3] in Jewish demonology, the 'dancing roof-top demons' are out on the nights of Wednesday and the Sabbath;[4] God created light on the fourth day and sun-light has healing properties according to the Talmud,[5] (the Arabic for Wednesday is *al-arba'a'*, 'the fourth'). The same process can be discerned in the case of the evil eye: this primitive and ubiquitous superstition is given religious legitimacy by specific and biased interpretations of certain verses in the Quran,[6] and by recourse to numerous sayings attributed to the Prophet Muhammad.[7]

[2] Ibid., and Canaan, *Aberglaube und Volksmedizin im Lande der Bibel* (Abhandlung der Hamburgischen Kolonialinstituts 20, Hamburg, 1914); see also, R. Campbell Thompson, *Semitic Magic its Origins and Development* (London, 1908), pp. 57–60.   [3] Canaan, 'Demons as an aetiological factor', p. 5.

[4] *The Jewish Encyclopaedia* (12 vols., New York and London, 1903), vol. 4, p. 516.

[5] Mal. 4: 2; Talmud, B.B. 16b.; *The Jewish Encyclopaedia*, vol. 11, p. 590.

[6] Quran, Sura 113 and Sura 114, both of which refer to deliverance from 'the mischief of the envious' and 'the mischief of the whisperer who slyly withdraweth, who whispers evil suggestions into the breasts of men'. These two Suras supposedly refer to the bewitchment of Muhammad by Lobeid the Jew and his daughters. See note to Sura 113 in George Sale's translation of the Quran (London, 1921).

[7] References to the evil eye and its effects occur in many places in the collection of the Prophet's sayings on health (most of them almost certainly apocryphal)

In general, though, the sort of folk medicine which uses magic and religion tended to remain historically distinct from main-stream traditional medicine in the Arab world. This is reflected in the existence of two types of practitioner: the one practising 'Arabic medicine' and the other, who was often either a religious sheikh or wise-woman, using spells and amulets for treating a variety of emotional ailments and incurable afflictions. This paper is concerned with the former type of practitioner and with the modern survival of classical Arabic medicine as revealed by a field-survey of the traditional medicine of Syria and Jordan which the author undertook at the end of the 1970s. The study was set up to investigate the survival of classical Arabic medicine among the rural population of Syria and Jordan. This medical system first became established in the Islamic world during the seventh century and reached its zenith in the ninth, tenth and eleventh centuries – the age of Rhazes, Avicenna and Averroes. Its influence stretched at one time from Spain to Samarkand. By way of Spain, it crossed into mediaeval Europe where, in Latin dress, it continued to influence medical ideas and medical education until the sixteenth century and beyond. And yet, standard histories of Arabic medicine have tended to regard it, even at its zenith, as no more than an exotic landing-stage on the journey from classical antiquity to mediaeval Europe, and its later centuries have been labelled 'the age of decline' and then conveniently forgotten.[8] But, as our study showed, this was far from the case; classical Arabic medicine, in fact, continued as a practical system well into this century, in spite of the efforts that the Arabs themselves have made to annihilate it. For, the Arab world of today is passionately bent on 'modernisation'; technology, ideas and insti-

---

known as *The Prophet's Medicine* (al-Tibb al-Nabawi). See for example, Ibn Qayyim al-Jawziyya's *al-Tibb al-Nabawi*, ed. Abd al-Ghani 'Abd al-Khaliq (Cairo, 1980), pp. 150, 155, 157, 161.

[8] There are in fact very few histories of Arabic medicine *per se*; it would be more accurate to say that the chapters on Arabic medicine in standard histories of medicine treat the subject in the dismissive and patronising way referred to in the text; for example, the chapters in M. Neuburger, *History of Medicine*, trans. E. Playfair (2 vols., London, 1910), vol. 1, pp. 346–84; F. Garrison, *An Introduction to the History of Medicine*, 4th edn. (Philadelphia, 1929), pp. 73–8; A. Castiglioni, *A History of Medicine*, 2nd edn. (London, 1947), pp. 258–87. The few histories of Arabic medicine which exist are limited in scope, as for example, E. G. Browne, *Arabian Medicine* (Cambridge, 1921), and C. Elgood, *A Medical History of Persia* (Cambridge, 1951), both of which confine themselves to Persian medicine; most recently, M. Ullmann's *Islamic Medicine* (Edinburgh, 1978) has appeared. This is the best of them and the most extensive in scope, but nevertheless, the book is a collection of essays and not a comprehensive history.

tutions have been imported at an unprecedented rate, and this process has begun to leave its mark. The old Arabic medicine as it had been practised for centuries is dying away, replaced by the new medicine and the new pharmacology. Yet, enough of it remained to allow us observation of its practice as a living system which made sense of what would otherwise have been no more than dry and obsolete ancient theory. At the same time, it was possible to investigate the responses of the patient to the two types of medicine and thereby to trace historical developments in and around Arabic medicine.

The history of Arabic medicine, whether in appreciative or unappreciative hands, has been the history of great men and great books. Roy Porter's plea in the Introduction to this book for a history of the patient can be echoed by the modern historian of Arabic medicine. There is extraordinarily little evidence about what medicine ordinary people practised, what they felt about illness, what they thought about their doctors, or how they responded to the medical institutions which the state provided. The historical sources, where they exist, are unpublished, and it will be some painstaking scholar's task one day to unravel the mystery. The printed sources are, alas, unsuitable: Goitein's fascinating revelations of the daily lives of the Jewish community of Cairo in the thirteenth century[9] could have been of great value in this context, but it deals exclusively with a special community and is unrepresentative. Arabic history has no Samuel Pepys or even diarists as modest as those in Lucinda Beier's paper who could help, but there is on the other hand a wealth of anecdotes, stories and poetry which could throw light on the problem. No scholar has so far appeared willing to investigate this potentially important source.

II

The areas chosen for study were the villages around A'zaz, a large town of three thousand inhabitants in the north-west of Syria near the Turkish border, and the Jarash region in the north-east of Jordan, which has a comparable population. Both regions were agricultural and relatively inaccessible, the Syrian more so than the Jordanian; the peasants of Syria were sedentary, but in Jordan the population included a fair number of nomadic bedouins whose customs were also studied. The inquiry was centred on certain practices, in particular cautery, cupping and venesection, but much other material was gathered on

---

[9] S. D. Goitein, *A Mediterranean Society: The Jewish Communities of the Arab World as Portrayed in the Documents of the Cairo Geniza* (Berkeley, 1967–78).

the way. Local folk practitioners were identified and interviewed and their techniques, rationale for treatment and medical ideas were recorded. The patient population was easier to make contact with, since all of them, except the very old, came sooner or later to the government health clinics which were held daily in the major towns.

The traditional techniques of cauterisation, cupping and venesection were essentially the same in both countries. Cupping, with or without scarification, was especially common, used for all chest ailments where it 'drew out the illness'. It was relatively harmless and, as in other parts of the world, will probably outlive all other folk practices.[10] More dramatic were the practices of cautery and venesection. The aim of most cauterisation was to effect a full-thickness skin burn and then to induce suppuration at the site. A red-hot iron was used for this or, alternatively, a piece of cotton which was ignited and left to burn slowly down to the skin; thereafter, a foreign body was inserted into the burn and left to produce 'laudable pus'[11] for seven to ten days. Such burns could be quite deep and leave much scarring; the subject often had to be held down forcibly in order to tolerate the 'treatment'. But not all cautery was so painful. In the superficial type, particularly indicated for cases of sciatica, the skin was touched lightly in several places with the cautery iron. Many people resorted to cautery despite its brutality for chronic ailments such as arthritis, ill-defined stomach pains and debility, usually after the clinic medicine had failed to bring relief; most of these claimed that it was greatly superior. It 'drew out the illness and the pain with the pus'.

Venesection as a practice had virtually died out, but where it was still to be found (the heartland of the Syrian villages) it was a fascinating relic of the past. The 'needle' was a triangular piece of broken glass

[10] S. Bayfield, *A Treatise on Practical Cupping* (London, 1823); P. S. Maloof, 'Medical beliefs and practices of Palestinian Americans' (Ph.D. Thesis, Catholic University of America, Washington, D.C., 1979), p. 101; A. Green, 'Scarification, cupping, and other traditional measures with reference to folk medicine in Greece and elsewhere', *Australian Journal of Dermatology*, XII (1971), 89–96; J. L. Turk and E. Allen, 'Bleeding and cupping', *Annals of the Royal College of Surgeons of England*, LXV (1983), 128–31.

[11] This was not in fact their phrase for it, but rather what their own description ('leaving the wound to work'), irresistibly evoked. The concept of laudable pus – even to the exact Arabic rendering of laudable as *mahmud* – was very familiar to classical Arabic medicine. See J. D. Latham, '"Mahmud" and "laudable"', *Journal of the Royal Asiatic Society*, I (1977), 31–40. Other descriptions which I have quoted represent exact translations from the original Arabic of the people seen during the study.

wedged into the side of a short stick and tied in place with string. When
blood was to be drawn, the upper arm was tied with a scarf acting
as a tourniquet and the needle-point was poised over the swollen vein.
The head of the needle was then struck with a spoon to make it
penetrate the vein and the 'black blood' was let out until it changed
to red. The veins of the forehead were also bled, the tourniquet/scarf
being then applied to the neck. The indications for venesection were
recognisably humoral: 'over-fullness' (which must correspond to the
condition of *plethora* described in the classical Greek and Arabic books),
the 'black diseases' such as epilepsy and madness, and also for the
preservation of health in spring when the blood 'increases and froths
and jumps about'. 'The blood decreases in autumn which is also the
season when madness is worse.' Madness and epilepsy were caused by
a collection of 'black blood' over the brain, although *jinn* were also
responsible for madness. The insane and epileptics must avoid certain
foods: goats' flesh, onions, lentils, eggs and hot spicy things, for all
these excite the disease and increase the 'psychic wind' (see below).
Epilepsy was also treated with nasal fumigation using a spice from the
spice-seller (*al-'attar*).

Herbal medicines were used for many conditions, and were often
compound preparations; their ingredients were strikingly familiar
from the mediaeval Arabic medical books. Of particular interest was
the use of women's milk as a therapy. This practice was well-known
in antiquity and was perpetuated during the Arabic period (as well as
in the West) when women's milk was instilled into the nose, or milked
over the head, or taken by mouth, especially for cases of consumption.[12]
In Jordan, bone-setters were still important practitioners. They set
fractures and dislocations with a manual skill which must have survived
intact for a thousand years at least, and which owed nothing to a formal
knowledge of anatomy or pathology, even in humoral terms. The
relationships of bones and joints to each other had been learned by
touch alone, and experience dictated the length of time in plaster and
when bones united. The 'plaster' consisted of gauze impregnated with
a mixture of olive-oil soap and egg-white which was said by the

[12] 'Ali b. al-'Abbas al-Majusi, *Kamil al-Sina'a fi'l Tibb* (hereafter *Kamil*) (2 vols.,
Cairo, 1877), vol. 2, p. 134, 1.5–6; Hippocrates, *Oeuvres complètes d'Hippocrate*,
ed. E. Littré (10 vols., Paris, 1839–61), vol. 7, p. 121, vol. 8, p. 167; Galen,
De Simplicium Medicamentorum Temperamentis ac Facultatibus, Book 10, and *De
Methodo Medendi*, Book 5 (vol. 2, p. 265 and vol. 10, p. 366 respectively in
Claudii Galeni Opera Omnia, ed. C. G. Kuhn, 20 vols., Hildesheim, 1821–33).

bone-setters to be more comfortable for the patient than the hard, solid plaster of the modern hospital.

The findings of the survey showed that 'Arabic medicine' had a considerable and similar prevalence in both countries. Most of the larger villages had an Arabic medicine practitioner, and the people of the smaller villages went to the nearest 'centre'. However, nearly every one of these practitioners was aged over fifty and often they were over seventy. The younger generation were not being trained for the same job in the way their parents in many 'medical families' had been. There was much more Arabic medicine some fifty years ago, but it was now dying out; this was most evident in the case of venesection. Part of the reason for this decline was the introduction of laws in Syria specifically designed to deter the practice of Arabic medicine; one practitioner was known to be in prison at the time of the study, convicted of causing a man's death with this medicine, and this had clearly intimidated the rest.

In essence, the study revealed that the folk medicine of the rural people of Syria and Jordan is no typical folk medicine, within the usual meaning of that term, but rather a residual form of classical Arabic medicine, in that it contains recognisable traces of a medical system which is known to us from a written tradition. For example, cauterisation is described in al-Zahrawi's (Albucasis) tenth century treatise on surgery and, although the instruments differ and the range of conditions for which cauterisation was indicated is more extensive, yet the essential features are recognisably the same.[13] According to the humoral theory, epilepsy and madness were both 'black diseases' because they were caused by black bile. This collects in the brain or putrefies in the stomach and its vapour ascends to the ventricles of the brain – hence the 'psychic wind' of our village doctors.[14] Certain foods

[13] Abu'l-Qasim al-Zahrawi (d. 1009), *Albucasis on Surgery and Instruments* (hereafter *Albucasis*), ed. M. S. Spink and G. L. Lewis (London, 1973), pp. 8–165.

[14] 'Psychic wind' is the exact translation of the Arabic the natives used, *al-rih al-nafsani*. There is a possible confusion here between the word *rih*, meaning wind or vapour, and the word *ruh*, meaning spirit or pneuma. The psychic pneuma or *al-ruh al-nafsani* was, according to humoral ideas, elaborated in the ventricles of the brain. Interference with it, as for example if its exit from the brain was blocked by phlegm, was one of the mechanisms which led to epilepsy. Whether the natives' use of the term referred to the vapour of black bile, or whether to the disturbance of psychic pneuma, in either case there are well-established classical written traditions for these concepts. See al-Majusi

were believed to give rise to the production of black bile in the body, and hence were to be avoided in the treatment of black bile diseases, as was found in our survey.[15] Venesection was the treatment of choice for these: the black blood containing an excess of black bile was released and the system was thus returned to a state of equilibrium (of the humours).[16] Venesection from the veins of the forehead was also indicated for disease of the face and the head, the method being the same as is used today.[17] Blood was usually let in the spring for the preservation of health; otherwise the body became prone to sanguine diseases when the blood increased. In the same way, black bile increased during the autumn, when this humour preponderated.[18] Epilepsy could also be treated by nasal fumigation according to classical writers; the ancient Greek recommendation of the use of peony for the treatment of epileptics was taken over by the Arabic physicians, who even transcribed the Greek word into the Arabic *fawania*.[19] Although this plant was not mentioned by name by the Syrian healers, yet the reference must have been to the same practice. Another form of fumigation practised in Jordan for the diagnosis of infertility was another example of an almost perfect survival of a similar method from classical times. Garlic is inserted into the vagina of the infertile woman last thing at night; if garlic can be smelt on her breath the next morning, she is pronounced fertile.[20] Even in the least theoretical type of traditional medicine, namely bone-setting, the ingredients of plasters

on vapour and psychic pneuma in *Kamil*, vol. 1, p. 331, 1.9–10, and vol. 1, p. 332, 1.23. The Galenic system of pneumatology which anteceded this is well expounded by O. Temkin, *The Double Face of Janus* (Baltimore, 1977), pp. 154–62.

15 Majusi, *Kamil*, vol. 1, p. 333.

16 The technique of venesection is given in detail in *Albucasis*, pp. 640–54; see also Ibn al-Tilmidth (d. 1154), *Maqala fi'l-Fasd* (A treatise on venesection), Well. Hist. Lib. MS. Or. 9 (description in A. Z. Iskandar, *A Catalogue of Arabic Manuscripts on Medicine and Science in the Wellcome Historical Library*, London, 1967, pp. 130–1).   17 *Albucasis*, p. 628.

18 This theory is lucidly explained in Majusi, *Kamil*, vol. 1, pp. 43–8; see also Ullmann's exposition of Arabic humoralism in his *Islamic Medicine*, pp. 57–60. There is a specific reference to blood-letting for the preservation of health in *Albucasis*, p. 640.

19 O. Temkin, *The Falling Sickness*, 2nd edn. (Baltimore, 1971), pp. 13, 25, 68; al-Qamari (d. 990), *K. al-Ghina wal-Muna* (The book of riches and desires), Br. Lib. MS. Or. 6623, fo. 21v. 'Blow powdered peony into his nose, for it has a special effect in curing this malady [epilepsy], such that it will often cure boys if a piece of it is hung around their necks' (my translation).

20 An identical procedure is to be found described in the Hippocratic works, see Littré's edn., vol. 8, p. 417.

were the same as those recommended by the greatest mediaeval Arabic writer on orthopaedics.[21]

Thus, our study showed the survival of a fairly pure form of classical humoral medicine, albeit attenuated and sometimes mixed with magic and folk-belief, that had been handed down over the centuries, not through the learned tomes and compendia of the mediaeval physician, but through the daily practice of illiterate peasants. Despite the widespread use of humoral terms among them, as has been seen, they were clearly unaware of the classical past or of the medical compendia or the famous physicians of Islam. Most, but not all, of the people seen in the study could not read or write, but those of them who could still transmitted their medical knowledge through oral channels. How had this situation come about? How did the scholastic achievements of the Arabs reach these humble peasants? Was Graeco/Arabic medicine once the preserve of an educated class and did it afterwards percolate downwards, converted from a literate to an oral tradition? If so, when and how did this happen? Or was it the case that this 'official' medicine did not have 'far down' to go, for already the Near East was considerably hellenised and therefore familiar with Greek medical ideas at the time of the Arab conquest? I am making an implicit assumption here that the mode of transmission, whether humoral medicine had far to go or not, went from books to oral culture. Once the literate Graeco/Arabic medicine had been established, the written tradition eventually reached the people where it may or may not have mixed with some similar concepts and practices already present. This can only be an assumption, since oral traditions are, by their very nature, impossible to document historically.[22] However, there are arising out

---

[21] The large section on bone-setting in *Albucasis* describes the reduction of fractures and dislocations and includes much humoral pathology. Olive oil and egg-white are standard ingredients of the plasters he lists, pp. 690–4.

[22] The issue of oral transmission, its implications and problems, has been addressed by a number of authors and in a variety of ways for the West. See for example, J. Blackman, 'Popular theories of generation: the evolution of *Aristotle's Works*, the study of an anachronism', in *Health Care and Popular Medicine in Nineteenth Century England*, ed. J. Woodward and D. Richards (London, 1977), pp. 56–8; V. Rippere, 'The survival of traditional medicine in lay medicine: an empirical approach to the history of medicine', *Medical History*, xxv (1981), 411–4; C. G. Helman, '"Feed a cold, starve a fever" – folk models of infection in an English suburban community and their relation to medical treatment', *Medicine and Society*, ii (1978), 107–37; J. Goody, *The Domestication of the Savage Mind* (Cambridge, 1977); P. Burke, *Popular Culture in Early Modern Europe* (London, 1978); E. L. Eisenstein, *The Printing Revolution in Early Modern Europe* (Cambridge, 1983).

324   *Ghada Karmi*

of the survey some grounds for believing that the mode of transmission
here is indeed that suggested. It is hard to explain the use of certain
specific technical terms in any other way, as, for example, the 'psychic
wind' (whether that alludes to vapour or to pneuma), or the
'over-fullness' or repletion (Arabic, *al-tukhma*) which is one technical
Arabic translation for *plethora*.

III

In fact, little is known of the medicine of the people in the areas newly
conquered by the Muslims in the seventh century: to note that the
Alexandrian school was teaching a syllabus of Galenic and Hippocratic
works in synopsis at the time of the Islamic conquest[23] is to say nothing
about the medicine which people practised or the way in which they
dealt with illness. It is certainly true that the medical literature of late
antiquity which the Arabs came across and later translated and used
was Greek and may be assumed to have been the dominant literature,
but none of this indicates how far down it went. Such evidence as there
is seems to show that its influence may have been quite limited. The
hellenisation of even the most 'Greek' of cities in the Near East –
Damascus, Antioch, Caesarea, Jerusalem, and Alexandria itself – seems
to have been only skin-deep for a very long time. To be sure, official
business was conducted in Greek; those aspiring to high office had to
learn Greek; and the intelligentsia used Greek as their everyday
language, but the ordinary people continued to speak Coptic in Egypt
and Aramaic (later Syriac) in Syria.[24] The hellenisation of these areas
was greatly accelerated by the establishment of the Christian Church,[25]
and it is very likely that urban dwellers were directly affected by this.
But the population of the rural areas remained culturally distinct, and
some historians have even seen an underlying anti-Greek nationalism
in the revolt of the Syrian church against the church at Byzantium
during the fifth and sixth centuries.[26] Indirect evidence for the weak
hold that hellenism had on the lands of Syria and Mesopotamia at the
time of the Arab conquests also comes from eighth and nineth century
Arabic historical accounts of these conquests. Syria, Palestine and

[23] A. Z. Iskandar, 'An attempted reconstruction of the late Alexandrian medical
curriculum', *Medical History*, xx (1976), 135–58.
[24] De Lacy O'Leary, *How Greek Science Passed to the Arabs* (London, 1949),
pp. 7–8.
[25] *Ibid.*, chs. 4 and 5, pp. 36–73.
[26] P. Hitti, *History of the Arabs from the Earliest Times to the Present*, 10th edn.
(London, 1970), p. 153.

Mesopotamia were overcome by the Arabs within a very short time and with little difficulty, in striking contrast to the conquest of Persia which took them ten years to accomplish. Arabs had been settled in the former countries in any case for centuries before Islam, and there was a racial affinity with the new conquerors which must have played a part.[27] With the exception of the hellenised cities of Jerusalem and Caesarea, the records indicate that elsewhere the people welcomed the Muslims as deliverers from Byzantine oppression.[28]

All this would seem to argue against a widespread familiarity with Greek medicine at the popular level. In fact, there is a suggestion that the everyday medicine of the time included a great deal of magic and superstition. The sixth century Greek physician, Alexander of Tralles, has left a compendium of medicine which, as well as setting down the usual summary of Galenic humoral medicine familiar from all the other writers of late antiquity, also includes numerous magical practices and remedies which were current in his day.[29] Such a situation would not have struck the conquering Arabs as in the least bit strange, for their own desert medicine was no different. It is true that some of their own physicians at the beginnings of Islam had acquired some knowledge of Greek medicine,[30] but this had little effect on the medicine of Arabia, in which magic played a major part. Cautery, cupping, animal products (particularly those of the camel), honey, oil and simple herbs were used, none of which could have done much to counter the effects of the variety of lethal diseases endemic to the area.[31] The early caliphs, who took over a Byzantine administrative system in the Near East, also took over Greek physicians. Little is known about the court physicians whom the caliphs appointed, but they seem to have practised a sort of Greek medicine; one of this kind was a certain Tiyaduq who attained considerable fame and was said to have had many pupils.[32]

[27] D. R. Hill, *The Termination of Hostilities in the Early Arab Conquests* (London, 1971), pp. 70, 74, 75, 84.   [28] *Ibid.*, p. 98.

[29] Alexander of Tralles, *Alexander Trallianus Opera*, ed. and trans. into German by T. Puschmann (2 vols., Vienna, 1878–9), vol. 1, pp. 562, 564, 566; vol. 2, p. 584.

[30] Al-Harith b. Kalada, for example, who was an older contemporary of the Prophet, is said to have studied Greek humoral medicine at Jundi-Shapur in Persia. See his biography in Ibn Abi Usaybi'a, *K. 'Uyun al-Anba fi Tabaqat al-Atibba'* (hereafter *IAU*), ed. A. Müller (2 vols., Cairo, 1882–4), vol. 1, pp. 110–13.

[31] Ullmann, *Islamic Medicine*, pp. 1–5; A. Wensinck, *A Handbook of Early Muhammadan Tradition* (Leiden, 1927).

[32] Tiyaduq is a mysterious figure about whom little is known. He was the court physician to the governor of Iraq, al-Hajjaj b. Yusuf, in the late seventh

At the beginning of the eighth century, the Abbasid caliphs invited Syriac-speaking physicians from the school of Jundi-Shapur in Persia to Baghdad, and thus paved the way for the massive translation movement of medical works from Greek into Arabic which established Greek medicine in its dominant position. The school of Jundi-Shapur, about which little is known but much has been written,[33] was developed by the Persian emperor, Kisra Anushirawan, in the mid-sixth century. This emperor had a great interest in learning and attracted a large number of Greek scholars to his academy. By the time of the Arab conquest, Jundi-Shapur had a hospital and a flourishing academy, staffed by Syriac-speaking Christian doctors practising Greek medicine. Its fame was so great that the caliph invited its director and his colleagues to set up something similar at Baghdad. In this way, Greek influence through Syriac began to make itself felt in Arabic medical circles, and this in turn led to the subsequent flourishing of Greek medicine among the Arabs and to the creation of an Arabic medical literature based on Greek medicine.

Nevertheless, and even if the real story were as simple as that, we are little the wiser as to the medical practice of ordinary people in the cities, let alone in the countryside. We may suppose, however, that urban dwellers, whatever their familiarity with Greek medicine had been before the advent of the Muslims, would eventually have gained reasonable access to it under Islam, whereas the situation was very different for the country areas. The latter remained isolated. The fact that most, if not all, 'good' doctors practised in the major cities may be inferred from the regulation brought in by the wazir to the caliph al-Muqtadir during the early part of the tenth century, that the physicians of Baghdad would be obliged to visit the country areas around the city in travelling clinics, so bad was the state of medicine there.[34] During the ninth century a type of medical book appeared, apparently catering specifically for those people who had no access to a doctor, either because they lived outside major cities or because they

century and left a compendium of medicine, fragments of which survive in later Arabic writings. See M. Ullmann, *Die Medizin im Islam* (Leiden, 1970), pp. 22–3; Ibn al-Qifti, *Ta'rikh al-Hukama'*, ed. J. Lippert (Leipzig, 1903), p. 105.

[33] Al-Qifti, *Ta'rikh al-Hukama'*, gives a page-long description of the academy at Jundi-Shapur which all later historians have used, p. 133; see also Browne, *Arabian Medicine*, pp. 19–22; O'Leary, *How Greek Science Passed to the Arabs*, p. 71; most recently, H. H. Schoffler has put together all the bibliography relating to Jundi-Shapur in his *Die Akademie von Gondischapur* (Stuttgart, 1979).   [34] *IAU*, vol. 1, p. 221, 1.13–27.

could not afford the doctor's fees; hence such titles as 'The poor man's medicine', or 'For him who has no physician to attend him'.[35] To the same genre belong the numerous books of 'traveller's medicine' which purported to help those who had no access to a doctor because of distance from their homes or unfamiliarity with new countries.[36] Such books had had their precedents in late antiquity: Rufus, the second century Greek physician and contemporary of Galen, left a large book entitled *Medicine for the Layman*, fragments of which survive in quotations from Arabic writers;[37] and there may have been others.

For whom were such books really written? Did they help to disseminate medical ideas to the masses? A similar question has been raised with a parallel, although much later case in the Western tradition. Rosenberg has argued persuasively that Buchan's *Domestic Medicine* and others of the same ilk were intended for the educated English middle classes who used them within a long-standing tradition of medical self-help.[38] (Ginnie Smith discusses this tradition for the same period elsewhere in this volume.) We simply do not know the answer for the Arabic case. The educated Arabic-speaking layman certainly read medical books for intellectual interest, much in the way

35 Al-Razi (d. 925) wrote such a book, *Man la Yahduruhu al-Tabib* (He who has no physician to attend him) in whose introduction he says: 'When I saw that the most notable [among physicians] wrote at length in their books and mentioned medicines and types of food which can scarcely be found except in the store-houses of kings, I wanted to compose a concise treatise on the treatment of disease with well-known medicines and nutriments which the common people possess, so that the book would be more appropriate for the needs of most people' (my translation), Well. Hist. Lib. MS., see Iskandar, *A Catalogue of Arabic Manuscripts*, pp. 128–9; Ibn al-Jazzar (d. 980), the famous Tunisian doctor, also wrote *Tibb al-Fuqara' wal-Masakin* (The medicine of the poor and wretched), see Ullmann, *Die Medizin im Islam*, p. 148.

36 Such a book, celebrated in the Latin West throughout the Middle Ages, was Ibn al-Jazzar's *Zad al-Musafir wa Qut al-Hadir*, Latin, *Viaticum Peregrinantis*. See Ullmann, *Die Medizin im Islam*, p. 148; also, my 'The Arabic medical *Kunnash* in the 10th century: its status, significance, and tradition, a study mainly based on the book *Ghina wa Muna* by Abu Mansur al-Qamari (al-Qumri)' (Ph.D. Thesis, University of London 1978), pp. 287, 314–35.

37 Fragments of this survive in al-Razi's medical encyclopaedia, *K. al-Hawi*. It is probably the same as *Tadbir man la Yahduruhu al-Tabib* (The management of him who has no physician to attend him), which is also cited by al-Razi in *K. al-Hawi* and listed by *IAU*, vol. 1, p. 34, 1.2. See Ullmann, *Die Medizin im Islam*, p. 74.

38 C. E. Rosenberg, 'Medical text and medical context: explaining William Buchan's "Domestic Medicine"', *Bulletin of the History of Medicine*, LVII (1983), 22–42; also, C. J. Lawrence, 'William Buchan: medicine laid open', *Medical History*, XIX (1975), 20–35.

of the educated Romans whom Vivian Nutton discusses in his paper. Many medical books from the Golden Age of Islamic civilisation carry dedications to famous persons and were specifically commissioned by such people to satisfy their curiosity, and a knowledge of medicine was considered a desirable part of a general education: a glance at any of the mediaeval Arabic bibliographies of learned men will show how many of these combined a knowledge of medicine with philosophy, logic, astronomy, theology, and a host of other things.[39] Medical knowledge was not the preserve of a professional group, although, as we shall see later, doctors were a definable class in a legal and objective sense.

Graeco/Arabic medicine had therefore been thoroughly adopted by the new urban intelligentsia, but Islamic society had a medical alternative which might have appealed to the ordinary man, not least because it did not require the services of a doctor. This was the so-called *Prophet's Medicine*, a collection of injunctions about health and the cure of disease, all purportedly going back to the Prophet Muhammad. They originated in part from the books of Prophetic *Hadith* (the sayings of the Prophet),[40] and in part from ancient pre-Islamic magical practices and beliefs which had been dressed in religious guise and dignified with the Prophet's authority.[41] There were several collections of the *Prophet's Medicine* by different authors which mostly came into prominence after 1300. The influence of humoral medicine is clearly to be discerned in them, despite the fact that the men of religion promoted the Prophet's medicine as the only medicine fit for the believer who must shun the heathen Graeco/Arabic medicine.

If honey is drunk before breakfast, it dissolves phlegm, washes staleness out of the stomach, clarifies the viscid matter within it, expels the superfluities

---

[39] For example, Ibn al-Nadim (fl. 987), *K. al-Fihrist* (The index), ed. G. Flugel (Leipzig, 1871–2); al-Qifti (d. 1248), *K. Ta'rikh al-Hukama'* (The history of physicians); Yaqut al-Rumi (fl. thirteenth century), *Irshad al-Arib ila Ma'rifat al-Adib*, ed. and trans. as *Yaqut's Dictionary of Learned Men*, D. S. Margoliouth (London, 1936–8). All these books contain biographies of learned men from all parts of the Islamic state and span several centuries.

[40] The *Hadith* (tradition) is an account of what the Prophet said or did, or of his approval of what was said and done, collected in several volumes. These are supposed to guide Muslims in all matters moral, spiritual and practical. Inevitably, as in all oral histories, many traditions of dubious authenticity were incorporated. Many such formed the substance of the *Prophet's Medicine*.

[41] See Ullmann, *Islamic Medicine*, p. 5; C. Elgood, 'Tibb ul-Nabi or Medicine of the Prophet', *Osiris*, XIV (1962), 33–192; J. C. Bürghel, 'Secular and religious features of medieval Arabic medicine', in *Asian Medical Systems*, ed. C. Leslie (Berkeley, 1976), pp. 54–61.

from it, warms it to a moderate degree...but it harms the bilious patient because it is hot and so is yellow bile and the honey may agitate the bile.[42]

The authenticity of the Prophet's medicine was called into question early on in Arabic circles: the fourteenth century social historian, Ibn Khaldun, drew attention to its secular, bedouin origins,[43] but this did not deter religious zealots from urging the faithful to adopt it. How much they succeeded is a matter of conjecture, for, although it may have provided a real alternative for some devout Muslims (particularly today, when it is enjoying something of a revival), nevertheless, it is clear that mainstream Arabic medicine remained significantly free from religious influences. The great Arabic medical texts of the classical period are faithful to the Greek rational tradition and contain no compromises with religious dogma. For example, the Muslim prohibition on wine is nowhere allowed to intrude or to amend the many prescriptions which contain it, and, although most of the writers would have been familiar with the religious sayings on health, this never appears in medical tracts. Maimonides, the prominent Jewish doctor who was also a rabbi, never drew on Talmudic medicine (with which he, more than any other, had reason to be familiar) in any of his medical works.

But even though a non-religious rationalism permeated medical writing and medical treatment, religious influences played a strong part in lay people's attitudes towards illness and its cure. In the Muslim view of these things, disease was not considered a punishment for sin, and hence was generally not amenable to religious healing. (This has not been true for Shi'a Islam which incorporated many Christian and Persian elements and in which saints, shrines and miracles feature strongly.) Death could not be postponed, for the exact span of each human life was predestined by God – 'to every people is a term appointed; when their term is reached, not an hour can they delay it nor an hour advance it'[44] – and so prayer in this context is of no avail. The Muslim idea of illness is encapsulated in the Prophetic saying, 'God has created no disease for which He has not also created the cure'; the disease is God-sent but as a part of creation and man must pray for guidance to cure it. During the plague epidemics which attacked Syria and Palestine in the mid-fourteenth century, several writers left

---

[42] Ibn Qayyim al-Jawziyya, *al-Tibb al-Nabawi*, p. 204.
[43] Ibn Khaldun, *The Muqaddimah: An Introduction to History*, trans. F. Rosenthal, 2nd edn. (3 vols., Princeton, 1967), vol. 3, p. 150.
[44] Quran, Sura 10, verse 49.

accounts in which the plague is put down to impurity of the air, contagion, to the simple fact of God's creation, but rarely to divine anger or retribution.[45] In fact, the idea was current that victims of the plague would be deemed martyrs and would go to Paradise. So much so, that one fifteenth century writer welcomed the plague as a means to martyrdom.[46]

The great plagues aside, the picture of lay medicine under Islam is far from complete. From the extensive *hisba* literature, however, we do know something of what the urban layman could expect in medical standards from his doctors; whether his expectations were met and how often is another matter. *Hisba* was a system of surveillance instituted by the Islamic state during the ninth century and administered by *muhtasibs* in order to regularise transactions in the market. Among other things, the *muhtasib* was to guard the public against malpractice from doctors and pharmacists. Manuals of guidance for *muhtasibs* came into being, many of which survive, containing instructions for the examination and licensing of physicians, surgeons ophthalmologists, and bone-setters, as well as a variety of para-medical practitioners such as blood-letters and druggists.[47] Only if the examiners whom the *muhtasib* called to his aid were satisfied with the practitioner could he be licensed to practise. There had, in any case, been numerous tracts written in Arabic on the examination of physicians,[48] and licensing laws to distinguish *bona fide* doctors from quacks had appeared in Baghdad in the tenth century.[49] And yet, it seems that malpractice (presumably defined against the background of this *hisba* legislation) was widespread. Itinerant doctors, whose practice was impossible to control, abounded;

[45] Ullmann, *Islamic medicine*, pp. 92–5; M. Dols, *The Black Death in the Middle East* (Princeton, 1977), pp. 109–13; and *ibid.*, pp. 114–15 for a discussion on the instances when plague was seen by Muslims as a punishment.

[46] Ibn Hajr al-'Asqalani (d. 1448), *K. Badhl al-Ma'un fi Fadl al-Ta'un*, Zahiriyya Lib. Damascus MS. 3158; see Ullmann, *Die Medizin im Islam*, p. 248; also Dols, *The Black Death in the Middle East*, pp. 110–13.

[47] S. K. Hamarneh, 'Origins and functions of the Hisba system in Islam and its impact on the health professions', *Sudhoffs Archiv*, XLVIII (1964), 157–73; see also my 'State control of the physician in the Middle Ages: an Islamic model' in *The Town and State Physician in Europe from the Middle Ages to the Enlightenment* (Wolfenbüttel, 1981), pp. 63–85.

[48] Al-Razi, for example, wrote twice on this subject: a short chapter in his famous *K. al-Mansuri* and again in a separate tract, *On the Examination of the Physician*, ed. A. Z. Iskandar, *al-Mashriq*, LIV (1960), 502–14.

[49] Al-Qifti, *Ta'rikh al-Hukama'*, p. 190, relates that the caliph al-Muqtadir ordered the *muhtasib* of Baghdad to prohibit all doctors from practising until they had been examined and licensed by his court physician, Sinan b. Thabit. A total of 860 physicians were examined by Sinan in this way.

charlatans posing as doctors were a real menace, and adulterated drugs were a constant hazard to the public.[50] Nevertheless, the inference must be that in places where the *hisba* was in force, people received a certain measure of protection from the most extreme forms of malpractice. But this was almost certainly confined to the larger cities and even then, only during the early years of the *hisba* office; for, in later Islam, the *hisba* office fell into decay and a licence could simply be purchased for a small consideration.[51] Indeed, the license to practise medicine could also be bought in the 1740s 'for a few sequins'.[52]

But even with these limitations, the institution of *hisba* and its emphasis on setting and maintaining medical standards must, if nothing else, have had the effect of disseminating the 'new medicine' to a large number of the lay public in the cities. Hospitals also would have served a similar function. By the tenth century, every major city and many minor ones had its own hospital or hospitals where treatment and drugs were dispensed free of charge.[53] All sections of the population used these amenities and would therefore have been exposed to official medicine on a mass scale. Thus, although the question of how and when the ordinary man first became acquainted with the precepts of humoral medicine remains uncertain, it is a reasonable inference that the people at large, whether in urban centres or in the countryside, had, by the later mediaeval period, become familiar with this medicine to some degree. And it proved remarkably enduring, at least among the lower classes. Dr John Fryer, a physician with the East India Company, writing of the medical situation in Persia in 1677 (which seems to have been dismal) had this to say:

Physic which, though it be here in good repute, yet its sectators are too much wedded to antiquity, not being at all addicted to find out its improvements by new enquiries; wherefore they stick to the Arabian method as devoutly

---

[50] There is a detailed account of the tricks of charlatans in the major *hisba* work, *Nihayat al-Rutba fi Talab al-Hisba* by the twelfth century writer 'Abd al-Rahman b. Nasr al-Shayzari, ed. al-Sayyid al-Baz al'-Arini (Cairo, 1946), p. 102. Likewise, al-Razi 'On the tricks of charlatans', from his *K. al-Mansuri*, ed. Iskandar, *al-Mashriq*, pp. 487–92.

[51] See the *Encyclopaedia of Islam*, 2nd edn. (4 vols., Leiden and London, 1971), vol. 3, p. 488.

[52] Alexander Russell, *A Natural History of Aleppo and Parts Adjacent* (London, 1756, reprinted 1856), p. 97.

[53] Elgood, *A Medical History of Persia*, p. 398: apparently, during the seventeenth century every large town in Persia had one or two hospitals; see also Ahmad Isa Bey, *Les Bimaristanes a l'Epoque Islamique* (Cairo, 1929); and S. K. Hamarneh, 'Development of hospitals in Islam', *Journal of the History of Medicine*, XVII (1962), 366–84.

as to the sacred tripod, which they hold as infallible as of old that Delphic oracle was accounted.[54]

Similarly, in Aleppo some seventy years later, the Scottish physician Alexander Russell, who was physician to the British factory there for twenty years, while also noting the bad state of medicine among the natives, observed that:

The Europeans, of whom there are several, practise medicine in their own way and are greatly respected by the inhabitants; though partly to save money, and partly from a notion of their giving violent medicines, they seldom apply to them till they have tried their own doctors to no purpose.[55]

During the plague epidemics of the 1740s, the people of Aleppo even attempted to dissuade the Europeans from taking precautions against it because it contradicted their own practice.[56]

There is evidence to show that Arabic medicine, as the medicine of a privileged class, had begun to decline by the sixteenth century, if not before. In 1530, for example, neither the sultan of North Africa's wazir nor his wife had a physician of their own, and had to call on the Portuguese doctors to attend them.[57] During the next century, Arabic medical works began to show the influence of Western medicine, as for example with Ibn Sallum, the physician to the Ottoman sultan Mehmet IV, who included a section on 'the chemical medicine of Paracelsus' in his book *Ghayat al-itqan fi tadbir badan al-insan* (The most precise information on the regimen of the human body).[58] During an epidemic of plague in the eighteenth century, the sultan Mustafa III commissioned his court physician to translate Boerhaave's *Institutiones medicinae* and his *Aphorismi de cogniscendis et curandis morbis*, in the hope that they might have something more to offer against the plague than Arabic medicine had.[59] Although neither Paracelsus nor Boerhaave became influential in the East, yet their introduction is symptomatic of the change that was taking place at the top. This change became virtually complete by the nineteenth century with the

54 Quoted by Elgood, *A Medical History of Persia*, pp. 401–2.
55 Russell, *History of Aleppo*, p. 100.
56 *Ibid.*, p. 253.
57 R. Ricord, 'Médecine et médecins à Arzila (1508–1539)', *Hespèris*, xxvi (1939), 171–8.
58 For Ibn Sallum's life, see Ullmann, *Die Medizin im Islam*, pp. 182–4, and *idem*, *Islamic Medicine*, p. 182; for a description of his book, still in manuscript form, see Iskandar, *A Catalogue of Arabic Manuscripts*, pp. 96–9, 203–6.
59 C. E. Daniëls, 'La version orientale Arabe et Turque de deux premiers livres de Herman Boerhaave', *Janus*, xvii (1912), 295–312.

establishment of the first modern medical school in Cairo in 1828; French, Italian and German professors taught there.[60] In Iran, meanwhile, the Dar al-Funun was founded in 1850 where medicine was taught by Austrians and Italians and the language of instruction was French.[61] Gallagher has thrown further light on this subject for North Africa in her recent study of medicine there in the eighteenth and nineteenth centuries.[62] She shows that in Tunis, the ruling Beys had patronised European doctors since the early eighteenth century, although they still retained the native *amin al-atibba'* or chief of physicians.[63] The latter's function was to license local practitioners, while the former was used by the Bey not only as a personal physician but also as his representative in commercial and diplomatic negotiations with Europe.[64] The Beys sought, just as the Ottoman sultans had done, to solve the urgent medical problems with new scientific European ideas. The influence of Western medicine finally became supreme among these ruling classes in the latter half of the nineteenth century. During the cholera epidemic in Egypt in 1883, the French mission which came to study the epidemic found that all the leading doctors of Cairo and Alexandria were Europeans.[65] In Tunis, after 1856, all licenses to practise were issued not by the Muslim chief of physicians, but by the Bey's European doctor.[66] The maristan (hospital) of Tunis had its last native chief in 1876. The new chief was the first European-trained Algerian doctor.[67]

The drift away from the pure Arabic medicine of classical Islam, which began in the Arab East after 1500, was only a drift at the top and, even then, it was half-hearted for a long time thereafter. The eighteenth century translator of Boerhaave tried to harmonise the ideas in the book with those of traditional Arabic medicine. Throughout most of the eighteenth and nineteenth centuries, the European doctors

[60] F. M. Sandwith, 'The history of Kasr-el-Aini and the modern school of medicine in Egypt', *British Medical Journal*, ΙΙ (1902), 909–10.

[61] Elgood, *A Medical History of Persia*, pp. 501–3; K. Hummel, 'Die Entwicklung der neuzeitlichen Naturwissenschaft in Iran', *Die Welt des Oriens*, VI (1971), 240–54.

[62] N. E. Gallagher, *Medicine and Power in Tunisia 1780–1900* (hereafter *Tunisia*) (Cambridge, 1983). I am greatly indebted to this excellent study for much of the information on North Africa in the rest of my paper.

[63] Gallagher, *Tunisia*, p. 17.

[64] *Ibid.*, p. 18.

[65] J. B. Picot Bey, 'La mission Pasteur de 1883 pour l'étude du choléra en Egypte', *Bulletin de l'Institut d'Egypte*, V (1923), 1–7.

[66] Gallagher, *Tunisia*, p. 84.　　　　[67] *Ibid.*, p. 87.

at the Bey's court in Tunisia shared power with the Muslim chief of physicians; there is even a record of a French surgeon seeking employment at the hospital of Tunis.[68] The people, meanwhile, remained largely unaffected and continued to practise Arabic medicine just as they had done since mediaeval times. It is significant in this context that, just as the changeover of medical manpower was taking place in official circles and the first European-type medical school was being established in the Egypt of the nineteenth century, so the first printed editions of the great Arabic medical textbooks of Ibn Sina (Avicenna), al-Majusi (Haly Abbas), and Ibn al-Baitar appeared, published by the newly founded Bulaq Press of Cairo.[69] In any case, there had been numerous manuscript copies of these and other Arabic medical books made throughout the eighteenth century. There is no question that this signified a continuing practical need for these books and not a mere interest in the history of Arabic medicine. Here again, the Tunisian records attest to the existence of a widespread local, indigenous Arabic medical practice throughout the nineteenth century.[70] It was officially brought to an end by the decree of 1888 when doctors could practise only if they had completed three years of medical school.[71] The number of European-trained doctors was, however, very small, and the majority of the population continued to turn to Arabic medicine[72] – a situation which is not unlike that in other Arab countries, as the study showed, even today.

And therein may lie one of the major reasons for the survival of Arabic medicine well into the present century. For, in a way, the most remarkable thing about the findings in Syria and Jordan was not that Arabic medicine was dying out, but rather that it was there at all. It had survived many centuries and many historical and political changes. The fact that it has done so calls for some explanation. Of course, for a very long time there was no alternative. The European invasions of the nineteenth century did not bring with them a more effective form of medicine into the countries of the Middle East, had it even been available to the ordinary man and woman. The latter would have continued to use traditional medicine for that reason alone. However, there are other factors. In the Syrian study it was clear that the demise

[68] *Ibid.*, p. 21.

[69] Ibn al Baitar's *K. al-Jami'li Mufradat al-Adwiya wal-Aghthiya* was published in 1874, Ibn Sina's *al-Qanun fi'l-Tibb* (The Canon) and al-Majusi's *Kamil al-Sina'a fi'l-Tibb* were both published in 1877.

[70] Gallagher, *Tunisia*, p. 87.

[71] *Ibid.*, p. 93.   [72] *Ibid.*, p. 94.

of indigenous medicine was being hastened by pressure from above. The government had outlawed Arabic medicine and its practitioners, a measure that has historical precedents. In North Africa, towards the end of the nineteenth century, local medical practitioners became a debased class, the best among them no better than 'médecins tolerés', as the official designation went.[73] The attitude of the French, the major occupying power in North Africa at the time, is summed up in the words of the French doctor who made a study of Arabic medicine in Algeria in 1855, when he concluded that French medicine had 'errors to correct, ignorance to dissipate, misery and apathy to destroy'.[74]

Much earlier, in Spain, the medicine of the Arabs (Moriscos) there had been forced underground by pressure from the Christians.[75] Up till the time of the Christian reconquest in the fourteenth century, the medicine of Southern Spain had been the classical Arabic medicine familiar from elsewhere in the Islamic state. The Spanish reconquest brought with it a savage intolerance of the Arab presence in Spain in all its manifestations. It was this that led to the dispersal of the Moriscos and, more importantly from our point of view, to the banning of their form of medicine. This imposed termination of a medical system that had been dominant for centuries in Spain did no more than force it underground. From 1400 onwards, Morisco (or Arabic) medicine was practised secretly in the villages rather than in the major cities so as to evade official vigilance. Arabic medical books were passed from hand to hand, and later, as this became more and more difficult, medical lore was transmitted by word of mouth. There is evidence to show that this medicine was still alive at the end of the sixteenth century in different parts of Spain.[76]

The story of Arabic medicine in Spain provides a particularly good example of the forceful transfer of a medical system from one class to another for political reasons and of the consequent creation of an oral tradition in what had previously been a highly literate one. It also demonstrates the importance of this medicine as an aspect of cultural identity. For the Moriscos, their medicine, like their religion, was uniquely their own. They clung to it at least partly as an expression of political resistance to their annihilation as a group. Likewise, it is not difficult to see how European medicine, which was imposed as a

---

[73] *Ibid.*, p. 93.   [74] *Ibid.*, p. 95.
[75] L. Garcia Ballester gives an account of this in his study of the Moriscos in Spain, *Medicine, Ciencia y Minoras Marginadas: Los Moriscos* (Granada, 1976).
[76] *Ibid.*, p. 87.

'civilising force' onto the indigenous population in the wake of modern colonialism in the Middle East, might have been resisted for the same reason. Some light was thrown on this matter by the modern studies in Syria and Jordan. The very fact that the people designated their traditional medicine 'Arabic medicine', while that of the government clinics was called 'Western medicine' or sometimes 'clinic medicine' or 'government medicine', is significant. Assertions that Arabic medicine was superior to 'the other medicine', often said with defiance, were commonplace, even among the young. That the issue is a real one could also be inferred from the reverse point of view, particularly among Jordanians: traditional Arabic medicine was obsolete and dangerous and must be displaced in favour of modern, technological Western medicine.

The survival of classical Arabic medicine and its revival for reasons of cultural identity is explicit in Pakistan. Arabic medicine, or Unani medicine as it is called there, had in any case never died out in India, perpetuated by the Bahmanid dynasty from the fourteenth to the sixteenth century and later by the Mogul emperors from 1525 to 1857. In 1954 the Hamdard National Foundation was founded in Karachi. This was done with the avowed aim of strengthening national Islamic identity through the preservation and teaching of Eastern medicine, which of course included Arabic medicine.[77]

Eastern medicine began to languish when Afro-Asian countries became colonies of Western Powers and consequently Western culture, science and medicine were superimposed on indigenous culture, science, and medicine.[78]

In the hope of changing this 'painful' situation, and of restoring the national heritage, an academy was also built for the training of *hakims* or traditional practitioners. Their four-year syllabus includes the *Canon* of Ibn Sina, which had in any case remained in continuous use in India for centuries. The Hamdard Foundation is very active today and produces its own herbal medicines, has a large number of clinics in the country as well as a few in India, and edits a number of journals. In recent years, Kuwait has established an institute for the study of classical Islamic medicine with the aim of reviving it as a living discipline; the decision was a governmental one, in line with the general promotion of Islam and Islamic values as a political policy, but also with the intention of demonstrating that classical Islamic medicine

[77] See *Hamdard Foundation Pakistan, Twenty-Five Years of Service 1954–1979* (Karachi, 1979).   [78] *Ibid.*, p. 17.

has something practical to offer. In the same way, the Eastern medicine of Hamdard was promoted as a useful and legitimate part of health care, not just a gesture towards the glorious past.

Nor can the issue of efficacy be ignored as a factor in the survival of traditional medicine. After all, the remedies and treatments of traditional medicine have been tried by the centuries and have proved their worth, whether that be real or imagined, over generations. Such a legacy is not easily jettisoned and especially not for something as alien in spirit and concept as Western medicine.[79] Something of a compromise was reached between the two systems in Syria and Jordan, whereby an arbitrary division had been made between those diseases which responded better to traditional methods and those which were best treated by the clinic doctors. (Kleinman found the same compromise in the popular medicine of Taiwan.)[80] But, efficacy aside, traditional therapy has other advantages over Western medicine. Firstly, there is the individual attention that the patient receives from the traditional doctor as opposed to the hurried, often unsympathetic consultation with the clinic doctor. Secondly, there is the immediacy of diagnosis and treatment – no X-rays, no bacteriology, no investigations; cautery, cupping, venesection are instant and visible experiences in contrast to the slow and silent action of antibiotics, anti-inflammatory drugs and antacids. Furthermore, there is little mystique left in these age-old remedies: everyone knows what most treatment consists of and why it is prescribed. There is a sharing of management between the practitioner and the patient. The practitioner is a part of the community: no better, no worse. He has a skill that neither puts him above the rest nor makes him responsible for them. Those who go for help to such practitioners are not called 'patients', and the individual remains in charge of his disease and his body throughout.

There was a striking difference between the behaviour of people attending the clinic and those seeing their local practitioners. Already, despite (and perhaps because of) the recent arrival of modern medicine among them, they were diffident, afraid to express themselves, and docile when they first went to the clinic. None of them knew what medicines they were being given nor why; at the same time, they had

---

[79] See *Biocultural Aspects of Disease*, ed. H. Rothschild (New York, 1981), pp. 512–25.

[80] See the various contributions made by A. Kleinman in *Medicine in Chinese Cultures: Comparative Studies of Health Care in Chinese and Other Societies*, ed. A. Kleinman (Washington, 1975).

expectations of a perfect cure and were querulous or demanding on subsequent visits to the clinic. The doctor regarded them as inferiors and they had begun to fear and resent him. The fact that medicine was free did not help either; this only increased the dependency and resentment. All this was in striking contrast to the dignity and control of the transaction between the same people and their folk doctors. It was clear that the helplessness, which is a characteristic of the modern patient in Western society, had begun to emerge as an important factor among these backward peasants, and herein lay one of the fascinating features of the study: for, it permitted observation of a historical process in the making. One could conjecture that until the arrival of Western medicine in recent years, the people had practised the self-help medicine that was once typical of Europe from the Middle Ages onwards. Joan Lane's paper analyses this phenomenon for England in the eighteenth century. In similar fashion, the Syrian peasants medicated themselves for many simple ailments or applied to their folk doctors or wise-women for certain remedies and operations, which is an extension of self-help, since it was they who usually made the diagnosis, defined the appropriate treatment, and only then sought the 'doctor's' help in prescribing it. This ancient tradition was now being rapidly eroded and replaced by a new form of doctor–patient relationship.

Ironically enough, it has come about just at the time when Western medical thinkers have begun to analyse and criticise the phenomenon of the passive patient created by scientific and social changes in the nineteenth and twentieth centuries,[81] when the view of the body as an object 'containing fascinating pathology'[82] was formulated. In the Western case, this process and its rebound response were indigenous, evolving out of the same society which contained the patient and the doctor and their critics. By contrast, in the Middle East, the creation of the passive, helpless patient has been an instant import, and where it might be possible to argue that in England the nineteenth century transition from self-medication and self-help to control by the medical establishment was not resisted by the patient, at least initially, it is certain that the parallel transition among the Arabs, imposed as it is from outside and through agents more in sympathy with it than with them, has been met with a mixture of hostility and bewilderment. Even

[81] D. Armstrong, *The Political Anatomy of the Body* (Cambridge, 1983), pp. 2–6, 101–12.
[82] This concept is discussed by M. Foucault in *Discipline and Punish: The Birth of the Prison* (London, 1977), part III.

though the government doctors with whom they were dealing were fellow countrymen and often originally came from the same villages, a Western-style medical training had served to distance them from their clients and had imbued them with an overwhelming sense of superiority, where scientific knowledge became a tool with which to subdue and mystify. Not only had this alienated the people, but, as practical medicine, it was not very effective either. The standard of medical practice was poor, drugs dispensed freely and without adequate rationale or investigation. Not surprisingly, the results were often disappointing, and many patients reverted to their own traditional treatments after trying the clinic medicine. Nevertheless, this will not halt the steady advance of modern medicine and the 'civilising mission' of modern technology. Even as this research study was being undertaken, traditional medicine was dying out and a whole network of social and psychological attitudes to health and disease, preserved through countless generations, was coming to an end.

INDEX

Aberdeen, University of, 5, 6, 167
abstergent lotion, 271
accidents,
  to adults, 85, 86, 88, 116, 120, 122,
    208, 237, 305
  to children, 103, 107ff, 110
accoucheurs, 219
acute disorders, 111, 124
Adair, James Mackittrick, 272, 276
Addington, Anthony, 223, 240
Adlam, Thomas, 154
advertising, 310
advice books, 62, 187, 188, 250, 255,
  282, 304
aether
  electrical, 269
  occult, 268
after-birth, 151
ague, 108–28 passim
ailments
  minor, 110
  morbid obsession with, 91, 181
  most feared, 125
  multiple, 120
air
  country, 265
  fresh, 281
  hot, 264
  infected, 126
  natural air best physick, 241
  simple, 266
  universal spirit of, 268, 269
alchemy, 156, 180
alcohol, 38, 224
Alexander of Abonuteichos, 46
Alexander, Disney, 272, 276
Alexander of Tralles, 325
Alexandria, 30, 31, 35, 36, 50, 324, 333
Alexio, 39
Algeria, 333, 335

allopathic cures, 41
alternative medicine, 8, 16
al-tukhma, 324
al-Zahrawi, 321
Ambrose, Isaac, 67n, 68, 69, 82
American colonists, 87, 208
Amphiaraus, 46
amputation, 305, 306
amulets, 315
Anabaptists, 260
Anastasius of Sinai, 45
anatomical demonstrations, 32
anatomical dissection, 306, 307
anatomy, 295
Ancien Regime, 289
ancient medicine, 23–53 passim
anecdotes, medical, 318
angels, 157
Angier, John, 64
Anglicanism, 56, 57, 68, 75, 76, 78, 96,
  133, 154, 161, 162, 163, 164, 165,
  172
Anglican Tories, 173
Anglican Trinitarians, 165
animal magnetism, 156, 157n, 171
anointing the stomach, 92
anthropology, 21n
  medical, 13, 20, 83, 288
anti-arthritic powder, 265
Anti-Slave Trade Movement, 148
Anushirawan, Kisra (Persian emperor),
  326
anxiety, 98
Apollo, 45, 46
Apollonius, 33
apoplexy, 72, 224
apothecaries, 73, 117, 119, 120, 121, 130,
  152, 169, 208, 221, 310
  surgeon-, 312
apparitions, 157

Printed in the United States
By Bookmasters